Atrial Fibrillation

Fundamental and Clinical Cardiology

Editor-in-Chief
Samuel Z. Goldhaber, M.D.
Harvard Medical School
and Brigham and Women's Hospital
Boston, Massachusetts

Associate Editor, Europe
Henri Bounameaux, M.D.
University Hospital of Geneva
Geneva, Switzerland

ADDITIONAL VOLUMES IN PREPARATION

Atrial Fibrillation

edited by

Peter Kowey

Jefferson Medical College
Philadelphia
and the
Lankenau Hospital and Main Line System
Wynnewood, Pennsylvania, U.S.A.

and

Gerald V. Naccarelli

Pennsylvania State University
College of Medicine
and the
Milton S. Hershey Medical Center
Hershey, Pennsylvania, U.S.A.

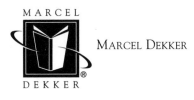

MARCEL DEKKER

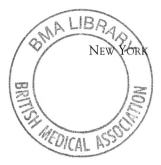

NEW YORK

Library of Congress Cataloging-in-Publication Data
A catalog record for this book is available from the Library of Congress.

ISBN: 0-8247-5410-7

This book is printed on acid-free paper.

Headquarters
Marcel Dekker, 270 Madison Avenue, New York, NY 10016, U.S.A.
tel: 212-696-9000; fax: 212-685-4540

Distribution and Customer Service
Marcel Dekker, Cimarron Road, Monticello, New York 12701, U.S.A.
tel: 800-228-1160; fax: 845-796-1772

World Wide Web
http://www.dekker.com

The publisher offers discounts on this book when ordered in bulk quantities. For more information, write to Special Sales/Professional Marketing at the headquarters address above.

PRINTED IN THE UNITED STATES OF AMERICA

Series Introduction

Marcel Dekker, Inc., has focused on the development of various series of beautifully produced books in different branches of medicine. These series have facilitated the integration of rapidly advancing information for both the clinical specialist and the researcher.

My goal as editor-in-chief of the Fundamental and Clinical Cardiology series is to assemble the talents of world-renowned authorities to discuss virtually every area of cardiovascular medicine. In the current monograph, *Atrial Fibrillation*, Peter Kowey and Gerald Naccarelli have edited a much-needed and timely book. Future contributions to this series will include books on molecular biology, interventional cardiology, and clinical management of such problems such as coronary artery disease and ventricular arrhythmias.

Samuel Z. Goldhaber

Foreword

Twenty years ago atrial fibrillation (AF) was said to affect some 0.4% of the general population; now it is present in well over 1%, and by the year 2050 it will affect more than 2% of the population of the industrialized world. Although AF may occur as an arrhythmic expression of long-standing cardiac disease of all types, it may also occur in the setting of pulmonary disease, postthoracotomy, thyroid overactivity, alcohol toxicity, and autonomic disturbance. Although it may occasionally be due largely to a genetic cause, in most instances the link to genetic factors is weak. The overwhelming factor that contributes to its occurrence is age, either because of degenerative mechanisms or coexisting cardiopulmonary disease. It is therefore no surprise that increasing longevity, particularly of those surviving cardiac problems that might previously have killed them, is leading to the meteoric rise in the prevalence of this condition.

At one time AF was thought to be almost normal; its very common presentation in otherwise seemingly well individuals contributed to this mistaken view. More recently it has been realized that AF accounts for a very high proportion of thromboembolic strokes and aggravated heart failure. It is probably associated with a 50% increase in the risk of death, is often highly symptomatic and is associated with a distinct degradation of the quality of life. AF is therefore a disease rather than a second-best alternative to sinus rhythm.

AF is not only the most common sustained cardiac arrhythmia but also the most written about rhythm disturbance. PubMed searches reveal over 13,500 references to atrial fibrillation, compared with only 10,000 references to ventricular fibrillation and 6000 to ventricular tachycardia. Numerous theses, reviews, guidelines, and book chapters have also been published.

Surprisingly, very few books have been devoted to atrial fibrillation and no modern book has concentrated on this arrhythmia.

This volume was compiled by two experts in this arena. They have assembled a galaxy of authors, all well known for their original scientific contributions to this field and for their ability to synthesize, communicate, and educate. The book is a *tour de force* that has successfully sifted the most cogent and relevant information from the endless pages that have been written about this arrhythmia. Within this volume, the reader will find new and important knowledge about this condition. All the contributions should prove helpful for the management of patients who suffer from atrial fibrillation.

A. John Camm
St. George's Hospital Medical School
London, United Kingdom

Preface

Atrial fibrillation is by far the most frequently diagnosed cardiac arrhythmia in humans, accounting for tens of thousands of hospital admissions and millions of doctor visits. It is responsible for significant morbidity and mortality independent of the myriad of disease states with which it commonly coexists. Though given a common appellation, what we call atrial fibrillation represents a cornucopia of diseases extending from a focally activated pulmonary vein generator in patients with normal hearts to the diffuse degenerative disease process seen in the very old. It is this diversity of mechanism, combined with our primitive knowledge of its pathophysiology, which has rendered this arrhythmia so resistant to a myriad of interventions. It is the rare patient who can be "cured." For the vast majority, palliation is the goal, whether achieved with drugs or nonpharmacological therapy. The appropriate use of warfarin anticoagulation has had a positive impact on stroke, the most feared complication of the disease, but widespread implementation remains a thorny issue.

Given these facts, it is not surprising that we are in the midst of a massive effort to improve therapy and outcomes of patients stricken with atrial fibrillation. This includes symptom relief with the development of new and improved drugs for suppression of atrial fibrillation, better methods of rate control and anticoagulation, and the advent of several novel nonpharmacological therapies. The field is fast-moving and the information highly complex. Thus there is a need for a compendium, digestible by physicians in practice, in which the very latest data are adequately but succinctly summarized. Since information presented in book form can become outdated soon after publication, we organized this book in such a way as to make the time to publication short and to allow for a rapid preparation of subsequent editions.

This book is organized along traditional lines, moving from general epidemiological information through a discussion of pathophysiology and then several forms of management. However, for each chapter, we sought to enlist contributors who are working at the cutting edge of their discipline. They were given explicit instructions to include only new and evolving information from recent trials and to avoid more conventional dissertations. We requested that the new information, however, be placed in clinical context, with realistic appraisals of the potential applicability of each new therapy.

We believe that we have succeeded in assembling a book that should be useful to clinical scientists, arrhythmologists, practicing cardiologists and internists, cardiac surgeons, physician extenders, physicians-in-training, nurses, and students. Since it is our intention to update this information fairly often and on a regular basis, we welcome constructive criticism and suggestions for new material. Our ultimate goal is to create a renewable source of solid information in an accessible format so as to keep the medical public current in all of the many aspects of caring for patients with this very common arrhythmia.

Contents

Contributors

Maurits A. Allessie, M.D., Ph.D. Professor, Department of Physiology, Cardiovascular Research Institute Maastricht, Maastricht University, Maastricht, The Netherlands

Emelia J. Benjamin, M.D., Sc.M. Associate Professor, Department of Cardiology, Boston University School of Medicine, Boston, and Director, Echocardiography and Vascular Laboratory, The Framingham Heart Study, Framingham, Massachusetts, U.S.A.

Yuri Blaauw, M.D. Department of Physiology, Cardiovascular Research Institute Maastricht, Maastricht University, Maastricht, The Netherlands

Shih-An Chen, M.D. Professor of Medicine, Division of Cardiology, Department of Medicine, National Yang-Ming University, and Taipei Veterans General Hospital, Taipei, Taiwan

Mina K. Chung, M.D. Department of Cardiovascular Medicine, The Cleveland Clinic Foundation, Cleveland, Ohio, U.S.A.

Harry J. G. M. Crijns, M.D. Professor, Department of Cardiology, Maastricht University, and University Hospital Maastricht, Maastricht, The Netherlands

Joachim R. Ehrlich, M.D.   Division of Cardiology, Department of Medicine, Johann Wolfgang Goethe-University, Frankfurt, Germany

Kenneth A. Ellenbogen, M.D.   Kontos Professor of Medicine, Department of Medicine, Medical College of Virginia, Virginia Commonwealth University, Richmond, Virginia, U.S.A.

Andrew E. Epstein, M.D.   Professor, Division of Cardiovascular Diseases, Department of Medicine, The University of Alabama at Birmingham, Birmingham, Alabama, U.S.A.

Greg C. Flaker, M.D.   Professor, Department of Medicine, University of Missouri, Columbia, Missouri, U.S.A.

Stefan H. Hohnloser, M.D.   Professor, Departments of Cardiology and Electrophysiology, Johann Wolfgang Goethe-University, Frankfurt, Germany

Lai Chow Kok, M.B.B.S.   Assistant Professor, Division of Cardiology, Department of Internal Medicine, Medical College of Virginia, Virginia Commonwealth University, and Codirector, Cardiac Electrophysiology, Cardiology Section, Hunter Holmes McGuire, Veterans Affairs Medical Center, Richmond, Virginia, U.S.A.

Peter R. Kowey, M.D.   Professor, Division of Cardiology, Department of Medicine, Jefferson Medical College, Philadelphia, Pennsylvania, U.S.A.

Paul A. Levine, M.D.   Vice President and Medical Director, St. Jude Medical Cardiac Rhythm Management Division, Sylmar, and Loma Linda University School of Medicine, Loma Linda, California, U.S.A.

Mohammed Murtaza, M.D.   Postdoctoral Fellow, Division of Cardiology, Department of Medicine, University of Missouri, Columbia, Missouri, U.S.A.

Gerald V. Naccarelli, M.D.   Bernard Trabin Chair in Cardiology; Chief, Division of Cardiology; Professor, Department of Medicine; and Director, Cardiovascular Center, Pennsylvania State University College of Medicine and the Penn State Milton S. Hershey Medical Center, Hershey, Pennsylvania, U.S.A.

Philip J. Podrid, M.D.   Professor, Section of Cardiology, Department of Clinical Cardiology, and Associate Professor of Pharmacology and Experimental Therapeutics, Department of Pharmacology and Experimental Therapeutics, Boston University School of Medicine, Boston, Massachusetts, U.S.A.

James A. Reiffel, M.D. Professor, Division of Cardiology, Department of Medicine, Columbia University College of Physicians and Surgeons, and New York Presbyterian Hospital, New York, New York, U.S.A.

Luz-Maria Rodriguez, M.D., Ph.D. Associate Professor, Department of Cardiology, Maastricht University, and University Hospital Maastricht, Maastricht, The Netherlands

Ulrich Schotten, M.D., Ph.D. Department of Physiology, Cardiovascular Research Institute Maastricht, Maastricht University, Maastricht, The Netherlands

Bramah N. Singh, M.D., Ph.D. Department of Cardiology, Veterans Affairs Medical Center of West Los Angeles and the David Geffen School of Medicine at UCLA, Los Angeles, California, U.S.A.

Ching-Tai Tai, M.D. Division of Cardiology, Department of Medicine, National Yang-Ming University, and Taipei Veterans General Hospital, Taipei, Taiwan

Carl Timmermans, M.D., Ph.D. Associate Professor, Department of Cardiology, Maastricht University, and University Hospital Maastricht, Maastricht, The Netherlands

Thomas J. Wang, M.D. Instructor, Cardiology Division, Massachusetts General Hospital, Boston, and The Framingham Heart Study, Framingham, Massachusetts, U.S.A.

D. George Wyse, M.D., Ph.D., F.R.C.P.C., F.A.C.P., F.A.C.C., F.A.H.A. Professor, Department of Cardiac Sciences, Libin Cardiovascular Institute of Alberta, University of Calgary, and Calgary Health Region, Calgary, Alberta, Canada

Introduction

Atrial fibrillation (AF) is a multifaceted arrhythmia; like few other clinical entities, it challenges the physician to address multiple management issues for each new patient he or she evaluates. Because AF is a multifaceted disease state, we felt that a multichapter, multiauthored, contemporary textbook would provide a compendium of information that would be of practical use to physicians, trainees, and other health care professionals. What has emerged is a comprehensive and yet relatively succinct treatise on the many components of the diagnosis and treatment of this common arrhythmia, organized along traditional lines.

We start with a consideration of the epidemiology of the disease by Dr. Benjamin. In discussing this, she has drawn heavily on the Framingham experience, about which she is very knowledgeable. She has provided detailed information about the incidence and prevalence of the disease and its demography as well as its complications, including stroke and other thromboembolic events.

Dr. Podrid follows with a discussion of the etiology and pathogenesis of atrial fibrillation. He considers the diseases that are associated with this arrhythmia and posits how they participate in the genesis of the arrhythmic substrate. Dr. Podrid's chapter underscores the fact that AF has diverse etiologies, which is why we should consider this arrhythmia to be a collection of diseases grouped under a single name rather than a single, distinct clinical entity.

Dr. Singh delves further into the issue of pathogenesis, with a presentation of the perturbations of the cellular electrophysiology that give rise to AF. Of particular importance here are emerging data regarding abnormalities of specific ion channels ("channelopathies") that have been identified. It is now clear that abnormal channel function causes disturbances in conduction and repolarization that ultimately give rise to AF in its many forms.

Obtaining accurate information about mechanisms of disease in humans is predicated on the development and use of adequate animal models, and Dr. Allessie covers this matter in his chapter on preclinical testing. Though he focuses on the well-developed goat model from his own laboratory, which has taught us so much, it is clear that several types of models are necessary to study various aspects of this disease in order to generate appropriate hypotheses for clinical study.

For many years, we suspected that rate control and anticoagulation would serve as adequate therapy for many patients with AF. We have had that clinical impression "affirmed" by a number of clinical trials recently reported and summarized by Dr. Wyse, who also provides an interesting historical perspective on the subject.

Since rate control is a very important component of the management of AF, we asked Dr. Epstein to review the pharmacological and nondrug options for accomplishing that goal. He includes information related to acute and chronic management and highlights the advantages and disadvantages of each approach, including complete interruption of atrioventricular (AV) nodal conduction using ablation techniques, followed by ventricular pacing.

The most feared complication of AF is stroke and other thromboembolic events; therefore a detailed chapter on anticoagulation is essential. Dr. Flaker reports and analyzes all of the major primary and secondary prevention trials that have been carried out in patients with valvular and nonvalvular AF. These trials used an assortment of treament methods, including aspirin and other antiplatelet agents, unfractionated and low-molecular-weight heparins, warfarin, and new and more specific antithrombotic agents.

For many patients for whom restoration of sinus rhythm is the chosen strategy, the first step may be cardioversion. Dr. Crijns outlines the technique of electrical conversion including aspects of selecting the proper waveform, shock energy, and technique. He incorporates a thorough discussion of methods to prevent thromboembolic events, including anticoagulation and the use of transesophageal echocardiography, as well as the studies that support their use.

Though very effective, electrical cardioversion is not the only option for conversion of AF to sinus rhythm. There are several pharmacological options that are identified and described by Dr. Hohnloser. In this chapter, he lists drugs that can be used orally or parenterally for this purpose as well as their utility for prevention of early recurrence and for facilitating electrical conversion when indicated.

Once sinus rhythm has been restored, either iatrogenically or spontaneously, the challenge is to maintain that rhythm over the intermediate and long term. Dr. Reiffel lists and evaluates the many drugs that have been used, approved, recommended, and investigated for this purpose, drawing on a wealth of clinical trial data to do so. He highlights not only their efficacy but also their potential adverse effects, which are so important in assessing the relative value of any therapy.

Given the overall lack of satisfaction with drug therapy for AF suppression, alternative approaches have great potential value. One such approach is the use of devices both for prevention and termination of AF. Dr. Ellenbogen describes these therapies, including their use in combination with antiarrhythmic drugs, or so-called hybrid therapy.

Catheter ablation of many arrhythmias, most especially reentrant supraventricular tachycardia (SVT), has been enormously successful; thus it is logical that this technique should be applied to AF as well. Dr. Chen takes on this topic in his chapter, in which he reviews the various techniques that have emerged in the last decade. He includes in this discussion the potential for using ablation in concert with cardiac surgery.

AF that occurs after cardiac surgery is an interesting clinical entity that appears to have its own unique pathogenesis and natural history, distinct from those of other AF syndromes. Dr. Chung defines the syndrome and outlines several therapeutic approaches that have been used to prevent and treat this problem and its complications.

Finally, Dr. Naccarelli and I provide the "last word," in which we attempt to summarize the diverse information provided by our distinguished contributors and then go on to offer a glimpse into the future and how we think drugs, devices, anticoagulants, and other therapies may be employed to treat this very complex and unique disease state.

1

The Epidemiology of Atrial Fibrillation

Thomas J. Wang
Massachusetts General Hospital, Boston and The Framingham
Heart Study, Framingham, Massachusetts, U.S.A.

Emelia J. Benjamin
Boston University School of Medicine, Boston, and The Framingham
Heart Study, Framingham, Massachusetts, U.S.A.

I. INTRODUCTION

In the United States, atrial fibrillation (AF) accounts for approximately 400,000 annual hospital discharges and affects an estimated 2.3 million adults at any given time, more than any other abnormality of heart rhythm (1,2). From an epidemiological standpoint, AF is predominantly a disease of elderly individuals with cardiovascular disease. As a consequence, two trends affecting industrialized countries are expected to raise the prevalence of AF in the coming decades: the growth of the elderly population and improved survival with cardiovascular conditions such as myocardial infarction and heart failure.

This chapter reviews the prevalence, incidence, risk factors, and prognosis of AF and atrial flutter. We also summarize some novel epidemiological data concerning AF, including the lifetime risk and genetics of AF. It is important to recognize that most epidemiological investigations of AF have been conducted in North American and European Caucasians (3). The etiology and epidemiology of AF may differ in other regions and ethnicities. In addition, most studies preceded the International Consensus Conference on nomenclature and classification of AF, so definitions of AF subtypes have varied from study to study (4).

II. PREVALENCE AND INCIDENCE OF AF

A. Prevalence

Estimates of the overall adult prevalence of AF in the United States range from 1 to 6% (Table 1) (2,5–8). Because the prevalence of AF rises sharply with age, these estimates must be interpreted in the context of the age distribution in the samples studied. Most studies indicate that the overall prevalence of AF exceeds 5% in individuals aged 70 and above. Age-specific prevalences from a recent investigation in a large health maintenance organization (ATRIA cohort) are shown in Figure 1. AF is more prevalent among men than women, but approximately half the individuals with AF are women, given the higher proportion of women in older age groups.

B. Incidence

The incidence of AF has been reported in the Framingham Heart Study and the Cardiovascular Health Study (9,10). The Framingham Heart Study is a longitudinal, epidemiological investigation that was initiated in 1948 to study risk factors for cardiovascular disease. Among 4731 participants aged 55 to 94 who were free of AF in 1948, a total of 562 developed AF during follow-up of up to 38 years. Because participants were examined every 2 years, the incidence rates were reported as biennial rates. In men, the biennial incidence ranged from 6 per 1000 person-examinations in those 55 to 64 years old (approximately 0.3% per year), to 76 per 1000 person-examinations in those 85 to 94 years old (approximately 3.8% per year). In women, corresponding incidences were 4 per 1000 person-examinations (approximately 0.2% per year) and 63 per 1000 person-examinations (approximately 3.2% per year). As shown in Figure 2, the incidence of AF doubled for each successive decade

Table 1 Prevalence of AF in the United States

Study	Setting	Case Ascertainment	Age	Prevalence
ATRIA study (2)	Health maintenance organization	Claims data and ECG database	≥20 years	1.0%
Framingham Heart Study (5)	Community-based cohort	Biennial examinations	≥50 years	2.1%
Rochester Epidemiology Project (8)	Population sample	Medical record review	≥35 years	2.8%
Cardiovascular Health Study (7)	Cohort in four communities	ECG and self-report	≥65 years	5.4%

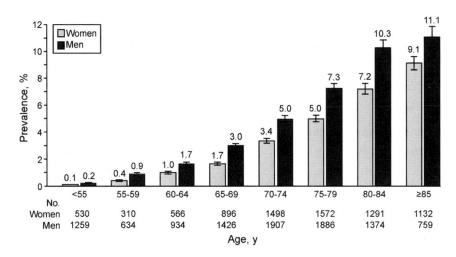

Figure 1 Prevalence of AF by age and sex. Bars represent 95% confidence intervals. (From Ref. 2.)

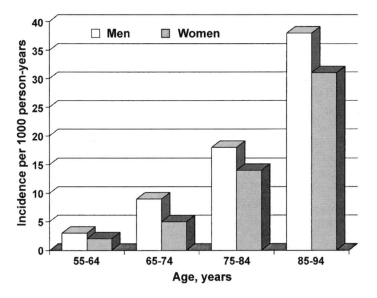

Figure 2 Incidence of AF in the Framingham Heart Study by age and sex. Biennial incidence rates are shown by dark bars for men and light bars for women. (From Ref. 9.)

of age in both men and women. The incidence of AF was about 50% higher in men than in women, even after adjusting for other risk factors for AF. The Cardiovascular Health Study is a longitudinal cohort study focusing on older individuals (at least 65 years old) who were enrolled at four centers in the United States beginning in 1990. The incidence of AF in this study was higher than that reported in Framingham, even after accounting for differences in the age of the study sample (10). Incidence rates ranged from 1.2% per year in men aged 65 to 69 to 5.9% in men aged 80 years and older. In women, corresponding incidence rates ranged from 1.1 to 2.5%. The inclusion of self-reported cases of AF, yearly electrocardiographic (ECG) examinations (rather than biennial examinations), and the more contemporary time period may have contributed to the higher incidence rates reported by the Cardiovascular Health Study (10).

C. Trends in Prevalence

Several studies indicate that the prevalence of AF has been increasing in the past several decades. Estimates from the National Ambulatory Medical Care Survey indicate that office visits for AF increased from 1.3 to 3.1 million between 1980 and 1992 (11). Hospital discharges for AF in individuals over age 65 increased from 30.6 to 59.5 per 10,000 between 1982 and 1993 (12). The increasing prevalence has been confirmed by more recent data published in the National Heart, Lung, and Blood Institute's *Chartbook* (13). Between 1980 and 1999, AF hospitalizations increased 80% for patients aged 45 to 65 and doubled for patients 65 years of age and older.

The aging of the population alone is expected to raise the number of individuals with AF from just over 2 million in 1995 to more than 3 million by 2020 and 5.6 million by 2050 (Fig. 3) (2). However, increases in the prevalence of AF may also be driven by factors other than aging. Framingham Heart Study investigators reported that the age-adjusted prevalence of AF nearly tripled in men between 1968 and 1989, rising from 3.2 to 9.1% (12). In women, a more modest, statistically nonsignificant increase was observed (2.8 to 4.7%). Recently, investigators from Rochester, Minnesota, reported similar magnitudes of increase in prevalence, using data from a case-cohort study of stroke patients and age-matched controls (mean age 75) (14). The increased prevalence of coronary artery disease, heart failure, and hypertension may be contributing to this trend (14,15).

D. Lifetime Risk of AF

Another measure of disease burden is the residual lifetime risk, which describes the probability of an individual developing a given disease over his or

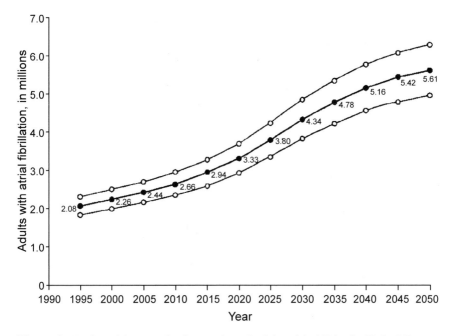

Figure 3 Projected increase in the number of adults with AF in the United States. Estimates based on U.S. Census projections of changing age and sex demographics. (From Ref. 2.)

her remaining lifetime. Framingham data indicate that men and women at age 40 have a residual lifetime risk of approximately 1 in 4 of developing AF (Table 2) (16). This risk remains relatively constant for individuals attaining older ages free of AF, as the shorter lifespan is balanced by the sharp age-related increase in the risk of AF. Thus, the lifetime risk of AF is substantial and higher than the risk of other, noncardiovascular conditions that affect elderly individuals, such as breast cancer (1 in 9) and hip fracture (1 in 6 for white women, 1 in 20 for white men) (17,18).

E. AF in Different Ethnicities

There are limited data regarding the epidemiology of AF in white versus nonwhite individuals. The report from the ATRIA cohort noted a lower prevalence of AF in blacks than in whites (1.5 vs. 2.2%, $p < 0.001$) among participants aged 50 and older (2). The Cardiovascular Health Study also noted a trend toward a lower incidence of AF in blacks than in whites (RR

Table 2 Lifetime Risk of Developing AF at Selected Index Ages[a]

Index age	Men	Women
40	26.0% (24.0–27.0%)	23.0% (21.0–24.0%)
50	25.9% (23.9–27.0%)	23.2% (21.3–24.3%)
60	25.8% (23.7–26.9%)	23.4% (21.4–24.4%)
70	24.3% (22.1–25.5%)	23.0% (20.9–24.1%)
80	22.7% (20.1–24.1%)	21.6% (19.3–22.7%)

[a] Values represent residual lifetime risk of AF (with 95% confidence intervals) for individuals attaining various index ages free of AF.
Source: Ref. 15.

0.47, 95% CI 0.22 to 1.01), a finding that achieved statistical significance in AF subjects without cardiovascular disease (RR 0.21, 95% CI 0.05 to 0.86) (10). The increased propensity for whites to develop AF has also been observed in heart failure cohorts (19) and stroke cohorts (20). Ethnic differences in AF have also been noted in British studies (20,21). Given the higher prevalence of many AF risk factors (e.g., hypertension) in blacks vs. whites, the lower prevalence of AF is puzzling and requires further study.

F. International Burden of AF

The estimated prevalence of AF in studies from Europe and Scandinavia ranges from 0.6 to 5.4% (3,22–28). Some of this variation is attributable to different ages in the study populations and different methods of case ascertainment. Estimates from other parts of the world and nonwhite populations are limited (3). One study reported that 1.3% of individuals in an elderly health survey in Hong Kong had AF (29). Similarly, AF was detected in 1.3% of individuals in a Japanese cohort of men and women >40 years of age (30). In one Himalayan village in India, the prevalence of AF was only 0.1% (31). All of these estimates were based on a single electrocardiogram, however, and the Himalayan study contained very few individuals older than 65 years. More studies are needed to examine global variation in the epidemiology of AF.

III. EPIDEMIOLOGY OF PAROXYSMAL AF

AF often presents as an intermittent condition known as "paroxysmal AF." The frequency of paroxysmal vs. chronic AF has not been established, partly because definitions of paroxysmal AF have varied until recently (4). Furthermore, it may be difficult to establish temporality in clinical studies because participants may be followed for short periods, as in hospital-based studies, or seen once every few years, as in epidemiological studies. In individuals prone to AF, asymptomatic atrial arrhythmias may also be common (32).

In the Stroke Prevention in AF trials, 28% of patients were classified as having intermittent AF (33). In this study, intermittent AF was defined as the presence of at least one ECG showing sinus rhythm at follow-up visits 1 and 3 months after enrollment. Compared with constant AF, those individuals with intermittent AF were younger, more likely to be women, and less likely to have hypertension, heart failure, left atrial enlargement, or left ventricular dysfunction. In a hospital-based Japanese study, 94 (40%) of 234 individuals with AF had paroxysmal AF, defined as conversion to sinus rhythm without electrical or chemical cardioversion (34). The frequency of paroxysmal AF in community-based studies is also variable. The Framingham Heart Study investigators reported that 41% of individuals with AF were found to have sinus rhythm at a subsequent biennial examination (35). A study from the Mayo Clinic reported a much higher prevalence of paroxysmal AF (62%) (8).

Recently, a clinical classification for AF was proposed that defines paroxysmal AF as an episode which spontaneously terminates within 7 days and usually lasts less than 48 hr (4). In this scheme, persistent AF is considered AF that lasts more than 7 days or requires cardioversion, whereas permanent (accepted) AF includes AF that fails to terminate with cardioversion or terminates and relapses within 24 hr. Using the above definition, French investigators studied 756 patients with AF in office practices and found that paroxysmal AF was present in 22% (36).

An intriguing area that has received little study is the temporal variability in paroxysmal AF. A transtelephonic study reported that 9989 recorded episodes of paroxysmal AF were not randomly distributed but were more likely to occur in the morning and the evening (37). Significantly fewer episodes were noted on Saturday compared with other days of the week, and more episodes were observed during the last months of the year. The authors concluded that there was a circadian and seasonal variation of paroxysmal AF events reminiscent of that noted with other cardiovascular diseases.

There are limited data regarding the natural history of paroxysmal AF. Studies indicate that the recurrence risk of AF is high, ranging from 49 to 90% (33,38). In the Stroke Prevention in AF studies, independent predictors of recurrent AF were left atrial enlargement and history of myocardial infarction (33). In hospital-based studies, 18 to 33% of patients appear to develop permanent AF (34,39,40). An investigation based in a university practice found that advancing age (hazard ratio per decade of age, 1.8, 95% CI 1.3 to

2.5) and AF at presentation (hazard ratio 3.6, 95% CI 1.7 to 7.3) predicted transition from intermittent to permanent AF (40).

IV. AF IN ASYMPTOMATIC INDIVIDUALS

Part of the difficulty in studying AF is that a substantial proportion of AF events are asymptomatic. A transtelephonic ECG monitoring study found that asymptomatic paroxysmal AF events (of at least 30-sec duration) were 12 times more frequent than symptomatic events; the mean event rates per 100 days per patient were 62.5 vs. 5.2 ($p < 0.01$) (32). In a drug study, 13% of subjects randomized to azimilide and 18% of subjects randomized to placebo had asymptomatic events documented on intermittent transtelophonic monitoring (41). Similarly, in the Cardiovascular Health Study, 12% of participants with AF were unaware of this rhythm, which was detected by a routine clinic ECG (10).

V. EPIDEMIOLOGY OF ATRIAL FLUTTER

As with paroxysmal AF, knowledge about the epidemiology of atrial flutter is incomplete. Most epidemiological studies include atrial flutter in the definition of AF, in part because subsequent conversion to AF is common (42). However, there is controversy over whether the risk of stroke and other adverse outcomes is the same for the two arrhythmias. Also, in contrast to AF, atrial flutter is often curable with ablative therapy. These developments have generated increased interest in the epidemiology and clinical correlates of atrial flutter.

One of the few studies on this topic is based on data from the Marshfield Epidemiologic Study Area. Investigators identified 181 cases of atrial flutter in a catchment area encompassing 58,820 resident in central Wisconsin. Based on these data, they estimated an overall incidence of 0.88 per 1000 person-years for atrial flutter (43). Not surprisingly, the incidence was age-dependent, ranging from 0.05 per 1000 person-years in individuals aged less than 50 years, to 5.9 per 1000 person-years in individuals above age 80. Compared to age- and sex-matched controls, individuals with atrial flutter had a higher prevalence of heart failure (RR 3.5, 95% CI, 1.7 to 7.1) and chronic obstructive pulmonary disease (RR 1.9, 95% CI, 1.1 to 3.4). A recent study examined the clinical characteristics and outcome of patients with atrial flutter from the Canadian Registry of Atrial Fibrillation (44). Of 881 eligible patients with AF, 94 had atrial flutter. Those with atrial flutter tended to have a higher prevalence of heart failure ($p = 0.08$) and were marginally more likely to be male ($p = 0.07$), but they were otherwise similar to the AF patients. During follow-up of up to 10 years, 28% subsequently converted to AF. The risk of stroke (1.33 vs 1.24 per 100 person-years; $p = 0.99$) and the risk of death (3.51 vs. 2.91 per 100 person-years; $p = 0.29$) did not differ significantly in the atrial flutter group compared with the AF group (44).

VI. RISK FACTORS FOR AF

A. Clinical Risk Factors

A wide variety of cardiovascular and noncardiovascular diseases have been associated with AF. These etiologies are covered in Chapter 2. AF is also a common complication of cardiovascular surgery, as discussed in Chapter 13. While hospital-based studies are important for establishing the spectrum of diseases that may lead to AF, epidemiological data provide insights into the conditions that most frequently predispose to AF in unselected individuals. These are conditions most likely to affect the burden of AF in the general population.

Data from epidemiological studies reinforce the notion that AF usually occurs in people with cardiovascular disease or cardiovascular disease risk factors. Risk factors for developing AF in the Framingham Heart Study are shown in Table 3. Older age, diabetes, left ventricular hypertrophy on ECG, hypertension, prior myocardial infarction, prior heart failure, and valvular disease were associated with incident AF (9). Multivariable analyses are necessary to examine the independent contribution of these individual risk factors, because risk factors commonly occur together. In multivariable analyses based on the Framingham data, age, diabetes, hypertension, myocardial infarction (in men), heart failure, and valvular disease remained significantly associated with the risk of developing AF. Myocardial infarction in women and left ventricular hypertrophy on ECG in both sexes were not significant predictors, probably because of their lower prevalences and their association with other characteristics. Male gender was also a significant predictor of incident AF (adjusted OR 1.5, 95% CI 1.3 to 1.8; $p < 0.0001$) (9).

Similar findings have been reported in the Cardiovascular Health Study (10). In multivariable analyses, age, systolic blood pressure, blood glucose, coronary disease, valve disease, and heart failure were associated with incident AF. In contrast to the Framingham Heart Study, male sex and congestive heart failure were not associated with AF. The Cardiovascular Health Study analyses adjusted for left atrial size on echocardiography, which may have attenuated associations in which left atrial enlargement was in the causal pathway. Lung disease (low forced expiratory volume in 1 sec) was also

Table 3 Risk Factors for Developing AF

Variables	Men				Women			
	AF	No AF	Age-Adjusted OR	Fully Adjusted OR	AF	No AF	Age-Adjusted OR	Fully Adjusted OR
Age, per 10 years	–	–	–	2.1[a]	–	–	–	2.2[a]
Cigarette smoking	35%	34%	1.0	1.1	29%	23%	1.4[a]	1.4
Diabetes	16%	10%	1.7[a]	1.4[a]	16%	8%	2.1[a]	1.6[a]
ECG LVH	11%	4%	3.0[a]	1.4	14%	4%	3.8[a]	1.3
Hypertension	44%	31%	1.8[a]	1.5[a]	52%	41%	1.7[a]	1.4[a]
Myocardial infarction	26%	13%	2.2[a]	1.4[a]	13%	5%	2.4[a]	1.2
Heart failure	21%	3%	6.1[a]	4.5[a]	26%	3%	8.1[a]	5.9[a]
Valvular disease	17%	7%	2.2[a]	1.8[a]	30%	9%	3.6[a]	3.4[a]
Body mass index, kg/m^2	26.2	26.0	1.03	–	26.0	25.7	1.02	–
Ethanol, oz/wk	5.4	5.1	1.01	–	1.5	1.8	0.95	–

Key: ECG LVH, electrocardiographic left ventricular hypertrophy; OR, odds ratios; values are age-adjusted percents (categorical data) or means (continuous data). Age-adjusted and multivariable-adjusted odds ratios are from 2-year pooled logistic regression.
[a] $p < 0.05$.
Source: Ref. 9.

an independent correlate, a finding confirmed by the Copenhagen City Heart Study (45).

The concept of population-attributable risk provides additional information regarding the impact of a risk factor on the societal burden of disease, because this index integrates the prevalence of a risk factor and the strength of its association with the disease. Population-attributable risks for AF from the Framingham Heart Study are shown in Table 4. Hypertension, congestive heart failure, and valvular disease (in women) are associated with the highest population-attributable risks for AF (9).

Although alcohol use ("holiday heart") may be an important precipitant of AF in some individuals, it does not appear to contribute substantially to the risk of AF on a community level (46–48). Paradoxically, alcohol use was associated with a reduced risk of AF in the Cardiovascular Health Study (RR 0.96 for an additional drink per week, CI 0.96 to 0.99), perhaps reflecting the low levels of alcohol consumption in the elderly (10). In an analysis of the Framingham cohort using long-term data on alcohol use, moderate alcohol consumption was not associated with AF risk in either gender (48). However, heavy consumption (more than three drinks per day) appeared to increase the risk of AF in men. Thyrotoxicosis is another uncommon but established precipitant of AF (49). Interestingly, even in clinically euthyroid individuals, a low serum thyrotropin was associated with a higher risk of AF (50).

B. Echocardiographic Predictors

Several studies have examined the relations between baseline echocardiographic findings and the development of AF. In these studies, left atrial size is

Table 4 Population-Attributable Risks for Atrial Fibrillation[a]

Variable	Men	Women
Cigarette smoking	2%	8%
Diabetes	4%	4%
Left ventricular hypertrophy on ECG	2%	1%
Hypertension	14%	14%
Myocardial infarction	5%	1%
Heart failure	10%	12%
Valve disease	5%	18%

[a] Based on coefficients from 2-year pooled logistic regression.
Source: Ref. 9.

the most consistent predictor of AF (10,51,52). In the Framingham Heart Study, individuals in the highest quartile of left atrial diameter (≥44 mm) had approximately 2.5 times the risk of developing AF compared with individuals in the lowest quartile of left atrial diameter (≤35 mm) after adjusting for age and sex (51). There was a multivariable-adjusted 1.4-fold increase in the risk of AF for every 5 mm increase in left atrial diameter. An effect of similar magnitude was observed in the Cardiovascular Health Study cohort (10). Investigators from the Mayo Clinic reported that left atrial volume, using a biplane area length method, predicted the development of AF over and above left atrial diameter (52). These studies have provided the valuble insight that left atrial enlargement can precede the development of AF, because AF itself may lead to left atrial dilation (53,54). Nonetheless, it is not known whether interventions that reduce left atrial size also decrease the risk of AF.

Although AF is an arrhythmia of atrial origin, echocardiographic abnormalities in the left ventricle have been associated with AF. These abnormalities may correlate with higher left atrial filling pressures, which may predispose to AF independently of structural atrial dilation. The Framingham investigators reported that both left ventricular wall thickness and endocardial fractional shortening were related to the development of AF (Fig. 4) (51). These associations persisted even after adjustment for left atrial

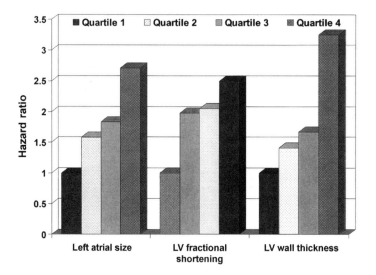

Figure 4 Hazards ratios for developing AF according to quartile of echocardiographic predictors. Hazards ratios were age-stratified and sex-adjusted. (From Ref. 51.)

size and clinical risk factors. The Mayo Clinic and Framingham investigators have found that abnormalities of diastolic filling by Doppler echocardiography were independently associated with incident AF (55,56).

C. AF and Heart Failure

AF and congestive heart failure (CHF) are closely linked disorders, both epidemiologically and pathophysiologically. Braunwald has labeled them "the two new epidemics of cardiovascular disease," in recognition of the increasing public health importance of AF and CHF (57). Because both disorders predominantly affect elderly individuals with preexisting cardiovascular disease, their epidemiological features are strikingly similar. Indeed, the demographic trends leading to increases in AF prevalence are likely to affect CHF prevalence as well. Their lifetime risks are also very similar (16,58).

The association between AF and CHF reflects more than common demographic features. They share common risk factors, including older age, hypertension, myocardial infarction, and valvular heart disease (9,59). Furthermore, each condition may directly predispose to the other. CHF may precipitate AF by acutely elevating left atrial filling pressures and by chronically causing atrial fibrosis and excessive sympathetic activation (60,61). Conversely, AF may cause a reduction in cardiac output through loss of atrial transport; prolonged tachycardia is an unusual but well-described etiology of dilated cardiomyopathy (62).

As shown in Figure 5, which is based on a report from the Framingham Heart Study, there is a high incidence of new-onset AF after a diagnosis of CHF, and vice versa (63). Rates of developing AF in individuals with CHF are 54 per 1000 person-years. Rates of developing CHF after AF are 33 per 1000 person-years. A retrospective analysis from the SOLVD trial suggests that angiotensin converting enzyme (ACE) inhibition with enalapril reduces the incidence of AF in CHF patients (64).

D. Lone AF

A small proportion of individuals have AF in the absence of any known cardiovascular disease. The prevalence of this entity ("lone AF") in community-based cohorts ranges from 2 to 11%, depending on the definition and the age of the sample studied (65–67). Approaches to stroke prophylaxis in individuals with lone AF are described in Chapter 7. As medical knowledge advances, it is likely that lone AF will represent an increasingly small percentage of overall AF cases. Investigators have implicated genetic factors in the etiology of some cases of lone AF, particularly in the very young (see below) (68).

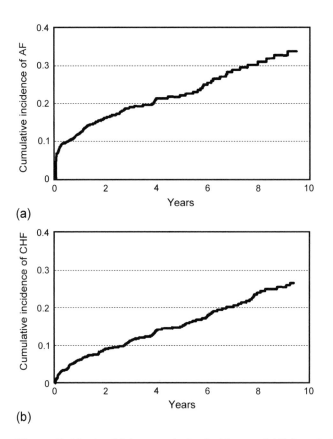

Figure 5 Kaplan-Meier cumulative incidence of AF (panel a) in individuals with CHF, and Kaplan-Meier cumulative incidence of CHF (panel b) in individuals with AF. (From Ref. 63.)

E. Genetic Epidemiology of AF

Familial transmission of AF was first reported in 1943 (69). In 1997, a report from Brugada and colleagues stimulated renewed interest in the genetic underpinnings of this arrhythmia (68). The investigators described three families with apparent autosomal dominant transmission of AF, and linkage to a locus on chromosome 10q22-24 was demonstrated in all three families. Subsequent studies have identified families with AF mapping to loci on chromosomes 6q14-16 and 11p15 (70,71). In the family with linkage to chromosome 11p15, a causative gain-of-function mutation was identified in the KCNQ1 gene, which encodes a subunit of several types of potassium channels expressed in the heart (70,71).

Despite the existence of familial AF, the contribution of genetic factors to AF in the general population is unknown. A recent study found a positive family history in 5% of AF patients referred to an arrhythmia clinic, including 15% of patients with lone AF, suggesting that familial AF may be more common than previously thought (72). In the Framingham Heart Study, individuals with a parental history of AF had an increased risk of developing AF themselves (multivariable-adjusted odds ratio, 1.85, 95% confidence interval, 1.12–3.06) (73). This finding was stronger when the age of AF was limited to less than 75 years (multivariable-adjusted odds ratio, 3.23, 95% confidence interval, 1.87–5.58). These data support a genetic predisposition to AF, even in unselected individuals, although the specific genetic factors responsible remain to be elucidated.

VII. COMPLICATIONS AND PROGNOSIS OF AF

A. Stroke and AF

One of the most serious complications of AF is systemic embolism, particularly stroke. The association between AF and stroke in rheumatic heart disease was recognized at least 70 years ago (47). The concept that nonrheumatic AF is also a major risk factor for stroke was slower to gain acceptance (74,75). In 1978, investigators from the Framingham study reported a 5.6-fold increased rate of stroke in participants with nonrheumatic AF after adjustment for age, sex, and hypertensive status (76). Subsequently, numerous investigations in different countries have supported the independent association between nonrheumatic AF and stroke risk (22,30,77).

The population-attributable risk of stroke associated with AF and various other conditions is shown in Table 5, based on 34-year follow-up data from the Framingham study (5). For AF, the population-attributable risk

Table 5 Population-Attributable Risks for Stroke[a]

Condition	Age group (years)			
	50–59	60–69	70–79	80–89
Hypertension	48.8%	53.2%	48.6%	33.4%
Coronary heart disease	11.1%	12.4%	12.6%	0.0%
Heart failure	2.3%	3.1%	5.6%	6.0%
Atrial fibrillation	1.5%	2.8%	9.9%	23.5%

[a] A significant increase in attributable risk with age was observed for atrial fibrillation ($p < 0.01$) but not other conditions.
Source: Ref. 5.

rises from 1.5% in 50 to 59-year-olds to 24% in 80-to 89-year-olds. In contrast, the population-attributable risk for hypertension, coronary artery disease, and heart failure does not exhibit a significant increase with age. In the same study, the multivariable-adjusted relative risk of stroke in 80-to 89-year-olds was 4.5 ($p < 0.001$) for participants with AF vs. those without AF. The relative risk for other stroke risk factors was substantially less (1.7 for hypertension, 0.7 for coronary artery disease, and 1.7 for heart failure). The attributable risk is highest for hypertension because of the high prevalence of hypertension, but these data suggest that AF is the second most important contributor to stroke in the very elderly.

In addition to increasing stroke risk, AF is associated with greater stroke severity. In the Copenhagen Stroke Study, patients with stroke due to AF had higher mortality, longer hospitalizations, and greater neurological and functional disability than patients with stroke and no AF (78). Similar findings have been reported from the Framingham study (79) and a hospital-based study in northern Spain (80).

The powerful independent influence of AF on the risk of stroke is supported by data from numerous randomized trials, which show an approximately 60% reduction in stroke events with warfarin prophylaxis (81). Because the stroke risk in AF is heterogeneous, studies have attempted to define clinical predictors of stroke in AF (82–87). The use of these predictors for risk stratification in AF and for making decisions about anticoagulation is discussed in Chapter 7.

B. Other Embolic Complications of AF

AF is also associated with embolism to other arterial beds. In a recent Danish study, the relative risk of peripheral thromboembolism was 4.0 (95% CI, 3.5 to 4.6) in men and 5.7 (95% CI, 5.1 to 6.3) in women with AF compared with age-matched controls (88). The most common sites of embolism were the upper and lower extremities (61%), followed by the mesenteric arteries (29%), the pelvic arteries (9%), the aorta (7%), and the renal arteries (2%).

C. AF and Dementia

Several recent studies have reported that AF may be a risk factor for dementia. Investigators from the Rotterdam Study noted that dementia was approximately twice as common in individuals with AF than in those without AF (23). This association did not appear attributable to differences in age, cardiovascular risk factors, or prior stroke. In a study of 69- to 75-year-old men in Uppsala, Sweden, scores on cognitive tests were lower in those with AF than in those without AF after adjustment for age, diabetes, diastolic blood pressure, and educational status (89). Several smaller studies have reported similar findings (90,91).

One potential mechanism for these findings is the occurrence of silent brain infarcts after AF. Participants in the Veteran Affairs Stroke Prevention in Non-rheumatic AF Study underwent computed tomography scans of the head at the time of entry (92). Nearly 15% of AF patients had evidence of a silent brain infarct despite a normal neurological examination. In a separate investigation using magnetic resonance imaging, investigators found an association between AF and white matter hyperintensities, which are a possible marker of cerebral hypoperfusion (93).

D. AF and Mortality

A number of studies have documented increased mortality in individuals who develop AF (94–98). In the Framingham study, AF was a predictor of mortality in both genders, even after adjusting for age and cardiovascular disease risk factors (97). Interestingly, however, the influence of AF was stronger in women (adjusted OR 1.9, 95% CI, 1.5 to 2.2) than in men (adjusted OR 1.5, 95% CI, 1.2 to 1.8), such that AF appeared to diminish the female survival advantage. The elevated risk of death was not limited to those with clinical cardiovascular disease; AF was associated with a twofold increase in the risk of death in participants without prevalent cardiovascular disease.

Concomitant CHF in individuals with AF is associated with a particularly poor prognosis (99–101). In the Framingham study, a prior history of CHF was associated with an excess mortality risk of 2.2 in men and 1.8 in women with AF ($p < 0.001$ for comparison with AF subjects and no CHF history) (63). In those with AF and no history of CHF, the subsequent development of CHF was associated with an even greater relative risk of mortality (2.7 in men, 3.1 in women; both $p < 0.001$).

E. AF and Quality of Life

While AF is associated with substantial morbidity and mortality, its impact on quality of life is also an important consideration, particularly for examining therapies aimed at reducing episodes of paroxysmal AF. Most studies in this area have focused on patients undergoing atrioventricular nodal ablation (102). Using self-reported symptoms or standardized instruments to assess quality of life, the majority of these studies have demonstrated improvements in quality of life associated with nodal ablation (103,104). However, limitations of these studies include the highly selected nature of the patients and small sample sizes.

Recently, Dorian and colleagues reported on 152 consecutive AF patients referred to arrhythmia clinics in four countries (105). Compared with healthy controls, the AF patients had significantly worse quality-of-life scores across all scales of the SF-36, a widely used survey instrument. For instance, the general health score was more than a full standard deviation lower in the AF group compared with healthy controls ($p < 0.001$). In the Canadian Trial of AF, a subjective assessment of global well-being was higher in participants with no AF recurrence on antiarrhythmic therapy than in those with recurrence despite therapy (106).

F. Costs of AF

There are few data regarding the economic costs of caring for patients with AF. Hospitalizations for cardiac arrhythmias cost Medicare an estimated $2.1 billion in 1998 (1). Because AF accounts for more than half of arrhythmia hospitalizations, it is likely that the costs of hospitalizing patients with AF are substantial. A study using 1991 Medicare claims data estimated that total spending was 9 to 23% higher (depending on age and gender stratum) in individuals with AF compared with individuals without AF after adjusting for other comorbid diagnoses (107). Increases in hospitalizations for AF are likely to raise the economic burden of this condition even further (108).

VIII. FUTURE DIRECTIONS

The past two decades have seen major advances in knowledge about the epidemiology of AF. However, major gaps in understanding persist. Further study of the factors contributing to temporal increases in the prevalence and incidence of AF is warranted.

Additional investigations are needed to characterize the epidemiology of AF in nonwhites and in countries outside of North America and Europe. Risk factors for AF have been intensively studied, but relatively little is known about the contribution of genetic factors to the development of AF and its sequelae. Understanding the interplay between genetic and environmental factors in the pathogenesis of AF may provide targets for early intervention or therapeutic tailoring.

The prognosis of AF also requires further investigation. Differences in the presentation and prognosis between chronic AF and paroxysmal AF as well as between AF and atrial flutter remain poorly understood. Outcomes other than overt stroke—such as quality of life, silent stroke, and cognitive decline—have been incompletely investigated in large prospective studies.

AF is an arrhythmia of considerable public health importance because it is common, rising in prevalence, and associated with substantial morbidity and mortality. Because therapies for AF are toxic and in some cases controversial, prevention may be the most desirable strategy for dealing with this arrhythmia. Multiple epidemiological studies have established that cardiovascular disease contributes to the development of AF, which suggests that attention to traditional cardiovascular risk factors may reduce the incidence of AF in the general population.

REFERENCES

1. American Heart Association. Heart disease and stroke statistics—2003 updateDallas: American Heart Association, 2002.
2. Go AS, Hylek EM, Phillips KA, Chang Y, Henault LE, Selby JV, et al. Prevalence of diagnosed atrial fibrillation in adults: national implications for rhythm management and stroke prevention: the AnTicoagulation and Risk Factors in Atrial Fibrillation (ATRIA) Study. JAMA 2001; 285:2370–2375.
3. Ryder KM, Benjamin EJ. Epidemiology and significance of atrial fibrillation. Am J Cardiol 1999; 84:131R–138R.
4. Levy S, Camm AJ, Saksena S, Aliot E, Breithardt G, Crijns H, et al. International consensus on nomenclature and classification of atrial fibrillation: a collaborative project of the Working Group on Arrhythmias and the Working Group on Cardiac Pacing of the European Society of Cardiology and the North American Society of Pacing and Electrophysiology. Europace 2003; 5:119–122.
5. Wolf PA, Abbott RD, Kannel WB. Atrial fibrillation as an independent risk factor for stroke: the Framingham Study. Stroke 1991; 22:983–988.
6. Feinberg WM, Blackshear JL, Laupacis A, Kronmal R, Hart RG. Prevalence, age distribution, and gender of patients with atrial fibrillation: analysis and implications. Arch Intern Med 1995; 155:469–473.
7. Furberg CD, Psaty BM, Manolio TA, Gardin JM, Smith VE, Rautaharju PM. Prevalence of atrial fibrillation in elderly subjects (The Cardiovascular Health Study). Am J Cardiol 1994; 74:236–241.
8. Phillips SJ, Whisnant JP, OFallon WM, Frye RL. Prevalence of cardiovascular disease and diabetes mellitus in residents of Rochester, Minnesota. Mayo Clin Proc 1990; 65:344–359.
9. Benjamin EJ, Levy D, Vaziri SM, D'Agostino RB, Belanger AJ, Wolf PA. Independent risk factors for atrial fibrillation in a population-based cohort: the Framingham Heart Study. JAMA 1994; 271:840–844.
10. Psaty BM, Manolio TA, Kuller LH, Kronmal RA, Cushman M, Fried LP, et al. Incidence of and risk factors for atrial fibrillation in older adults. Circulation 1997; 96:2455–2461.
11. Stafford RS, Singer DE. National patterns of warfarin use in atrial fibrillation. Arch Intern Med 1996; 156:2537–2541.
12. Wolf PA, Benjamin EJ, Belanger AJ, Kannel WB, Levy D, D'Agostino RB. Secular trends in the prevalence of atrial fibrillation: the Framingham Study. Am Heart J 1996; 131:790–795.

13. Morbidity and Mortality: 2002 Chartbook on Cardiovascular, Lung, and Blood Diseases. Washington, DC: United States Public Health Service, National Institutes of Health, 2002.

14. Tsang TS, Petty GW, Barnes ME, O'Fallon WM, Bailey KR, Wiebers DO, et al. The prevalence of atrial fibrillation in incident stroke cases and matched population controls in Rochester, Minnesota: changes over three decades. J Am Coll Cardiol 2003; 42:93–100.

15. Hajjar I, Kotchen TA. Trends in prevalence, awareness, treatment, and control of hypertension in the United States, 1988–2000. JAMA 2003; 290:199–206.

16. Wang TJ, Larson MG, Lloyd-Jones DM, Leip EP, Levy D, Vasan RS, D'Agostino RB, Wolf PA, Massaro J, Benjamin EJ. Lifetime risk of atrial fibrillation: the Framingham Heart Study [abstr]. Circulation 2002; 106:II-456.

17. Feuer EJ, Wun LM, Boring CC, Flanders WD, Timmel MJ, Tong T. The lifetime risk of developing breast cancer. J Natl Cancer Inst 1993; 85:892–897.

18. Cummings SR, Black DM, Rubin SM. Lifetime risks of hip, Colles', or vertebral fracture and coronary heart disease among white postmenopausal women. Arch Intern Med 1989; 149:2445–2448.

19. Afzal A, Ananthasubramaniam K, Sharma N, al Malki Q, Ali AS, Jacobsen G, et al. Racial differences in patients with heart failure. Clin Cardiol 1999; 22:791–794.

20. Hajat C, Dundas R, Stewart JA, Lawrence E, Rudd AG, Howard R, et al. Cerebrovascular risk factors and stroke subtypes: differences between ethnic groups. Stroke 2001; 32:37–42.

21. Zarifis J, Beevers G, Lip GY. Acute admissions with atrial fibrillation in a British multiracial hospital population. Br J Clin Pract 1997; 51:91–96.

22. Boysen G, Nyboe J, Appleyard M, Sorensen PS, Boas J, Somnier F, et al. Stroke incidence and risk factors for stroke in Copenhagen, Denmark. Stroke 1988; 19:1345–1353.

23. Ott A, Breteler MM, de Bruyne MC, van Harskamp F, Grobbee DE, Hofman A. Atrial fibrillation and dementia in a population-based study. The Rotterdam Study. Stroke 1997; 28:316–321.

24. Langenberg M, Hellemons BSP, van Ree J, Vermeer F, Lodder J, Schouten HJA, et al. Atrial fibrillation in elderly patients: prevalence and comorbidity in general practice. BMJ 1996; 313:1534.

25. Sudlow M, Thomson R, Thwaites B, Rodgers H, Kenny RA. Prevalence of atrial fibrillation and eligibility for anticoagulants in the community. Lancet 1998; 352:1167–1171.

26. Wheeldon NM, Tayler DI, Anagnostou E, Cook D, Wales C, Oakley GD. Screening for atrial fibrillation in primary care. Heart 1998; 79:50–55.

27. Hill JD, Mottram EM, Killeen PD. Study of the prevalence of atrial fibrillation in general practice patients over 65 years of age. J R Coll Gen Pract 1987; 37:172–173.

28. Stewart S, Hart CL, Hole DJ, McMurray JJ. Population prevalence, incidence, and predictors of atrial fibrillation in the Renfrew/Paisley study. Heart 2001; 86:516–521.

29. Lok NS, Lau CP. Prevalence of palpitations, cardiac arrhythmias and their associated risk factors in ambulant elderly. Int J Cardiol 1996; 54:231–236.

30. Nakayama T, Date C, Yokoyama T, Yoshiike N, Yamaguchi M, Tanaka H. A 15.5-year follow-up study of stroke in a Japanese provincial city. The Shibata Study. Stroke 1997; 28:45–52.

31. Kaushal SS, DasGupta DJ, Prashar BS, Bhardwaj AK. Electrocardiographic manifestations of healthy residents of a tribal Himalayan village. J Assoc Physicians India 1995; 43:15–16.

32. Page RL, Wilkinson WE, Clair WK, McCarthy EA, Pritchett EL. Asymptomatic arrhythmias in patients with symptomatic paroxysmal atrial fibrillation and paroxysmal supraventricular tachycardia. Circulation 1994; 89:224–227.

33. Flaker GC, Fletcher KA, Rothbart RM, Halperin JL, Hart RG. Clinical and echocardiographic features of intermittent atrial fibrillation that predict recurrent atrial fibrillation. Stroke Prevention in Atrial Fibrillation (SPAF) Investigators. Am J Cardiol 1995; 76:355–358.

34. Takahashi N, Seki A, Imataka K, Fujii J. Clinical features of paroxysmal atrial fibrillation. An observation of 94 patients. Jpn Heart J 1981; 22:143–149.

35. Kannel WB, Abbott RD, Savage DD, McNamara PM. Coronary heart disease and atrial fibrillation: the Framingham Study. Am Heart J 1983; 106:389–396.

36. Levy S, Maarek M, Coumel P, Guize L, Lekieffre J, Medvedowsky JL, et al. Characterization of different subsets of atrial fibrillation in general practice in France: the ALFA study. The College of French Cardiologists. Circulation 1999; 99:3028–3035.

37. Viskin S, Golovner M, Malov N, Fish R, Alroy I, Vila Y, et al. Circadian variation of symptomatic paroxysmal atrial fibrillation. Data from almost 10,000 episodes. Eur Heart J 1999; 20:1429–1434.

38. Rostagno C, Bacci F, Martelli M, Naldoni A, Bertini G, Gensini G. Clinical course of lone atrial fibrillation since first symptomatic arrhythmic episode. Am J Cardiol 1995; 76:837–839.

39. Petersen P, Godtfredsen J. Embolic complications in paroxysmal atrial fibrillation. Stroke 1986; 17:622–626.

40. Al Khatib SM, Wilkinson WE, Sanders LL, McCarthy EA, Pritchett EL. Observations on the transition from intermittent to permanent atrial fibrillation. Am Heart J 2000; 140:142–145.

41. Page RL, Tilsch TW, Connolly SJ, Schnell DJ, Marcello SR, Wilkinson WE, et al. Asymptomatic or "silent" atrial fibrillation: frequency in untreated patients and patients receiving azimilide. Circulation 2003; 107:1141–1145.

42. Biblo LA, Yuan Z, Quan KJ, Mackall JA, Rimm AA. Risk of stroke in patients with atrial flutter. Am J Cardiol 2001; 87(3):346–349, A9.

43. Granada J, Uribe W, Chyou PH, Maassen K, Vierkant R, Smith PN, et al. Incidence and predictors of atrial flutter in the general population. J Am Coll Cardiol 2000; 36:2242–2246.

44. LeLorier P, Humphries KH, Krahn AD, Connolly SJ, Talajic M, Green M, et al. Prognostic differences between atrial fibrillation and atrial flutter. Am J Cardiol, 2003. In press.

45. Buch P, Friberg J, Scharling H, Lange P, Prescott E. Reduced lung function and risk of atrial fibrillation in the Copenhagen City Heart Study. Eur Respir J 2003; 21:1012–1016.

46. Thornton JR. Atrial fibrillation in healthy non-alcoholic people after an alcoholic binge. Lancet 1984; 2:1013–1015.

47. Ettinger PO, Wu CF, De La Cruz C Jr, Weisse AB, Ahmed SS, Regan TJ. Arrhythmias and the "holiday heart": alcohol-associated cardiac rhythm disorders. Am Heart J 1978; 95:555–562.

48. Djousse L, Levy D, Benjamin EJ, Blease S, Russ A, Larson MG, et al. Long-term alcohol consumption and the risk of atrial fibrillation in the Framingham Study. Am J Cardiol 2003. In press.

49. Osman F, Gammage MD, Sheppard MC, Franklyn JA. Clinical review 142: cardiac dysrhythmias and thyroid dysfunction: the hidden menace? J Clin Endocrinol Metab 2002; 87:963–967.

50. Sawin CT, Geller A, Wolf PA, Belanger AJ, Baker E, Bacharach P, et al. Low serum thyrotropin concentrations as a risk factor for atrial fibrillation in older persons. N Engl J Med 1994; 331:1249–1252.

51. Vaziri SM, Larson MG, Benjamin EJ, Levy D. Echocardiographic predictors of nonrheumatic atrial fibrillation. The Framingham Heart Study. Circulation 1994; 89:724–730.

52. Tsang TS, Barnes ME, Bailey KR, Leibson CL, Montgomery SC, Takemoto Y, et al. Left atrial volume: important risk marker of incident atrial fibrillation in 1655 older men and women. Mayo Clin Proc 2001; 76:467–475.

53. Sanfilippo AJ, Abascal VM, Sheehan M, Oertel LB, Harrigan P, Hughes RA, et al. Atrial enlargement as a consequence of atrial fibrillation. A prospective echocardiographic study. Circulation 1990; 82:792–797.

54. Petersen P, Kastrup J, Brinch K, Godtfredsen J, Boysen G. Relation between left atrial dimension and duration of atrial fibrillation. Am J Cardiol 1987; 60:382–384.

55. Tsang TS, Gersh BJ, Appleton CP, Tajik AJ, Barnes ME, Bailey KR, et al. Left ventricular diastolic dysfunction as a predictor of the first diagnosed non-valvular atrial fibrillation in 840 elderly men and women. J Am Coll Cardiol 2002; 40:1636–1644.

56. Vasan RS, Larson MG, Levy D, Galderisi M, Wolf PA, Benjamin EJ. Doppler transmitral flow indexes and risk of atrial fibrillation (the Framingham Heart Study). Am J Cardiol 2003; 91:1079–1083.

57. Braunwald E. Shattuck lecture: cardiovascular medicine at the turn of the millennium: triumphs, concerns, and opportunities. N Engl J Med 1997; 337:1360–1369.

58. Lloyd-Jones DM, Wang TJ, Leip EP, Larson MG, Levy D, Vasan RS, D'Agostino RB, Massaro JM, Wolf PA, Benjamin EJ. Lifetime risk for developing congestive heart failure: the Framingham Heart Study. Circulation 2002; 106:3068–3072.

59. Kannel WB, D'Agostino RB, Silbershatz H, Belanger AJ, Wilson PW, Levy D. Profile for estimating risk of heart failure. Arch Intern Med 1999; 159:1197–1204.

60. Li D, Fareh S, Leung TK, Nattel S. Promotion of atrial fibrillation by heart failure in dogs: atrial remodeling of a different sort. Circulation 1999; 100:87–95.
61. Crijns HJ, van den Berg MP, Van Gelder IC, van Veldhuisen DJ. Management of atrial fibrillation in the setting of heart failure. Eur Heart J 1997; 18(suppl C):C45–C49.
62. Shinbane JS, Wood MA, Jensen DN, Ellenbogen KA, Fitzpatrick AP, Scheinman MM. Tachycardia-induced cardiomyopathy: a review of animal models and clinical studies. J Am Coll Cardiol 1997; 29:709–715.
63. Wang TJ, Larson MG, Levy D, Vasan RS, Leip EP, Wolf PA, et al. Temporal relations of atrial fibrillation and congestive heart failure and their joint influence on mortality: the Framingham Heart Study. Circulation 2003; 107:2920–2925.
64. Vermes E, Tardif JC, Bourassa MG, Racine N, Levesque S, White M, et al. Enalapril decreases the incidence of atrial fibrillation in patients with left ventricular dysfunction: insight from the Studies Of Left Ventricular Dysfunction (SOLVD) trials. Circulation 2003; 107:2926–2931.
65. Brand FN, Abbott RD, Kannel WB, Wolf PA. Characteristics and prognosis of lone atrial fibrillation. 30-year follow-up in the Framingham Study. JAMA 1985; 254:3449–3453.
66. Kopecky SL, Gersh BJ, McGoon MD, Whisnant JP, Holmes DR Jr, Ilstrup DM, et al. The natural history of lone atrial fibrillation. A population-based study over three decades. N Engl J Med 1987; 317:669–674.
67. Godtfredsen J. Atrial fibrillation: course and prognosis- a follow-up study of 1212 cases. In: Kulbertus HE, Olsson SB, Schlepper M, eds. Atrial Fibrillation. Molndal, Sweden: AB Hassle, 1982:134–145.
68. Brugada R, Tapscott T, Czernuszewicz GZ, Marian AJ, Iglesias A, Mont L, et al. Identification of a genetic locus for familial atrial fibrillation. N Engl J Med 1997; 336:905–911.
69. Wolff L. Familial auricular fibrillation. N Engl J Med 1943; 229:396–397.
70. Ellinor PT, Shin JT, Moore RK, Yoerger DM, MacRae CA. Locus for atrial fibrillation maps to chromosome 6q14-16. Circulation 2003; 107:2880–2883.
71. Chen YH, Xu SJ, Bendahhou S, Wang XL, Wang Y, Xu WY, et al. KCNQ1 gain-of-function mutation in familial atrial fibrillation. Science 2003; 299:251–254.
72. Darbar D, Herron KJ, Ballew JD, Jahangir A, Gersh BJ, Shen WK, et al. Familial atrial fibrillation is a genetically heterogeneous disorder. J Am Coll Cardiol 2003; 41:2185–2192.
73. Fox CS, Parise H, D'Agostino RB, et al. Parental Atrial Fibrillation as a Risk Factor for Atrial Fibrillation in Offspring. JAMA 2004; 291:2851–2855.
74. Harris AW, Levine SA. Cerebral embolism in mitral stenosis. Ann Intern Med 1941; 15:637–643.
75. Fisher CM. Embolism in atrial fibrillation. In: Kulbertus HE, Olsson SB, Schlepper M, eds. Atrial Fibrillation: Kiruna, Sweden, 1981. Molndal, Sweden: AB Hassle, 1982:192–210.
76. Wolf PA, Dawber TR, Thomas HE Jr, Kannel WB. Epidemiologic assessment

of chronic atrial fibrillation and risk of stroke: the Framingham study. Neurology 1978; 28:973–977.

77. Manolio TA, Kronmal RA, Burke GL, O'Leary DH, Price TR. Short-term predictors of incident stroke in older adults. The Cardiovascular Health Study. Stroke 1996; 27:1479–1486.

78. Jorgensen HS, Nakayama H, Reith J, Raaschou HO, Olsen TS. Acute stroke with atrial fibrillation; The Copenhagen Stroke Study. Stroke 1996; 27:1765–1769.

79. Lin HJ, Wolf PA, Kelly-Hayes M, Beiser AS, Kase CS, Benjamin EJ, et al. Stroke severity in atrial fibrillation. The Framingham Study. Stroke 1996; 27:1760–1764.

80. Penado S, Cano M, Acha O, Hernandez JL, Riancho JA. Stroke severity in patients with atrial fibrillation. Am J Med 2002; 112:572–574.

81. Hart RG, Benavente O, McBride R, Pearce LA. Antithrombotic therapy to prevent stroke in patients with atrial fibrillation: a meta-analysis. Ann Intern Med 1999; 131:492–501.

82. Wang TJ, Massaro JM, Levy D, Vasan RS, Wolf PA, D'Agostino RB, et al. A risk score for predicting stroke or death in individuals with new-onset atrial fibrillation in the community: the Framingham Heart Study. JAMA 2003; 290:1049–1056.

83. Gage BF, Waterman AD, Shannon W, Boechler M, Rich MW, Radford MJ. Validation of clinical classification schemes for predicting stroke: results from the National Registry of Atrial Fibrillation. JAMA 2001; 285:2864–2870.

84. Patients with nonvalvular atrial fibrillation at low risk of stroke during treatment with aspirin: Stroke Prevention in Atrial Fibrillation III Study. The SPAF III Writing Committee for the Stroke Prevention in Atrial Fibrillation Investigators. JAMA 1998; 279:1273–1277.

85. Predictors of thromboembolism in atrial fibrillation: I. Clinical features of patients at risk. The Stroke Prevention in Atrial Fibrillation Investigators. Ann Intern Med 1992; 116:1–5.

86. Atrial Fibrillation Investigators. Risk factors for stroke and efficacy of antithrombotic therapy in atrial fibrillation: analysis of pooled data from five randomized controlled trials. Arch Intern Med 1994; 154:1449–1457.

87. van Walraven C, Hart RG, Wells GA, Petersen P, Koudstaal PJ, Gullov AL, et al. A clinical prediction rule to identify patients with atrial fibrillation and a low risk for stroke while taking aspirin. Arch Intern Med 2003; 163:936–943.

88. Frost L, Engholm G, Johnsen S, Moller H, Henneberg EW, Husted S. Incident thromboembolism in the aorta and the renal, mesenteric, pelvic, and extremity arteries after discharge from the hospital with a diagnosis of atrial fibrillation. Arch Intern Med 2001; 161:272–276.

89. Kilander L, Andren B, Nyman H, Lind L, Boberg M, Lithell H. Atrial fibrillation is an independent determinant of low cognitive function: a cross-sectional study in elderly men. Stroke 1998; 29:1816–1820.

90. O'Connell JE, Gray CS, French JM, Robertson IH. Atrial fibrillation and cognitive function: case-control study. J Neurol Neurosurg Psychiatry 1998; 65:386–389.

91. Sabatini T, Frisoni GB, Barbisoni P, Bellelli G, Rozzini R, Trabucchi M. Atrial fibrillation and cognitive disorders in older people. J Am Geriatr Soc 2000; 48:387–390.

92. Ezekowitz MD, James KE, Nazarian SM, Davenport J, Broderick JP, Gupta SR, et al. Silent cerebral infarction in patients with nonrheumatic atrial fibrillation. Circulation 1995; 92:2178–2182.

93. de Leeuw FE, de Groot JC, Oudkerk M, Kors JA, Hofman A, van Gijn J, et al. Atrial fibrillation and the risk of cerebral white matter lesions. Neurology 2000; 54:1795–1801.

94. Gajewski J, Singer RB. Mortality in an insured population with atrial fibrillation. JAMA 1981; 245:1540–1544.

95. Krahn AD, Manfreda J, Tate RB, Mathewson FA, Cuddy TE. The natural history of atrial fibrillation: incidence, risk factors, and prognosis in the Manitoba Follow-Up Study. Am J Med 1995; 98:476–484.

96. Lake FR, Cullen KJ, de Klerk NH, McCall MG, Rosman DL. Atrial fibrillation and mortality in an elderly population. Aust N Z J Med 1989; 19:321–326.

97. Benjamin EJ, Wolf PA, D'Agostino RB, Silbershatz H, Kannel WB, Levy D. Impact of atrial fibrillation on the risk of death: the Framingham Heart Study. Circulation 1998; 98:946–952.

98. Stewart S, Hart CL, Hole DJ, McMurray JJ. A population-based study of the long-term risks associated with atrial fibrillation: 20-year follow-up of the Renfrew/Paisley study. Am J Med 2002; 113:359–364.

99. Stevenson WG, Stevenson LW, Middlekauff HR, Fonarow GC, Hamilton MA, Woo MA, et al. Improving survival for patients with atrial fibrillation and advanced heart failure. J Am Coll Cardiol 1996; 28:1458–1463. Erratum appears in J Am Coll Cardiol 1997 Dec;30(7):1902.

100. Dries DL, Exner DV, Gersh BJ, Domanski MJ, Waclawiw MA, Stevenson LW. Atrial fibrillation is associated with an increased risk for mortality and heart failure progression in patients with asymptomatic and symptomatic left ventricular systolic dysfunction: a retrospective analysis of the SOLVD trials. J Am Coll Cardiol 1998; 32:695–703.

101. Middlekauff HR, Stevenson WG, Stevenson LW. Prognostic significance of atrial fibrillation in advanced heart failure. A study of 390 patients. Circulation 1991; 84:40–48.

102. Luderitz B, Jung W. Quality of life in patients with atrial fibrillation. Arch Intern Med 2000; 160:1749–1757.

103. Engelmann MD, Pehrson S. Quality of life in nonpharmacologic treatment of atrial fibrillation. Eur Heart J 2003; 24:1387–1400.

104. Weerasooriya R, Davis M, Powell A, Szili-Torok T, Shah C, Whalley D, et al. The Australian Intervention Randomized Control of Rate in Atrial Fibrillation Trial (AIRCRAFT). J Am Coll Cardiol 2003; 41:1697–1702.

105. Dorian P, Jung W, Newman D, Paquette M, Wood K, Ayers GM, et al. The impairment of health-related quality of life in patients with intermittent atrial fibrillation: implications for the assessment of investigational therapy. J Am Coll Cardiol 2000; 36:1303–1309.

106. Dorian P, Paquette M, Newman D, Green M, Connolly SJ, Talajic M, et al.

Quality of life improves with treatment in the Canadian Trial of Atrial Fibrillation. Am Heart J 2002; 143:984–990.

107. Wolf PA, Mitchell JB, Baker CS, Kannel WB, D'Agostino RB. Impact of atrial fibrillation on mortality, stroke, and medical costs. Arch Intern Med 1998; 158:229–234.

108. Wattigney WA, Mensah GA, Croft JB. Increasing trends in hospitalization for atrial fibrillation in the United States, 1985 through 1999: implications for primary prevention. Circulation 2003; 108:711–716.

2
Etiology and Pathogenesis of Atrial Fibrillation

Philip J. Podrid
Boston University School of Medicine, Boston, Massachusetts, U.S.A.

Atrial fibrillation (AF) is the most common sustained arrhythmia seen in clinical practice, and permanent or intermittent AF afflicts about 4% of the population (1–6). The prevalence of AF is increasing, resulting in part from the increase in the mean age of the population as well as the increase in the survival of patients with heart disease, especially those with heart failure. Although AF is frequently associated with atrial enlargement and ventricular dysfunction of any cause, it also occurs in the absence of any structural heart disease. However, regardless of the presence or absence of heart disease, AF has importance clinically because affected patients have an increased mortality; they are also at an increased risk for deterioration in hemodynamics due to the rapid and irregular heart rate, progressive dysfunction of the left atrium and left ventricle, and for embolic events resulting from left atrial and left atrial appendiceal thrombi (7,8).

I. ETIOLOGY OF ATRIAL FIBRILLATION

The frequency of AF in the population, its occurrence in those with and without cardiac disease, and its strong association with age suggest that there are many etiologies for this arrhythmia, which may share a common pathology and pathophysiology.

AF is associated with almost any type of underlying heart disease that causes changes of the atrial myocardium, including distention, inflammation, hypertrophy, ischemia, fibrosis, and infiltration (Table 1) (7,8). Additionally,

Table 1 Etiology of Atrial Fibrillation

Increased distention/pressure in atria and atrial hypertrophy
    Mitral or tricuspid valve disease
    Myocardial disease (primary or secondary) leading to diastolic or systolic
        dysfunction and heart failure
    Ventricular hypertrophy due to systemic or pulmonary hypertension or aortic
        or pulmonic valve disease
    Intracardiac tumors or thrombi
    Pulmonary disease
    Pulmonary embolism
Atrial ischemia
    Coronary artery disease
Inflammatory or infiltrative atrial disease
    Pericarditis
    Amyloidosis
    Myocarditis
    Lupus
Age-related atrial changes (fibrosis and amyloid deposits)
Intoxicants
    Alcohol
    Carbon monoxide
    Poison gas
Increased sympathetic activity
    Hyperthyroidism
    Exercise
    Pheochromocytoma
    Anxiety
    Alcohol
    Caffeine
    Sympathomimetic drugs (e.g., theophylline)
    Heart failure
    Pulmonary embolism
    Post–cardiac surgery
Increased parasympathetic activity
    Sleep
    Drugs (e.g., digoxin)
Primary or metastatic cancer in or adjacent to the atrial wall
Congenital heart disease
    Atrial septal defect
    Ebstein's anomaly
    Patent ductus arteriosus
    After surgical correction of tetralogy of Fallot, ventricular septal defect,
        transposition of great vessels
Neurogenic
    Subarachnoid hemorrhage
    Nonhemorrhagic stroke
Familial/genetic
Sick sinus syndrome
Idiopathic (i.e., lone AF)

there are normal age-related changes of the myocardium, including amyloid deposits and fibrosis, perhaps accounting for the increased incidence of AF in the elderly (9). Parasympathetic or sympathetic nervous system inputs alter atrial electrophysiological properties and can provoke AF (10). Systemic infections, pulmonary disease and infections, pulmonary embolism, hyperthyroidism, and certain toxins or metabolic abnormalities may promote AF even in the absence of underlying atrial disease (11). In up to 15% of cases, there is no structural heart disease and no identifiable cause for the arrhythmia; this has been termed "lone AF" (12–14).

Several autopsy studies have reported that the most common cardiac diseases associated with AF are coronary artery disease (CAD) with or without a prior myocardial infarction (MI), rheumatic heart disease, and hypertensive heart disease (9,17). However, clinical observation has emphasized that when AF occurs in those with CAD, left ventricular dysfunction or heart failure (HF) is usually present (7,8). Currently the most common underlying abnormalities associated with either intermittent or permanent AF are hypertensive heart disease, which increased the risk of AF almost 5-fold and 9-fold in men and women, respectively, during a 22-year follow-up, and HF of any etiology, which increased the risk by over 4-fold and 14-fold in men and women, respectively (15,16) (Table 2).

The more common causes for AF are discussed more fully below.

A. Hypertensive Heart Disease

In developed countries, hypertensive heart disease is the most common underlying disorder in patients with AF. Although the absolute percentage of patients with hypertension who develop AF is small, the very high

Table 2 Risk of Development of AF by Cardiovascular Disease in The Framingham Heart Study (2-year adjusted risk ratio)

Predisposing Cardiovascular Disease	Permanent AF		Intermittent AF	
	Men	Women	Men	Women
Coronary heart disease	2.2[a]	0.5	2.1[a]	4.5[a]
Hypertensive heart disease	4.7[a]	4.0[a]	4.4[a]	4.6[a]
Heart failure	8.5[a]	13.7[a]	8.2[a]	20.4[a]
Rheumatic heart disease	9.9[a]	27.5[a]	7.6[a]	24.3[a]
Any cardiovascular disease	3.2	4.8	4.4[a]	5.4[a]

[a] $p < 0.05$.
Source: Ref. 15.

prevalence of hypertension in the general population makes it the single most common cause of AF. Several population-based studies have found that 37 to 50% of patients with AF have a history of hypertension. For example, in The Framingham Heart Study of 4731 subjects followed for 38 years, the presence of hypertension was significantly associated with the risk of developing AF in both men and women (OR 1.8 and 1.7, respectively) (16). Approximately 50% of the subjects who developed AF had a history of hypertension, and hypertension was associated with a 50% excess risk of developing AF. In the AFFIRM trial of 4060 patients, 71% had a history of hypertension (17).

In the Framingham study, the population-attributable risk—which provides an estimate of the percentage of AF that would be eliminated if a risk factor were not present in the population—associated with hypertension was 14%. This risk remained stable over the 38-year follow-up period. In another study of 2482 patients with initially untreated essential hypertension who were followed for 38 years, a first episode of AF occurred at a rate of 0.46 per 100 person-years; AF became chronic in 33% of patients (18).

Hypertension may be of importance because it is a powerful predictor for the development of left ventricular hypertrophy (LVH) and left atrial enlargement, which are important factors associated with the development of AF. In the Framingham study, LVH on the ECG was significantly associated with the risk of developing AF in both men and women (odds ratio 3.0 and 3.8, respectively) (16). This may, however, be an underestimate, since the sensitivity of the ECG for establishing the presence of LVH is low. Two-dimensional echocardiography is a better method for establishing left ventricular mass and the presence of LVH. In an analysis of 1924 surviving subjects from the Framingham study cohort, the left ventricular wall thickness was associated with a multivariable relative risk for AF of 1.3 per 4-mm increment in wall thickness (19). In the study of 2482 subjects with essential hypertension mentioned above, age and left ventricular mass were the sole independent predictors of AF; the risk of AF was increased 1.2 times for every 1-SD increase in left ventricular mass (18).

Hypertension and associated LVH are also powerful predictors for left atrial enlargement on echocardiography. Regardless of the etiology, left atrial enlargement is another important factor associated with the development of AF. As an example, a retrospective analysis of 2200 adults found that the 5-year risk of AF was related to left atrial size (3, 12, 15, and 26% for each quartile of left atrial volume); after adjusting for other factors, a 30% larger left atrial volume was associated with a 43% greater risk of AF (20). A relationship between left atrial size and left ventricular hypertrophy was examined in the LIFE study, which evaluated 941 hypertensive patients with left ventricular hypertrophy on a baseline ECG (21). In logistic regression analysis, left atrial enlargement was related to ventricular hypertrophy and eccentric geometry. The SPAF trial of 3465 participants found that mean left atrial diameter was on average 6 mm larger in those with AF compared with those in sinus rhythm (48 vs. 42 mm, $p < 0.001$) (22). The presence of left atrial enlargement was related to multiple factors, including an increase in left ventricular mass and left ventricular dilatation; the presence of AF itself contributed approximately 2.5 mm to the left atrial diameter.

B. Coronary Disease

AF is not commonly associated with CAD unless it is complicated by acute MI or HF; the incidence of AF in CAD itself is low (2%); in the majority of these cases, the arrhythmia occurs in association with mitral regurgitation and left ventricular dysfunction (23–25). As an example, the Coronary Artery Surgical Study (CASS), which included over 18,000 patients with angiographically documented CAD, reported that only 0.6% of patients had AF, and it was associated with age >60 ($p < 0.001$), male sex ($p < 0.01$), and HF, which doubled the risk (25). In the Framingham Heart Study, the adjusted risk ratio for AF among men and women with CAD was 2.2 and 0.5, respectively, although women with CAD had an increased risk for developing intermittent AF (risk ratio 4.5) (15). However, because of the high prevalence of CAD in the population, CAD is a common cause of AF. As an example, in the AFFIRM trial, 38% of patients had underlying CAD (17).

Both the Framingham Heart Study and CASS found that AF was an independent predictor of mortality in patients with CAD (3,25). As an example, CASS reported that the 7-year survival was 38% among CAD patients with AF and 80% for those in sinus rhythm ($p < 0.001$); the relative risk was 1.98 at 7 years (25).

In summary, chronic stable CAD is an uncommon cause of AF unless there are associated factors such as mitral regurgitation, HF or hypertension.

C. Acute Myocardial Infarction

AF as a presenting rhythm during an acute MI is uncommon (26–29). Factors associated with its occurrence are older age, HF prior to admission, low systolic blood pressure, rales, cardiomegaly, wide P waves, left bundle branch block, left anterior hemiblock, marked ST-segment elevation, and PQ-segment depression. These clinical findings indicate more severe CAD, poorer left ventricular function, and higher left atrial pressure, suggesting that AF is due to the extent of the MI and its impact on left ventricular function. This is supported by the fact that an elevated pulmonary capillary wedge pressure and increased right atrial pressure are present prior to the onset of

AF. Another possible but infrequently associated cause is pericarditis, which is occasionally seen after an acute MI (30). A rare cause is atrial infarction.

Although AF as a presenting symptom of an acute MI is rare, the overall incidence of AF in the peri-infarction period ranges from 6 to 20% (31–33); this incidence has not been altered with the use of thrombolytic agents, and several large trials have reported an incidence of in-hospital AF ranging from 6 to 8.4% (34–37). AF occurs mainly within the first 72 hr after infarction; however, only 3% of such episodes are noted in the very early (less than 3 hr) phase (33). The major reason for AF in the post MI period is generally left ventricular dysfunction and HF.

The presence of AF during the peri-infarction period is associated with a higher mortality. As an example, one report of 4108 patients with an acute MI treated in the prethrombolytic era found that the overall incidence of new AF was 9.7%; the relative risk of dying when AF occurred was 1.7 (31). AF is more common in those with hemodynamic or other arrhythmic complications, and the arrhythmia is associated with indicators of a worse prognosis, including age >70, female sex, higher Killip class, previous MI, treated hypertension, high systolic blood pressure at admission, and HF (40). However, the outcome of patients treated with a thrombolytic agent who develop AF is better, although AF is still associated with an increased in-hospital (adjusted relative risk 1.98) and short-term mortality.

The negative impact of AF on mortality persists during long-term follow-up. In the GISSI-3 trial, for example, the mortality at 4 years remained higher in those with AF (adjusted relative risk 1.78 compared to no AF) (36). Similar findings were noted in the TRACE trial; those with AF had a higher mortality at 5 years (56 vs. 34% without AF, relative risk 1.3) (37). This association persisted even after adjusting for prognostic characteristics such as use of thrombolytic therapy, age, history of diabetes or hypertension, or prior MI. However, the association of AF with increased mortality appears to be related to factors such as heart failure, shock, or serious ventricular arrhythmias rather than AF itself (31,38–41).

The presence of AF is also associated with a higher mortality in patients presenting with an acute coronary syndrome (unstable angina or non-ST-elevation MI). As an example, in the PURSUIT trial, 6.4% of patients developed AF; these patients had a higher mortality at 30 days and 6 months (adjusted hazard ratio 4.4 and 3.0, respectively) (42).

Given the low incidence of AF in CAD and as a presenting arrhythmia in those with an acute MI, a common problem is the need for admission to the coronary care unit (CCU) for patients with AF of recent onset, in whom an MI is often considered to be causal (43,44). This issue was addressed in a series of 245 patients with new-onset AF admitted to CCU; only 5 had elevated cardiac enzymes diagnostic of an acute MI (43) All 5 had at least two of the following clinical features: LVH on the ECG, an old MI on the ECG, typical angina pectoris, or duration of symptoms less than 4 hr. However, it was not clear whether the MI precipitated the AF or AF and the rapid ventricular rate caused ischemia and an MI.

In a prospective cohort study of 255 patients who presented to a single-center emergency department with the primary diagnosis of AF, 190 were admitted to the hospital; 109 underwent a standard "rule-out MI" protocol, and 6 had an acute MI (45). The presence of ST-segment elevation or major ST-segment depression (>2 mm) was a reliable marker of an acute MI (sensitivity and specificity of 100 and 99%, respectively), while chest pain and ST-segment depression <2 mm were common but had limited use for predicting an MI.

In summary, AF is rarely a manifestation of an acute MI or ischemia in the absence of other signs or symptoms of an acute event (i.e., angina or ECG changes).

D. Cardiomyopathy and Heart Failure

AF occurs in 15 to 30% of patients with systolic or diastolic HF, although it may be as high as 50% in those with class IV HF (46–48). The loss of atrial contraction and, if present, a rapid heart rate can precipitate HF in patients with asymptomatic left ventricular dysfunction and cause hemodynamic deterioration, with worsening symptoms in those who already have HF (49–51). These changes can be reversed with rate control or reversion to sinus rhythm (52).

Both left ventricular dysfunction and HF are significant risk factors for AF (15,16,53,54). The Framingham Heart Study, which followed 2326 men and 2866 women for 24 years, found that the 2-year risk ratio for chronic AF in patients with HF was 8.5 for men and 13.7 for women; the values for transient AF were 8.2 and 20.4, respectively (15). At 38-year follow-up, HF remained the most powerful predictor of AF (16). Similar findings were noted in another series of 344 patients with HF who were followed for a mean of 19 months; 8% developed AF, which became chronic in 5% (51). Among patients with paroxysmal AF, the presence of HF and left ventricular dysfunction is an independent predictor for recurrent episodes of AF and the development of chronic AF (55).

It is unclear whether the patient with HF at risk for developing AF can be identified. It has been suggested that an abnormal P wave on a signal-averaged ECG may be helpful to predict paroxysmal AF in patients with HF. After a 21-month follow-up in one prospective study of 75 patients with HF who had no history of AF, those with an abnormal P wave on a signal-averaged ECG—defined as a P-wave duration >132 ms or late potential <2.3 µV—had a higher incidence of AF after a 21-month follow-up (32 versus 2%) (56).

An elevated level of plasma atrial natriuretic peptide (ANP) may also be helpful (56–58). In one study, an ANP level ≥60 pg/mL was predictive of AF (hazard ratio 8.6) (56). The association between ANP and AF was also found in another study, which examined 100 patients with and without AF (58). Patients with AF had higher levels of N-terminal ANP than those without AF (2.6 vs. 1.7 ng/mL); this association was independent of left atrial volume and left ventricular ejection fraction.

1. Dilated Cardiomyopathy

There is a high incidence of AF in patients with a dilated, congestive cardio-myopathy regardless of the etiology (7,46,59). In most cases AF is the result of HF and associated mitral or tricuspid regurgitation. The occurrence of AF in such patients often results in exacerbation of left ventricular dysfunction and HF due to the loss of atrial contraction, the rapid heart rate, and the irregularity of the RR intervals.

2. Hypertrophic Cardiomyopathy

AF is seen in 5% of patients with a hypertrophic cardiomyopathy at initial presentation and develops in an additional 10% during the 5 years after diagnosis (60). The overall incidence at 9 to 10 years is approximately 22 to 28%, or an incidence of 2% per year—a value that is four- to sixfold higher than that seen in the general population (61–63). Like AF in other conditions, the incidence increases with age.

There are several etiologies for AF in hypetrophic cardiomyopathy, including a significantly hypertrophied, stiffened, and noncompliant left ventricle, as in the situation with LVH due to hypertension; the presence of HF due to diastolic dysfunction; and in some patients associated mitral regurgitation (60,63–66). The occurrence of AF in patients with hypertrophic cardiomyopathy has a significant impact on the clinical course (63) and may result in rapid hemodynamic deterioration and cardiovascular collapse as well as the provocation of life-threatening ventricular tachyarrhythmias and sudden death (67,68).

Although it has been suggested that AF in hypertrophic cardiomyop-athy is of prognostic importance, this is a controversial issue. In one study, 52 patients with hypertrophic cardiomyopathy who had paroxysmal or chronic AF were compared with a matched population with hypertrophic cardiomy-opathy and sinus rhythm (60). While the arrhythmia resulted in a worsening of symptoms in 89% of patients, it was not associated with an increase in mortality during a 7-year follow-up. The estimated probability of survival at 5, 10, 15, and 20 years in those with AF was 0.86, 0.71, 0.65, and 0.50, respectively, compared with 0.92, 0.82, 0.71, and 0.41 when sinus rhythm was present. In contrast, another community-based study of 480 patients, 22% of whom developed AF during a 9 year follow-up, found that AF was associated with substantial risk for heart HF-related mortality, stroke, and severe functional disability, particularly in patients with outflow obstruction, those <50 years of age, or those developing chronic AF (62). However, the outcome was good in the 35% of patients with AF who did not have a stroke or severe symptoms.

3. Other Etiologies

Other etiologies of cardiomyopathy are also associated with AF. These include Chagas' disease, hemochromatosis, and tumor or amyloid infiltration, especially when these conditions involve the atrial myocardium (69). Indeed, senile amyloidosis of the left atrium has been implicated as a factor related to the increased incidence of atrial fibrillation in the elderly (70).

4. AF and Mortality in HF

The relationship between AF and mortality in HF is an area of controversy. One study of 409 patients, for example, found that AF was not associated with an adverse outcome after adjusting for important prognostic variables (71). In contrast, a 3-year follow-up of 6517 patients in the SOLVD trials found that those with AF had a significantly higher mortality compared with those without AF (34 vs. 23%, $p < 0.001$), including death due to pump failure (16.7 vs. 9.4%, $p < 0.001$), and the combined endpoint of death or hospitalization for HF (45 vs. 33%). There was no significant difference between the groups in arrhythmic events (72). After a multivariate analysis, AF remained significantly associated with each of these outcomes.

However, additional pharmacological therapy of HF may influence the relationship between AF and survival. This possibility is suggested by two observations from the same group at different points in time. In the first study of 390 consecutive patients with class III and IV HF followed between 1985 and 1989, overall survival was significantly lower for those with AF vs. those with sinus rhythm (52 vs. 71%, $p = 0.0013$) (46). Similarly, sudden death–free survival was significantly worse for those with AF (69 vs. 82%, $p = 0.0013$). In a study performed later, between 1990 and 1993, patients with AF had a lower survival rate, but the difference was smaller and not significant (47). These patients also had a higher 2-year survival rate than patients in the earlier time period (66 vs. 39%, $p = 0.001$)—a change that may have reflected more frequent use of angiotensin converting enzyme inhibitors and amiodarone and less frequent use of class I antiarrhythmic drugs. Support for this comes from another study of 234 patients evaluated for heart transplantation between 1993 and 1996; the presence of AF was not associated with a decreased event-free survival (death, placement of a left ventricular assist device, or transplantation) (73).

Another determinant of the prognostic importance of AF may be the severity of HF. Studies involving patients with class II or III HF, such as V-HeFT I and II, have not found a significant increase in mortality in patients with AF (74). Furthermore, AF was not associated with an increase in sudden death, hospitalization rate, or embolic events in these trials.

E. Rheumatic Heart Disease (RHD) Valvular Heart Disease

The association between AF and RHD, particularly mitral stenosis or mitral regurgitation, is well established (3). In the past, RHD and associated valvular abnormalities were the most common clinical causes for AF. However, since the prevalence of RHD in the population has declined, the actual number of cases due to this disease entity is small. It is, however, associated with a high prevalence of AF (75–77). In the Framingham study, the presence of rheumatic disease was the strongest predictor of AF; the 2-year age-adjusted risk ratio for chronic AF for men and women was 9.9 and 27.5, while for intermittent AF it was 7.6 and 24.3 (15). The population-attributable risk of AF from valvular disease in men and women is 5 and 18% (16).

1. Mitral Valve Disease

AF is estimated to occur in about 40% of patients with mitral stenosis and 75% of those with mitral regurgitation (78). There is, however, no association between AF and mitral valve area, pulmonary artery wedge pressure, and total pulmonary vascular resistance, but there is an association with age and duration of mitral stenosis (79,80). In such patients clinical factors associated with AF are increased left atrial size, P-wave abnormality on the ECG, PR-interval prolongation, and atrial premature beats (81). The occurrence of AF in patients with mitral valve disease often results in severe symptoms and a rapid clinical deterioration, often prompting surgical intervention.

AF is also common in patients with other nonrheumatic mitral valvular disease, including congenital heart disease, mitral valve prolapse, and chordal or papillary muscle rupture and a flail mitral leaflet. One study of patients with mitral regurgitation due to a flail mitral leaflet or mitral valve prolapse found that the incidence of AF at 10 years was 48 and 41%; independent baseline predictors of AF were age and left atrial (LA) diameter. In patients with a flail mitral leaflet, the development of AF during follow-up was independently associated with high risk of cardiac death or heart failure (adjusted risk ratio 2.23, $p = 0.025$) (82).

2. Aortic Valve Disease

Atrial fibrillation is less commonly seen with aortic valve disease; its occurrence suggests coexisting mitral valve disease or HF. The incidence of AF in isolated aortic stenosis is 1% and 8% in isolated aortic regurgitation (83). In general, AF is a late feature of aortic stenosis and regurgitation.

3. Other Valve Disease

Isolated right-sided valvular lesions are much less frequently associated with AF, although the prevalence of AF related to right-sided lesions is unknown. Endocarditis may provoke AF, especially when it causes mitral regurgitation. However, it has been reported that endocarditis occurring in patients with AF is unusual (84,85).

4. Multiple Valvular Abnormalities

The incidence of AF is particularly high in those with combined valvular abnormalities, especially involving the mitral valve. As an example, one study evaluated the frequency of AF in approximately 1100 patients with RHD (86). AF was present in 70% of those with mitral stenosis, mitral regurgitation, and tricuspid regurgitation, while it was present in 52% with mitral stenosis and mitral regurgitation. In contrast, the incidence for isolated mitral stenosis or mitral regurgitation was 29 and 16%.

5. Mitral Annular Calcification

Mitral annular calcification has also been associated with AF (87,88). It has been reported that LA enlargement was 2.4 times more prevalent and AF 1.9 times more prevalent in patients with mitral annular calcification vs. those without this finding (87).

6. Postoperative

AF occurs frequently after most types of cardiac surgery; the incidence is as high as 40% following conventional coronary artery bypass grafting (CABG) (89,90), 64% following valvular surgery (91,92), possibly lower with minimally invasive surgery (93–97), and about 24% after cardiac transplantation

(98). The incidence of AF after noncardiac surgery is low, approximately 4% in one series of 4181 patients (99). Most episodes of AF occur within the first few postoperative days, with peak incidence on days 2 to 3 (100). Although the arrhythmia is usually self-limited, it may be associated with embolic stroke or adverse hemodynamics. Postoperative AF is of importance largely because it increases morbidity, CCU stay, length of hospitalization, and medical costs (101–103).

The issue of postoperative AF is discussed more fully in Chapter 13.

F. Sick Sinus Syndrome

Sinus node dysfunction, commonly termed "sick sinus syndrome," involves a disorder of sinus node automaticity or sinoatrial conduction (104,105). It actually represents a spectrum of abnormalities presenting as an inappropriate and persistent sinus bradycardia, sinus arrest or pauses, or alternating periods of bradycardia and tachyarrhythmias that are temporarily related. One form, known as a "tachy-brady syndrome," presents with a tachycardia, most commonly AF, that terminates abruptly and is followed by a long offset pause prior to the resumption of sinus rhythm; as many as 50% of patients with a sick sinus syndrome have AF (106–108). It is during this offset pause and the resulting bradycardia that syncope may occur. Another form is a sinus bradycardia resulting in an escape tachyarrhythmia, often AF, known as a "brady-tachy syndrome."

Often a sick sinus syndrome is a part of generalized conduction system disease that also involves the atrioventricular (AV) node; AV-nodal conduction abnormalities are seen in 50% of patients with a sick sinus syndrome (109,110). When AV-nodal involvement is also present, AF is associated with a slow ventricular response, even in the absence of AV-nodal blocking drugs. It has been suggested that chronic AF is part of the natural history of a sick sinus syndrome, representing an "end stage" rhythm, and that many patients, especially the elderly, who are felt to have lone AF actually have a sick sinus syndrome as the underlying etiology (109,111,112).

Many etiologies for sinus node dysfunction are identical to those that can cause AF, therefore making it difficult to distinguish between these two conditions. However, the presence of underlying sinus and AV-nodal dysfunction does affect therapy for AF. The drugs that are often used to prevent AF (class 1A, 1C, and 3 antiarrhythmic drugs) or those used for slowing the ventricular rate by blocking the AV node (digoxin, beta blockers, calcium channel blockers) may exacerbate dysfunction of pacemaker tissue, resulting in a worsening of symptoms (113). Not infrequently, permanent pacemakers are inserted prior to therapy of AF (114,115). In some patients, AF as the rhythm of choice may be preferable so as to avoid symptoms during sinus bradycardia or to eliminate the need for a pacemaker.

G. Preexcitation Syndrome

It has been reported that 10 to 35% of patients with a preexcitation syndrome, particularly Wolff-Parkinson-White (WPW), develop AF, and there are several factor that predispose to its development (116–118). Closely coupled atrial premature beats are an appropriate trigger to initiate AF, but in WPW even spontaneous ventricular premature beats may be factors, since they are conducted retrogradely via the accessory pathway, activating the atria. Impulses conducted via the accessory pathway can collide with those originating from the sinus node, setting up the potential for multiple wavefronts and hence AF (117). Additionally, there is evidence that patients with WPW have intra-atrial conduction abnormalities (118). The presence of antegrade conduction over the accessory pathway that has a short refractory period facilitates the occurrence of AF (118,119). This is supported by the observation that surgical or catheter ablation of the pathway significantly reduces or eliminates AF episodes (119,120).

In patients with WPW, an AV reentrant tachycardia induced in the electrophysiology laboratory has been observed to degenerate into AF in approximately 15 to 35% of cases; it is often precipitated by a premature beat occurring during the tachycardia (118,121). Excitation contraction feedback has also been suggested as a possible mechanism (122). When a reentrant tachycardia occurs, there is an increase in atrial pressure and volume. This stretch shortens the atrial refractory period and increases intra-atrial conduction time, thus creating appropriate preconditions for establishing multiple reentrant circuits and AF.

H. Congenital Heart Disease

AF also occurs frequently in patients with congenital heart disease (123). The most common association is with an atrial septal defect, and AF occurs in up to 19% of adults with this condition (124). However, the incidence of AF is related to age, ranging in one series from 15% for those aged 40 to 60 to 61% for those over the age of 60 (125). AF also occurs in other forms of congenital heart disease affecting the atria, including Ebstein's anomaly and patent ductus arteriosus, as well as after surgical correction of some other abnormalities, including ventricular septal defect, tetralogy of Fallot, pulmonic stenosis, and transposition of the great vessels (123).

I. Other Cardiopulmonary Disease

AF occurs in up to 10% of patients with a documented pulmonary embolism
(126). Other cardiopulmonary diseases associated with AF include chronic
obstructive pulmonary disease (127); postpartum cardiomyopathy (128);
lupus myocarditis (129); the cardiomyopathy associated with severe obesity
(130); and in idiopathic, uremic, and post-MI and postbypass surgical
pericarditis, primarily when associated with myocarditis (131–133).

J. Alcohol

Alcohol has long been suspected as an etiological factor for AF in those with
and without heart disease (134–136). Alcohol has been reported to play a role
in up to 35% of patients with new-onset AF (134). Its role may be more
important among patients <65 years of age, while alcohol is less commonly
the sole factor in those over age 65 (135). One study observed that in patients
without heart disease who had a history of heavy alcohol use preceding AF,
the majority of hospital admissions or emergency room visits for atrial
arrhythmias occurred over weekends or holidays, when alcohol intake was
more marked. This was termed the "holiday heart syndrome" (136,137).
Mean alcohol consumption was found to be higher among young and middle-
aged patients who presented to an emergency room with recent-onset AF
compared to randomly selected age-matched control patients presenting to
the emergency room for other reasons and to randomly selected controls from
the local community (138).

Alcohol can cause AF by several mechanisms:

1. It may have acute effect on atrial refractoriness and conduction
    (139). There is, however, no universal agreement about any direct
    electrophysiological actions of alcohol. One electrophysiological
    study found that alcohol did not alter atrial electrophysiological
    parameters (139). However, when larger doses are used and blood
    levels are higher, there is an effect on atrial refractory periods.
2. Alcohol is toxic to the myocardium, and chronic alcohol consump-
    tion can cause cumulative depressive effects on myocardial function
    resulting from structural changes in the myocardial cells, includ-
    ing myofibrillar necrosis, interstitial fibrosis, and alterations in the
    sarcolemma and mitochondria (140–142). These changes are often
    heterogeneous, providing an appropriate substrate for arrhythmia.
3. Alcohol also interferes with myocardial metabolism, oxidative phos-
    phorylation, protein synthesis, fatty acid oxidation, sodium potas-
    sium ATPase activity, alignment of contractile proteins, and the
    reuptake of calcium by the sarcoplasmic reticulum (143).

4. Alcohol may alter sympathetic and parasympathetic inputs into the heart—important factors in arrhythmogenesis (144). While these may result from a direct effect of alcohol, autonomic changes, especially activation of the sympathetic nervous system, generally accompany alcohol withdrawal (145).

K. Hyperthyroidism

Thyroid dysfunction, specifically hyperthyroidism, is frequently associated with AF (146). Almost 3% of patients presenting to the emergency room with AF have hyperthyroidism as the etiology, although the overall incidence of hyperthyroidism in patients with AF varies from 10 to 30%. (147,148).

The risk of AF is increased up to fivefold in patients with subclinical hyperthyroidism (defined as a low level of thyroid-stimulating hormone [TSH] and normal level of thyroid hormone) (149,150). As an example, a study of 23,638 subjects found that the incidence of AF in those with clinical and subclinical hyperthyroidism was similar (14 and 13%, respectively) and higher than that in euthyroid subjects (2.3%) (150). Therefore serum TSH should be measured in all patients with AF, even if there are no symptoms suggestive of thyrotoxicosis. Those with low values (< 0.5 mU/L with the newer, more sensitive assays) and normal serum T4 probably have subclinical hyperthyroidism. One report assessed the frequency of hyperthyroidism by measuring serum TSH in 726 patients with recent-onset AF (151). Low TSH values were found in 39 (5.4%); 14 of these patients were taking thyroxine supplements for previous hyper- or hypothyroidism.

AF due to hyperthyroidism is more common in those over age 40 and still more so in the elderly (147,152). AF occurs in about 20 to 25% of older patients with hyperthyroidism, but it is unusual under the age of 30 (147,148). Hyperthyroidism in the elderly is often not obvious but is masked (apathetic hyperthyroidism). It has been suggested that many elderly patients with AF have occult or masked hyperthyroidism (153). It has been reported that an abnormal TSH infusion test was more frequent in elderly patients with AF than in elderly subjects without this arrhythmia (154). However, it is uncertain whether this abnormal response is a marker for hyperthyroidism, since an abnormal test may be seen in the normal elderly population (155).

The identification of hyperthyroidism as a precipitating factor for AF is of importance, since there is evidence that within 6 weeks of becoming euthyroid on antithyroid therapy, 60% of patients may have spontaneous reversion of AF and maintenance of sinus rhythm; older patients show an age-related decline in the frequency of spontaneous reversion (147,156). The conversion rate appears to be greater when hypothyroidism or a euthyroid state is produced more rapidly (157). Attempted electrical or pharmacological cardioversion is not indicated while the patient is thyrotoxic, since AF usually recurs in this setting.

The mechanism for AF in hyperthyroidism is multifactorial, including:

1. The direct effect of thyroxine on the myocardium, resulting in a shortening of the action potential duration and the refractory period and an increase in automaticity (158).
2. An associated hypercatecholamine state that can directly cause arrhythmia or may do so indirectly by the development of hypertension and an increase in LA pressure and dimension.
3. An increase in beta receptors and in adenyl cyclase activity with increased thyroxin; this sensitizes the heart to the effect of circulating catecholamines (159).

L. Medications

Certain medications—such as theophylline, caffeine, or other sympathomimetic agents—can cause or contribute to the development of AF (160). In addition, increased vagal tone can induce AF or prolong the duration of an episode (161,162); thus, drugs that increase vagal tone, such as digitalis, may share this effect (163,164).

M. Familial

A familial form of AF has been reported that is transmitted in an autosomal dominant fashion (165,166). Genetic linkage analysis found the responsible loci at 10q22-q24 and 11p15.5. The latter locus is associated with a gain-of-function mutation in the *KVLQT1* (*KCNQ1*) gene, the protein product of which is the alpha subunit of the slowly acting component of the outward-rectifying potassium current (IKs). A loss-of-function mutation associated with the same gene has been associated with the long-QT syndrome type 1 (166).

N. Inflammation

The high incidence of AF after cardiac surgery and in pericarditis suggests that an inflammatory process may play a role in the genesis of AF. In one case-control study that measured serum C-reactive protein (CRP) in 131 patients with atrial arrhythmia within 24 hr of testing and 71 control patients in sinus rhythm, serum CRP was significantly higher in patients with paroxysmal or persistent AF (167).

O. Other Supraventricular Arrhythmias

It has long been observed that there may be a transition from atrial flutter, which is due to a single reentrant circuit in the atrium, into AF, which is a result of multiple, simultaneously occurring circuits that produce multiple wavelets (168). AF may also be precipitated by other supraventricular tachycardias, such AV-nodal reentrant tachycardia and AV reentrant tachycardia, which occur in patients with the Wolff-Parkinson-White (WPW) syndrome (116,169). Enhanced vagal tone or an increase in dispersion of right atrial refractory periods may contribute to the development of AF associated with supraventricular tachycardias (170).

P. Lone AF

Some patients with intermittent or permanent AF have no evidence of structural heart defects or an obvious precipitating factor. This has been termed *idiopathic* or *lone AF* (11–14). In different reports, depending in part on the population studied, lone AF accounts for 2 to 31% of cases of AF overall and almost one-half of cases of intermittent AF. However, its incidence is lower than previously reported due to more sensitive techniques for the diagnosis of underlying heart disease, especially the echocardiogram, which has aided in the recognition of left ventricular hypertrophy resulting from hypertension. As an example, in the Framingham Heart Study, no cause for the arrhythmia was initially identified in 31% of the 100 patients who developed AF during a 22-year follow-up (13). However, cardiovascular disease subsequently occurred in all but 5 patients. Thus, in this outpatient group, only 5% of patients had lone AF.

In the majority of patients, lone AF is intermittent or paroxysmal (13,14). As an example, in a study from the Mayo Clinic that included 3623 patients with AF seen during a 30-year period, 2.7% had lone AF, which was chronic in only 9% (14). The conversion rate from intermittent to chronic AF was 18% over an 8-year period. Affected patients are younger than those with structural heart disease, are often male, have few symptoms, are refractory to maintaining sinus rhythm, and generally have a good prognosis, particularly if they are under the age of 60.

II. ATRIAL PATHOLOGY ASSOCIATED WITH AF

The normal atria have a thick layer of endocardium, consisting of a thin layer of endothelium, a delicate elastic layer of connective tissue, and a fibroelastic subendocardium that is composed of collagen, muscle cells, and elastic fibers (7,8). The atrial myocardium is similar to the ventricular myocardium but is more loosely arranged and composed of smooth muscle cells that are thinner and oriented in a chaotic fashion. Also present are elastic and collagen fibers. With age, there is an increase in the amount of fatty tissue within the atrial myocardium, and the muscle cells become atrophied. The epicardium over the atria is thicker than it is over the ventricle; it consists of collagen and fatty tissue. The conduction system of the atria consists of the sinus node, inter- and intra-atrial pathways (although their existence is still questionable), and the AV node.

While a number of pathological changes in the atria are associated with AF, none are specific. These include congenital changes, fibrosis, infiltration, fatty changes, acute and chronic inflammation, and tumor formation (7,8). As part of the normal aging process, there may be changes within the sinus or AV nodes or the nerves supplying these structures, atrial dilatation, or changes of the atrial myocardium, including amyloid deposition (9). Rarely seen are abnormalities of the atrial conduction system, while the most commonly noted changes are loss of atrial myocardial cells of the sinus node or the atrial tissue surrounding this structure, adipose infiltration of the atrial myocardium, and amyloid deposition in the atrial myocardium. Other changes seen in AF are associated with underlying disease states; these include atrial myocardial hypertrophy, disease of the small vessels serving the sinus and atrioventricular nodes, fibrofatty degenerative changes of the atrial conduction system, and degenerative changes of the atrial myocardium. Other changes may be evidence of acute or chronic inflammation, with necrosis, cellular infiltration, fatty metamorphosis, fibrosis, and calcification.

It has been reported that structural changes result from the arrhythmia itself, which may be associated with its persistence. Enlargement of either the right or left atrium is more commonly seen when the AF is acute in onset, while biatrial enlargement is more common when the arrhythmia is chronic (7).

Patients with lone AF have no gross structural abnormality, although patholgical studies demonstrate isolated atrial dilation, fibrosis of the internodal tracts, and occasinally abnormal sinoatrial nodal architecture.

III. ELECTROPHYSIOLOGICAL MECHANISMS

Several electrophysiological mechanisms are responsible for the occurrence of AF (171,172). When compared to the atrial tissue of patients without AF, tissue from those with AF has a resting membrane potential significantly less negative, which results in a decrease in upstroke velocity and action potential amplitude. This is associated with a reduction in impulse conduction velocity through the atrial myocardium, a precondition for reentry. In general, the effective atrial refractory period of atrial tissue from patients with a history of AF is shorter than it is in normal atrial tissue. Additionally, it has been reported that the refractory period of atrial tissue in patients vulnerable to AF shows no adaptation to changes in heart rate; i.e., it does not shorten appropriately to rapid rates nor does it prolong with slower rates (173,174). The tissue from patients with AF also has a higher percentage of cells that are partially depolarized, resulting in an increased heterogeneity or dispersion of action potential durations (175,176). All of these factors are preconditions for reentry.

It has been well established that there are differences in the velocity of impulse conduction in relation to muscle fiber orientation—i.e., anisotropic conduction. The velocity is two- to threefold faster when impulse direction is longitudinal or parallel to fiber orientation compared to a direction that is perpendicular to the long axis or transverse (177). Since the muscle cells of the atrial myocardium are arranged in a heterogeneous fashion, there is a great degree of anisotropy. This feature of the atrial myocardial cells causes reentrant excitation even when there is no structural abnormality and the electrophysiological properties are normal (178,179). The presence of fibrosis or other degenerative changes may enhance these differences.

In general, the incidence of AF is greater when the refractory period is shorter or the conduction slower. Normal and pathological changes of the atrial myocardium, a variety of drugs, and changes of the sympathetic and parasympathetic nervous systems can have effects on the conduction velocity and refractory periods that predispose to AF.

Studies have shown that there is no difference in atrial excitability between patients with AF or sick sinus syndrome compared with normals (180,181). However, patients with AF had a conduction time that becomes more significantly prolonged when a premature beat was added during early atrial diastole (i.e., during the relative refractory period). This was associated with the induction of repetitive atrial beats during premature stimulation and was observed in 43% of patients with AF but in none of the normals. Correlating with the increase in conduction time is fractionation of local atrial electrograms resulting from atrial premature beats (182,183).

Mapping of the atria during AF has led to the hypothesis that fibrillation is maintained by the presence of a number of independent wavelets (approximately six) that travel randomly through the myocardium around multiple islets or strands of refractory tissue (184,185). Each wavelet may accelerate or decelerate when it encounters tissue in a more or less excitable state. These multiple wavelets may collide with each other, divide, extinguish, or combine, resulting in continuous fluctuation in wavelet size, number, and direction. Since maintenance of fibrillation depends on the presence of a critical number of wavelets, a critical mass of atrial tissue is necessary.

It has been reported that there are electrophysiological or structural changes in the atrial myocardium that result from AF itself (173,174). This is known as electrical remodeling. In the normal situation, the atrial refractory period shortens with an increase in rate and prolongs when the rate decreases. AF, even after only a few minutes, induces transient changes in atrial electrophysiology that promote its perpetuation; there is a progressive decrease in atrial refractoriness and failure of the refractory period to lengthen appropriately at slow rates (e.g., with return to sinus rhythm). Electrical remodeling results from the high rate of electrical activation, which stimulates the AF-induced changes in refractoriness (174). These changes can increase the potential for AF. Hence paroxysmal episodes of AF may enhance the potential for more frequent episodes or sustained AF. It has also been noted that the longer the duration of a proxysmal episode, the greater the chance that the episode will be sustained (186). Electrical remodeling can be prevented by treatment with verapamil, suggesting a role for increased influx of calcium as a result of AF and the rapid atrial rate (187).

The sinus node may play an important role in the genesis of AF (188, 189). When the sinus node is destroyed or its function temporarily suppressed, sinus bradycardia occurs, and AF often develops spontaneously. This may be due to the development of multiple ectopic foci and waves of activation through the atrium, resulting in the loss of dominant pacemaker activity.

IV. ROLE OF THE AUTONOMIC NERVOUS SYSTEM

One of the most important inputs to the atrial myocardium is the autonomic nervous system; sympathetic and parasympathetic neural traffic can have significant effects on the atrial myocardium in addition to their known actions on the sinus and AV nodes (10,190,191). Alterations in autonomic tone may play an important role in some patients—for example, those with lone AF or patients observed to have multiple ectopic foci in the region of the pulmonary veins (192,193).

Both sympathetic and parasympathetic stimulation shorten atrial refractoriness and enhance conduction within the atrial myocardium (10). However, these effects are nonhomogenous, a result of no uniform anatomical distribution of the nerve endings as well as from temporal inhomogeneity of stimulation. Sympathetic stimulation augments the firing of automatic foci and enhances the amplitude of afterpotentials (194). When this occurs along with changes in atrial conduction and refractoriness, AF may be provoked. Vagal stimulation, known to provoke experimental AF, results in a shortening of the atrial refractory period and hyperpolarization of atrial fibers, causing an increase in conduction velocity (195,196). These changes occur in some but not all of the atrial tissue, and in this way reentry is promoted. This is especially important in the presence of an abnormal or diseased atrial myocardium.

It has been clinically observed that in some patients—for example, those with exercise-induced AF—the sympathetic nervous system plays a key role in the precipitation of this arrhythmia; in other patients—for example, those with nocturnal episodes of AF—the parasympathetic nervous system is the important factor (197,198). However, in most patients there is an interplay between the sympathetic and parasympathetic nervous systems, and the distinction is not clear.

Vagally mediated atrial fibrillation occurs more frequently in men than in women, with a ratio of 4 to 1 (198,199). The onset of the arrhythmia is usually between the ages of 40 and 50, and the duration may range from 2 to as long as 20 years. The arrhythmia tends to remain paroxysmal and generally does not become sustained. In most cases it is considered to be idiopathic; these patients are said to have lone AF. An important feature is the occurrence of the arrhythmia during periods of high vagal tone, such as at night or early in the morning. Other possible precipitating factors are rest, meals (especially dinner), and alcohol. Physical exertion and emotional stress are generally not associated factors in patients with vagally mediated AF.

Vagally mediated arrhythmia may present with alternating periods of atrial flutter and AF. This may result from a shortening of the refractory period and the increase in the velocity of impulse conduction due to vagal stimulation, which can cause an acceleration of the flutter rate, precipitating fibrillation. The arrhythmia is generally preceded by a period of sinus bradycardia due to enhanced vagal tone, which may be reproduced by the use of vagal maneuvers or vagotonic drugs.

Patients in whom the sympathetic nervous system plays a role in precipitating AF have the arrhythmia in association with hypercatecholamine states, as occurs in the morning hours, with exercise, or as a result of emotional stress and anxiety (198,199). Disorders associated with high catecholamine levels—such as hyperthyroidism, pulmonary embolism, or pheochromocytoma—may result in AF. Often there is acceleration of the sinus rate just prior to the occurrence of the arrhythmia. Sympathetically mediated AF is less common than AF provoked by enhanced vagal tone.

REFERENCES

1. Feinberg WM, Blackshear JL, Laupacis A, Kronmal R, Hart RG. Prevalence, age distribution, and gender of patients with atrial fibrillation. Analysis and implications. Arch Intern Med 1995; 155:469–473.

2. Majeed A, Moser K, Carroll K. Trends in the prevalence and management of atrial fibrillation in general practice in England and Wales, 1994–1998: analysis of data from the general practice research database. Heart 2001; 86:284–288.

3. Kannel WB, Abbott RD, Savage DD, McNamara PM. Epidemiology of atrial fibrillation: the Framingham study. N Engl J Med 1982; 306:1018–1022.

4. Go AS, Hylek EM, Phillips KA, Chang Y, Henault LE, Selby JV, Singer DE. Prevalence of diagnosed atrial fibrillation in adults: national implications for rhythm management and stroke prevention: the AnTicoagulation and Risk Factors in Atrial Fibrillation (ATRIA) Study. JAMA 2001; 285:2370–2375.

5. Krahn AD, Manfreda J, Tate RB, Mathewson FA, Cuddy TE. The natural history of atrial fibrillation: incidence, risk factors, and prognosis in the Manitoba Follow-up Study. Am J Med 1995; 98:476–484.

6. Benjamin EJ, Wolf PA, D'Agostino RB, McNamara PM. Impact of atrial fibrillation on the risk of death: the Framingham Heart Study. Circulation 1998; 98:946–952.

7. Davies MD, Pomerance A. Pathology of atrial fibrillation in man. Br Heart J 1972; 34:520–525.

8. Lie JT, Falk RH, James TN. Cardiac anatomy and pathologic correlates of atrial fibrillation. In: Falk RH, Podrid PJ, eds. Atrial Fibrillation: Mechanisms and Management. 2d ed. Philadelphia: Lippincott-Raven, 1997:23–52.

9. Lie TJ, Hammond PI. Pathology of the senescent heart: anatomic observations on 237 autopsy studies of patients 90 to 105 years old. Mayo Clin Proc 1988; 63:552–564.

10. Sopher SM, Malik M, Camm AJ. Neural aspects of atrial fibrillation. In: Falk RH, Podrid PJ, eds. Atrial Fibrillation: Mechanisms and Management. 2d ed. Philadelphia: Lippincott-Raven, 1997:155–167.

11. Kerr CR, Leather RA. Atrial fibrillation in the absence of overt cardiac disease. In: Falk RH, Podrid PJ, eds. Atrial Fibrillation: Mechanisms and Management. 2d ed. Philadelphia: Lippincott-Raven, 1997:169–182.

12. Evans W, Swann P. Lone atrial fibrillation. Br Heart J 1954; 6:189–194.

13. Brand FN, Abbott RD, Kannel WB, Wolf PA. Characteristics and prognosis of lone atrial fibrillation: thirty-year follow-up in the Framingham study. JAMA 1985; 254:3449–3453.

14. Kopecky SL, Gersh BJ, McGoon MD, Chu CP, Ilstrup DM, Chesebro JH, Whisnant JP. The natural history of lone atrial fibrillation. A population-based study over three decades. N Engl J Med 1987; 317:669–674.

15. Kannel WB, Abbott RD, Savage DD. Coronary heart disease and atrial fibrillation: the Framingham study. Am Heart J 1983; 106:386–396.

16. Benjamin EL, Levy D, Vairi SM, Agostino D'RB, Belanger AJ, Wolf PA. Independent risk factors for atrial fibrillation in a population-based cohort. The Framingham Heart Study. JAMA 1994; 271:840–844.

17. Wyse DG, Waldo AL, DiMarco JP, Domanski MJ, Rosenberg Y, Schron EB, Kellen JC, Greene HL, Mickel MC, Dalquist JE, Corley SD. A comparison of rate control and rhythm control in patients with atrial fibrillation. The Atrial

Fibrillation Follow-up Investigation of Rhythm Management (AFFIRM) investigators. N Engl J Med 2002; 347:1825–1833.

18. Verdecchia P, Reboldi G, Gattobigio R, Bentivoglio M, Borgioni C, Angeli F, Carluccio E, Sardone MG, Porcellati C. Atrial fibrillation in hypertension: predictors and outcome. Hypertension 2003; 41:218–223.

19. Vaziri SM, Larson MG, Benjamin EJ, Levy D. Echocardiographic predictors of nonrheumatic atrial fibrillation. The Framingham Study. Circulation 1994; 89:724–730.

20. Tsang TS, Barnes ME, Bailey KR, Leibson CL, Montgomery SC, Takemoto Y, Diamond PM, Marra MA, Gersh BJ, Wiebers DO, Petty GW, Seward JB. Left atrial volume: important risk marker of incidental atrial fibrillation in 1655 older men and women. Mayo Clin Proc 2001; 76:467–475.

21. Gerdts E, Oikarinen L, Palmieri V, Otterstad JE, Wachtell K, Boman K, Dahlof B, Devereux RB. Correlates of left atrial size in hypertensive patients with left ventricular hypertrophy: the Losartan Intervention For Endpoint Reduction in Hypertension (LIFE) study. Hypertension 2002; 39:739–743.

22. Dittrich HC, Pearce LE, Asinger RW, Mcbride R, Webel R, Zabalgiotia M, Pennock GD, Stafford RE, Rothbart RM, Halperin JL, Hart RG. Left atrial diameter in nonvalvular atrial fibrillation. An echocardiographic study. Stroke prevention in Atrial Fibrillation Investigators. Am Heart J 1999; 137:494–499.

23. Haddad AH, Pihkov VK, Dean DC. Chronic atrial fibrillation and coronary artery disease. J Electrocardiol 1978; 11:67–69.

24. Kramer RJ, Zeldis SM, Hamby RI. Atrial fibrillation, a marker for abnormal left ventricular function in coronary heart disease. Br Heart J 1982; 47:606–608.

25. Cameron A, Schwartz MJ, Kronmal RA, Kosinski AS. Prevalence and significance of atrial fibrillation in coronary artery disease (CASS Registry). Am J Cardiol 1988; 61:714–717.

26. Celik SV, Erdol C, Baykan M, Ian S, Kasap H. Relation between paroxysmal atrial fibrillation and left ventricular diastolic function in patients with acute myocardial infarction. Am J Cardiol 2001; 88:160–162.

27. Liem KL, Lie KI, Durrer D, Wellens HJ. Clinical setting and prognostic significance of atrial fibrillation complicating acute myocardial infarction. Eur J Cardiol 1976; 4:59–62.

28. Liberthson RR, Salesbury KW, Hutten AM, De Sanctis RW. Atrial tachyarrhythmias in acute myocardial infarction. Am J Med 1976; 60:956–960.

29. Cristal N, Scwarzberg J, Gueron M. Supraventricular arrhythmias in acute myocardial infarction: Prognostic importance of clinical setting: mechanism of production. Ann Intern Med 1975; 82:35–39.

30. Nagahama Y, Sugiura T, Takehana K, Hatada K, Inada M, Iwasaka T. The role of infarction-associated pericarditis on the occurrence of atrial fibrillation. Eur Heart J 1998; 19:287–292.

31. Goldberg RJ, Seeley D, Becker RC, Brady P, Chen ZY, Osganian V, Gore JM, Alpert JS, Dalen JE. Impact of atrial fibrillation of the in-hospital and long-term survival of patients with acute myocardial infarction: a community-wide perspective. Am Heart J 1990; 119:996–1001.

32. Jewitt DE, Balcon R, Raftery EB, Oram S. Incidence and management of supraventricular arrhythmias after acute myocardial infarction. Am Heart J 1969; 77:290–293.

33. James TN. Myocardial infarction and atrial arrhythmias. Circulation 1961; 24:761.

34. Wong CK, White HD, Wilcox RG, Criger DA, Califf RM, Topol EJ, Ohman EM. New atrial fibrillation after acute myocardial infarction independently predicts death: the GUSTO-III experience. Am Heart J 2000; 140:878–885.

35. Crenshaw BS, Ward SR, Granger CB, Stebbins AL, Topol EJ, Califf RM, for the GUSTO-1 Trial Investigators. Atrial fibrillation in the setting of acute myocardial infarction: the GUSTO-1 experience. J Am Coll Cardiol 1997; 30:40413.

36. Pizzetti F, Turazza FM, Franzosi MG, Barlera S, Ledda A, Maggioni AP, Santoro L, Tognoni G. Incidence and prognostic significance of atrial fibrillation in acute myocardial infarction: the GISSI-3 data. Heart 2001; 86:527–532.

37. Pedersen OD, Bagger H, Kober L, Torp-Pedersen C. The occurrence and prognostic significance of atrial fibrillation/flutter following acute myocardial infarction. TRACE Study group. TRAndolapril Cardiac Evaluation. Eur Heart J 1999; 20:748–754.

38. Behar S, Zahavi Z, Goldbourt U, Reicher Reiss H. Long-term prognosis of patients with paroxysmal atrial fibrillation complicating acute myocardial infarction. SPRINT study group. Eur Heart J 1992; 13:45–50.

39. Hod H, Lew AS, Keltae M, Cercek B, Geft IL, Shah PK, Ganz W. Early atrial fibrillation during evolving myocardial infarction. Circulation 1987; 75:146–150.

40. Sakata K, Kurihara H, Iwamori K, Maki A, Yoshino H, Yanagisawa A, Ishikawa K. Clinical and prognositc significance of atrial fibrillation in acute myocardial infarction. Am J Cardiol 1997; 80:1522–1527.

41. Eldar M, Canettii M, Rotstein Z, Boyko V, Gottlieb S, Kaplinsky E, Behar S, for the SPRINT and Thrombolytic Survey Groups. Significance of paroxysmal atrial fibrillation complicating acute myocardial infarction in the thrombolytic era. Circulation 1998; 97:965–970.

42. Al-Khatib SM, Pieper KS, Lee KL, Mahaffey KW, Hochman JS, Pepine CJ, Kopecky SL, Akkerhuis M, Stepinska J, Simoons ML, Topol EJ, Califf RM, Harrington RA. Atrial fibrillation and mortality among patients with acute coronary syndromes without ST-segment elevation: results from the PURSUIT trial. Am J Cardiol 2001; 88(A7):76–79.

43. Friedman HZ, Weber-Bornstein N, Deboe SF, Mancini GB. CCU admission criteria for suspected acute myocardial infarction in new onset atrial fibrillation. Am J Cardiol 1987; 59:866–869.

44. Shlofmitz RA, Hirsh BE, Meyer BR. New onset atrial fibrillation: is there a need for emergent hospitalization? J Gen Intern Med 1986; 1:139–192.

45. Zimetbaum PJ, Josephon ME, McDonald MJ, McClennen S, Korley V, Ho KK, Papageorgiou P, Cohen DJ. Incidence and predictors of myocardial

infarction among patients with atrial fibrillation. J Am Coll Cardiol 2000; 36:1223–1227.

46. Maisel WH, Stevenson LW. Atrial fibrillation in heart failure: epidemiology, pathophysiology, and rationale for therapy. Am J Cardiol 2003; 91:2D–8D.

47. Stevenson WG, Stevenson LW, Middlekauff HR, Fonarow GC, Hamilton MA, Woo MA, Saxon LA, Natterson DP, Steimle A, Walden JA, Tillisch JH. Improving survival for patients with atrial fibrillation and advanced heart failure. J Am Coll Cardiol 1996; 28:1458–1463.

48. Ehrlich JR, Nattel S, Hohnloser SH. Atrial fibrillation and congestive heart failure: specific considerations at the intersection of two common and important cardiac disease sets. J Cardiovasc Electrophysiol 2002; 13:399–405.

49. Van Gelder IC, Crijns JGM, Blanksma PK, Landsman ML, Posma JL, Van Den Berg MP, Meijler FL, Lie KI. Time course of hemodynamic changes and improvement in exercise tolerance after cardioversion of chronic atrial fibrillation unassociated with cardiac valve disease. Am J Cardiol 1993; 72:560–566.

50. Alam M, Thorstrand C. Left ventricular function in patients with atrial fibrillation before and after cardioversion. Am J Cardiol 1992; 69:694–696.

51. Pozzoli M, Cioffi G, Traversi E, Pinna GD, Cobelli F, Tavazzi L. Predictors of primary atrial fibrillation and concomitant clinical and hemodynamic changes in patients with chronic heart failure: a prospective study in 344 patients with baseline sinus rhythm. J Am Coll Cardiol 1998; 32:197–204.

52. Grogan M, Smith HC, Gersh BJ, Wood DL. Left ventricular dysfunction due to atrial fibrillation in patients initially believed to have idiopathic dilated cardiomyopathy. Am J Cardiol 1992; 69:1570–1573.

53. Furberg CD, Psaty BM, Manolio TA, Gardin JM, Smith VE, Rautaharju PM. Prevalence of atrial fibrillation in elderly subjects (the Cardiovascular Health Study). Am J Cardiol 1994; 74:236–241.

54. Krahn AD, Manfreda J, Tate RB, Mathewson FA, Cuddy TE. The natural history of atrial fibrillation: incidence, risk factors and prognosis in the Manitoba Follow-up Study. Am J Med 1995; 98:476–484.

55. Flaker GC, Fletcher KA, Rothbart RM, Halperin JL, Hart RG. Clinical and echocardiographic features of intermittent atrial fibrillation that predict recurrent atrial fibrillation. The Stroke Prevention in Atrial Fibrillation (SPAF) Investigators. Am J Cardiol 1995; 76:355–358.

56. Yamada T, Fukunami M, Shimonagata T, Kumagai K, Ogita H, Asano Y, Hirata A, Hori M, Hoki N. Prediction of paroxysmal atrial fibrillation in patients with congestive heart failure: a prospective study. J Am Coll Cardiol 2000; 35:405–413.

57. Hornestam B, Hall C, Held P, Carlsson T, Falk L, Karlson BW, Lundstrom T, Peterson M, for the Digitalis in Acute Atrial Fibrillation (DAAF) Trial Group. N-terminal proANF in acute atrial fibrillation: a biochemical marker of atrial pressures but not a predictor for conversion to sinus rhythm. Am Heart J 1998; 135:1040–1047.

58. Rossi A, Enriquez-Sarano M, Burnett JC, Lerman A, Abel MD, Seward JB.

Natriuretic peptide levels in atrial fibrillation. A prospective hormonal and Doppler-echocardiographic study. J Am Coll Cardiol 2000; 35:1256–1262.

59. Francis GS. Development of arrhythmias in the patient with congestive heart failure: pathophysiology, prevalence and prognosis. Am J Cardiol 1986; 57:3B–7B.

60. Robinson K, Frenneaux MP, Stockins B, Karatasakis G, Poloniecki JD, McKenna WJ. Atrial fibrillation in hypertrophic cardiomyopathy: a longitudinal study. J Am Coll Cardiol 1990; 15:1279–1285.

61. Cecchi F, Olivotto I, Montereggi A, Marconi P, Dolara A, Maron BJ. Hypertrophic cardiomyopathy in Tuscany: clinical course and outcome in an unselected regional population. J Am Coll Cardiol 1995; 26:1529–1536.

62. Savage DD, Seides SF, Maron BJ, Myers DJ, Epstein SE. Prevalence of arrhythmias during 24-hour electrocardiographic monitoring and exercise testing in patients with obstructive and nonobstructive hypertrophic cardiomyopathy. Circulation 1979; 59:866–875.

63. Olivotto I, Cecchi F, Casey SA, Dolara A, Traverse JH, Maron BJ. Impact of atrial fibrillation on the clinical course of hypertrophic cardiomyopathy. Circulation 2001; 104:2517.

64. Wigle ED, Sasson Z, Henderson MA, Ruddy TD, Fulop J, Rakowski H, Williams WG. Hypertrophic cardiomyopathy. The importance of the site and extent of hypertrophy. A review. Prog Cardiovasc Dis 1985; 28:1–83.

65. McKenna WJ, England D, Dor YL, Deanfield JE, Oakley C, Goodwin JF. Arrhythmia in hypertrophic cardiomyopathy: influence on prognosis. Br Heart J 1981; 46:168–172.

66. Gleaney DL, O'Brien KP, Gold HK. Atrial fibrillation in patients with idiopathic hypertrophic subaortic stenosis. Br Heart J 1970; 32:652–659.

67. Stafford WJ, Trohman RG, Bilsker M, Zaman L, Castellanos A, Myerburg RJ. Cardiac arrest in an adolescent with atrial fibrillation and hypertrophic cardiomyopathy. J Am Coll Cardiol 1986; 7:701–704.

68. Suzuki M, Hirayama T, Marumoto K, Okayama H, Iwata T. Paroxysmal atrial fibrillation as a cause of potentially lethal ventricular arrthythmia with myocardial ischemia in hypertrophic cardiomyopathy: a case report. Angiology 1998; 49:653–657.

69. Falk RH. Cardiac amyloidosis. Prog Cardiol 1989; 2:143–156.

70. Hodkinson HM, Pomerance A. The clinical pathology of heart failure and atrial fibrillation in old age. Postgrad Med 1979; 55:251.

71. Crijns HJ, Tjeerdsma G, de Kam PJ, Boomsma F, van Gelder IC, van den Berg MP, van Veldhuisen DJ. Prognostic value of the presence and development of atrial fibrillation in patients with advanced chronic heart failure. Eur Heart J 2000; 21:1238–1245.

72. Dries DL, Exner DV, Gersh BJ, Domanski MJ, Waclawiw MA, Stevenson LW. Atrial fibrillation is associated with an increased risk for mortality and heart failure progression in patients with asymptomatic left ventricular systolic dysfunction: a retrospective analysis of the SOLVD trials. J Am Coll Cardiol 1998; 32:695–703.

73. Mahoney P, Kimmel S, DeNofrio D, Wahl P, Loh E. Prognostic significance of atrial fibrillation in patients at a tertiary medical center referred for heart transplantation because of severe heart failure. Am J Cardiol 1999; 83:1544–1547.

74. Carson PE, Johnson GR, Dunkman WB, Fletcher RD, Farrell L, Cohn JN. The influence of atrial fibrillation on prognosis in mild to moderate heart failure. The V-HeFT Studies. The V-HeFT VA Cooperative Studies Group. Circulation 1993; 87:VI102–VI110.

75. Bentivoglio LG, Uricchio JF, Waldo A, et al. An electrocardiographic analysis of sixty five cases of mitral regurgitation. Circulation 1958; 18:572.

76. Rowe JC, Bland EF, Sprague HB, White PD. The course of mitral stenosis without surgery: ten and twenty year perspectives. Ann Intern Med 1960; 52:741.

77. Olesen KH. The natural history of 271 patients with mitral stenosis under medical treatment. Br Heart J 1962; 24:349.

78. Probst P, Goldschlager N, Selzer A. Left atrial size and atrial fibrillation in mitral stenosis: Factors influencing their relationship. Circulation 1973; 48:1282–1287.

79. Graham GK, Taylor JA, Ellis LB, Greenberg DJ, Robbins SL. Studies in mitral stenosis: a correlation of post-mortem findings with the clinical course in the disease in one hundred and one cases. Arch Intern Med 1951; 88:532–547.

80. Stone SJ, Feil HS. Mitral stenosis: a clinical and pathologic study of 100 cases. Am Heart J 1933; 9:53–62.

81. Podrid PJ, Falk RH. Management of atrial fibrillation: an overview. In: Falk RH, Podrid PJ, eds. Atrial Fibrillation: Mechanism and Management. New York: Raven Press, 1992:389–411.

82. Grigioni F, Avierinos JF, Ling LH, Scott CG, Bailey KR, Tajik AJ, Frye RL, Enriquez-Sarano M. Atrial fibrillation complicating the course of degenerative mitral regurgitation: determinants and long-term outcome. J Am Coll Cardiol 2002; 40:84–92.

83. Dujardin KS, Enriquez-Sarano M, Schaff HV, Bailey KR, Seward JB, Tajik AJ. Mortality and morbidity of aortic regurgitation in clinical practice. A long-term follow-up study. Circulation 1999; 99:1851–1857.

84. Rothschild MA, Sachs B, Libman E. The disturbances of the cardiac mechanism in subacute bacterial endocarditis and rheumatic fever. Am Heart J 1927; 2:316–374.

85. Fulton MN, Levine SA. Subacute bacterial endocarditis, with special references to the valve lesions and previous history. Am J Med Sci 1932; 183:60–77.

86. Diker E, Aydogdu S, Ozdemir M, Kural T, Polat K, Cehreli S, Erdogan A, Goksel S. Prevalence and predictors of atrial fibrillation in rheumatic heart disease. Am J Cardiol 1996; 77:93–98.

87. Aronow WS, Schomoetz KS, Koenigsberg M. Correlation of atrial fibrillation with presence or absence of mitral annular calcium in 604 patients older than 60 years. Am J Cardiol 1987; 59:1213–1214.

88. Savage DD, Garrison RJ, Castelli WP, McNamara PM, Anderson SI, Kannel

WB, Feinleib M. Prevalence of saturated (annular) calcium and its correlates in a general population-based sample. The Framingham study. Am J Cardiol 1983; 57:1375–1378.

89. Lauer MS, Eagle KA, Buckley MJ, DeSanctis RW. Atrial fibrillation following coronary artery bypass surgery. Prog Cardiovasc Dis 1989; 31:367–378.

90. Kowey PR, Taylor JE, Rials SJ, Marinchak RA. Meta-analysis of the effectiveness of prophylactic drug therapy in preventing supraventricular arrhythmia early after coronary artery bypass grafting. Am J Cardiol 1992; 69:963–965.

91. Asher CR, Miller DP, Grimm RA, Cosgrove DM III, Chung MK. Analysis of risk factors for development of atrial fibrillation early after cardiac valvular surgery. Am J Cardiol 1998; 82:892–895.

92. Creswell LL, Schuessler RB, Rosenbloom M, Cox JL. Hazards of postoperative atrial arrhythmias. Ann Thorac Surg 1993; 56:539–549.

93. Mueller XM, Tevaearai HT, Ruchat P, Stumpe F, von Segesser LK. Did the introduction of a minimally invasive technique change the incidence of atrial fibrillation after single internal thoracic artery-left anterior descending artery grafting? J Thorac Cardiovasc Surg 2001; 121:683–688.

94. Tamis-Holland JE, Homel P, Durani M, Iqbal M, Sutandar A, Mindich BP, Steinberg JS. Atrial fibrillation after minimally invasive direct coronary artery bypass surgery. J Am Coll Cardiol 2000; 36:1884–1888.

95. Asher CR, DiMengo JM, Arheart KL, Weber MM, Grimm RA, Blackstone EH, Cosgrove DM, Chung MK. Atrial fibrillation early postoperatively following minimally invasive cardiac valvular surgery. Am J Cardiol 1999; 84:744–749.

96. Ascione R, Caputo M, Calori G, Lloyd CT, Underwood MJ, Angelini GD. Predictors of atrial fibrillation after conventional and beating heart coronary surgery. A prospective, randomized study. Circulation 2000; 102:1530–1535.

97. d'Amato TA, Savage EB, Wiechmann RJ, Sakert T, Benckart DH, Magovern JA. Reduced incidence of atrial fibrillation with minimally invasive direct coronary artery bypass. Ann Thorac Surg 2000; 70:2013–2016.

98. Pavri BB, O'Nunain SS, Newell JB, Ruskin JN, William G. Prevalence and prognostic significance of atrial arrhythmias after orthotopic cardiac transplantation. J Am Coll Cardiol 1995; 25:1673–1680.

99. Polanczyk CA, Goldman L, Marcantonio ER, Orav EJ, Lee TH. Supraventricular arrhythmia in patients having noncardiac surgery: clinical correlates and effect on length of stay. Ann Intern Med 1998; 129:279–285.

100. Maisel WH, Rawn JD, Stevenson WG. Atrial fibrillation after cardiac surgery. Ann Intern Med 2001; 135:1061–1073.

101. Almassi GH, Schowalter T, Nicolosi AC, Aggarwal A, Moritz TE, Henderson WG, Tarazi R, Shroyer AL, Sethi GK, Grover FL, Hammermeister KE. Atrial fibrillation after cardiac surgery: a major morbid event? Ann Surg 1997; 226: 501–511.

102. Abreu JE, Reilly J, Salzano RP, Khachane VB, Jekel VF, Clyne CA. Com-

parison of frequencies of atrial fibrillation after coronary artery bypass grafting with and without the use of cardiopulmonary bypass. Am J Cardiol 1999; 83:775–776.

103. Kim MK, Deeb GM, Morady F, Bruckman D, Hallock LR, Smith KA, Karavite DJ, Bolling SF, Pagani FD, Wahr JA, Sonnad SS, Kazanjian PE, Watts C, Williams M, Eagle KA. Effect of postoperative atrial fibrillation on length of stay after cardiac surgery (the postoperative atrial fibrillation in cardiac surgery study). Am J Cardiol 2001; 87:881–885.

104. Bashur TT. Classification of sinus node dysfunction. Am Heart J 1985; 110:1251–1258.

105. Ferrer MI. The sick sinus syndrome. Cirulation 1973; 47:635–641.

106. Short DS. The syndrome of alternating bradycardia and tachycardia. Br Heart J 1954; 16:208.

107. Kaplan BM, Langendorf R, Lev M, Pick A. Tachycardia-bradycardia syndrome (so-called "sick sinus syndrome"). Pathology, mechanisms and treatment. Am J Cardiol 1973; 31:497.

108. Gomes JA, Kang PS, Matheson M, Gough WB, El-Sherif N. Coexistence of sick sinus rhythm and atrial flutter-fibrillation. Circulation 1981; 63:80–86.

109. Vallin H, Edhag V. Associated conduction disturbances in patients with symptomatic sinus node disease. Acta Med Scand 1981; 210:263–270.

110. Narula OS. Atrioventricular conduction defects in patients with sinus bradycardia. Analysis by His bundle recordings. Circulation 1971; 44:1096–1110.

111. Sutton R, Kenny RA. The natural history of sick sinus syndrome. PACE 1986; 9:1110–1114.

112. Ferrer MI. The etiology and natural history of sinus node disorders. Arch Intern Med 1982; 142:371–372.

113. Seipel L, Both A, Breithardt G, Loogen F. Action of antiarrhythmic drugs on His bundle electrogram and sinus node function. Acta Cardiol 1974; 48(suppl): 251–267.

114. Alt E, Volke R, Wirtzfeld A, et al. Survival and follow up after pacemaker implantation: a comparison of patients with sick sinus syndrome, complete heart block and atrial fibrillation. PACE 1985; 8:849–855.

115. Aeosty JM, Cohen SI, Marken E. Brady-tachycardia syndrome: results in twenty-eight patients treated by combined pharmacologic therapy and pacemaker implantation. Chest 1974; 66:257–263.

116. Bauernfiend RA, Wyndham CR, Swiryn SD, et al. Paroxysmal atrial fibrillation in the Wolff-Parkinson-White syndrome. Am J Cardiol 1981; 47:562–569.

117. Wellens HJJ, Smeets JLRC, Rodriguez LM, Gorgels APM. Atrial fibrillation in Wolff-Parkinson-White syndrome. In: Falk RH, Podrid PJ, eds. Atrial Fibrillation: Mechanism and Management. 2d ed. New York: Raven Press, 1997:205–217.

118. Fuijimura O, Klein GJ, Yee R, Sharma AD. Mode of onset of atrial fibrillation in the Wolff-Parkinson-White syndrome: how important is the accessory pathway? J Am Coll Cardiol 1990; 15:1082–1086.

119. Sharma AD, Klein GJ, Guirdauron GM, Milstein S. Atrial fibrillation in patients with Wolff-Parkinson-White syndrome: incidence after surgical ablation of the accessory pathway. Circulation 1985; 72:161–169.
120. Chen PS, Pressley JC, Tang ASL, Packer DL, Gallagher JJ, Prystowsky EN. New observations on atrial fibrillation before and after surgical treatment in patients with the Wolff-Parkinson-White syndrome. J Am Coll Cardiol 1992; 19:974–981.
121. Morady F, Sledge C, Shen E. Electrophysiologic testing in the management of patients with the Wolff-Parkinson-White syndrome and atrial fibrillation. Am J Cardiol 1973; 51:1623–1628.
122. Klein LS, Miles WM, Zipes DP. Effect of atrioventricular interval during pacing or reciprocating tachycardia in atrial size, pressure and refractory period: contraction excitation feedback in human atrium. Circulation 1990; 82:60–68.
123. Kanter RJ, Garson A. Arrhythmias in congenital heart disease. In: Podrid PJ, Kowey PR, eds. Cardiac Arrhythmias: Mechanisms, Diagnosis, and Management. 2d ed. Philadelphia: Lippincott, Williams & Wilkins, 2001:749–783.
124. Tikoff G, Schmidt AM, Hecht HH. Atrial fibrillation in atrial septal defect. Arch Intern Med 1968; 121:402.
125. Berger F, Vogel M, Kramer A, Alexi-Meskishvili V, Weng Y, Lange PE, Hetzer R. Incidence of atrial flutter/fibrillation in adults with atrial septal defect before and after surgery. Ann Thorac Surg 1999; 68:75–78.
126. Weber DM, Phillips JH. A reevaluation of electrocardiographic changes accompanying acute pulmonary embolism. Am J Med Sci 1966; 251:381.
127. Davidson E, Weinberger I, Rotenberg Z, Fuchs J, Agmon J. Atrial fibrillation: cause and time of onset. Arch Intern Med 1989; 149:457–459.
128. Walsh JJ, Burch GE, Black WC, et al. Idiopathic cardiomyopathy of the puerperium (post partum heart disease). Circulation 1965; 32:19.
129. Ansari A, Larson PH, Bates HD. Cardiovascular manifestations of systemic lupus erythematosus: current perspective. Prog Cardiovasc Dis 1985; 27:421–434.
130. Alexander JK. The cardiomyopathy of obesity. Prog Cardiovasc Dis 1985; 27:325–334.
131. Spodick DH. Arrhythmias during acute pericarditis. A prospective study of 100 consecutive cases. JAMA 1976; 235:39–41.
132. Levine HD. Myocardial fibrosis in constrictive pericarditis: electrocardiographic and pathologic observations. Circulation 1973; 48:1268.
133. Ristic AD, Maisch B, Hufnagel G, et al. Arrhythmias in acute pericarditis. An endomyocardial biopsy study. Herz 2000; 25:729–733.
134. Lowenstein AJ, Gaboer PA, Cramer J. The role of alcohol in new onset atrial fibrillation. Arch Intern Med 1983; 143:1882–1885.
135. Koskinen P, Kupari M, Leonine H. Alcohol and new onset atrial fibrillation: a case control study of a current series. Br Heart J 1987; 57:468–473.
136. Ettinger PV, Wu CF, De LaCruz C, Weisse AB, Ahmed SS, Regan TJ. Arrhythmias and the holiday: alcohol associated cardiac rhythm disorders. Am Heart J 1978; 95:555–562.

137. Menz V, Grimm W, Hoffmann J, Maisch B. Alcohol and rhythm disturbance: the holiday heart syndrome. Herz 1996; 21:227–231.
138. Koskinen P, Kupari M, Leonine H. Role of alcohol in recurrence of atrial fibrillation in persons less than 65 years of age. Am J Cardiol 1990; 66:954–958.
139. Engle TR, Luck JC. Effect of whisky on atrial vulnerability and holiday heart. J Am Coll Cardiol 1983; 1:816–818.
140. Gould L, Reddy LV, Becker W, et al. Electrophysiologic properties of alcohol in man. J Electrocardiol 1978; 11:219–226.
141. Gimeno AL, Bimeno MD, Webb JL. Effects of alcohol on cellular membrane potential and contractility of isolated atrium. Am J Physiol 1962; 203:194–196.
142. Hibbs RG, Ferrans VJ, Black WC. Alcohol cardiomyopathy: an electron microscopic study. Am Heart J 1965; 69:766–779.
143. Bing RJ. Cardiac metabolism: its contribution to alcoholic heart disease and myocardial failure. Circulation 1978; 58:965.
144. Thornton JR. Atrial fibrillation in healthy non-alcoholic people after an alcohol binge. Lancet 1984; 2:1013–1014.
145. Rich EC, Siebold C, Campion B. Alcohol-related acute atrial fibrillation: a case control study and review of 40 patients. Arch Intern Med 1985; 145:830–833.
146. Forfar JC, Toft AD. Thyrotoxic atrial fibrillation: an under diagnosed condition. Br Med J 1982; 285:909–910.
147. Woeber KA. Thyrotoxicosis and the heart. N Engl J Med 1992; 327:94–98.
148. Cobbler JL, Williams MC, Greenland P. Thyrotoxicosis in institutionalized elderly patients with atrial fibrillation. Arch Intern Med 1984; 144:1758–1770.
149. Sawin CT, Geller A, Wolf PA, Belanger AJ, Baker E, Bacharach P, Wilson PW, Benjamin EJ, D'Agostino RB. Low serum thyrotropin concentrations as a risk factor for atrial fibrillation in older persons. N Engl J Med 1994; 331:1249–1252.
150. Auer J, Scheibner P, Mische T, Langsteger W, Eber O, Eber B. Subclinical hyperthyroidism as a risk factor for atrial fibrillation. Am Heart J 2001; 142: 838–842.
151. Krahn AD, Klein GJ, Kerr CR, Boone J, Sheldon R, Green M, Talajic M, Wang X, Connolly S. How useful is thyroid function testing in patients with recent-onset atrial fibrillation? Arch Intern Med 1996; 156:2221–2224.
152. Iwasaki T, Naka H, Namatsu K, et al. Echocardiographic studies on the relationship between atrial fibrillation and atrial enlargement in patients with hyperthyroidism of Graves disease. Cardiology 1989; 76:10–17.
153. Thomas ES, Mozzferri EL, Skillman TK. Apathetic thyrotoxicosis: a distinct clinical and laboratory abnormality. Ann Intern Med 1970; 72:679–685.
154. Tajiri J, Hamasaki S, Shimade T, et al. Masked thyroid dysfunction among elderly patients with atrial fibrillation. Jpn Heart J 1986; 27:183–190.
155. Davies AV, Williams J, John R, et al. Diagnostic value of thyrotropin releasing hormone test in elderly patients with atrial fibrillation. Br Med J 1985; 291:773–776.
156. Fortar JC, Feck CM, Miller HC. Atrial fibrillation and isolated suppression of the pituitary thyroid axis to specific antithyroid therapy. Int J Cardiol 1981; 1:43–48.

157. Scott GR, Forfor JC, Toft AD. Graves disease and atrial fibrillation: the case for even high doses of therapeutic iodine-131. Br Med J 1984; 289:399–400.

158. Chen YC, Chen SA, Chen YJ, Chang MS, Chan P, Lin CI. Effects of thyroid hormone on the arrhythmogenic activity of pulmonary vein cardiomyocytes. J Am Coll Cardiol 2002; 39:366–372.

159. Williams LT, Lefkowitz RJ, Witanabe AM, et al. Thyroid hormone regulation of beta adrenergic receptor number. J Biol Chem 1977; 252:2787.

160. Varriale P, Ramaprased S. Aminophylline induced atrial fibrillation. Pacing Clin Electrophysiol 1993; 16:1953–1955.

161. Elvan A, Pride HP, Eble JN, Zipes DP. Radiofrequency catheter ablation of the atria reduces inducibility and duration of atrial fibrillation in dogs. Circulation 1995; 91:2235–2244.

162. Chiou CW, Eble JN, Zipes DP. Efferent vagal innervation of the canine atria and sinus and atrioventricular nodes. The third fat pad. Circulation 1997; 95:2573–2584.

163. Sticherling C, Oral H, Horrocks J, Chough SP, Baker RL, Kim MH, Wasmer K, Pelosi F, Knight BP, Michaud GF, Strickberger SA, Morady F. Effects of digoxin on acute, atrial fibrillation–induced changes in atrial refractoriness. Circulation 2000; 102:2503–2508.

164. Tieleman RG, Blaauw Y, Van Gelder IC, De Langen CD, de Kam PJ, Grandjean JG, Patberg KW, Bel KJ, Allessie MA, Crijns HJ. Digoxin delays recovery from tachycardia-induced electrical remodeling of the atria. Circulation 1999; 100:1836–1842.

165. Brugada R, Tapscott T, Czernuszewicz G, Marian AJ, Iglesias A, Mont L, Brugada J, Girona J, Domingo A, Bachinski LL, Roberts R. Identification of a genetic locus for familial atrial fibrillation. N Engl J Med 1997; 336:905–911.

166. Chen YH, Xu SJ, Bendahhou S, Wang XL, Wang Y, Xu WY, Jin HW, Sun H, Su XY, Zhuang QN, Yang YQ, Li YB, Liu Y, Xu HJ, Li XF, Ma N, Mou CP, Chen Z, Barhanin J, Huang W. KCNQ1 gain-of-function mutation in familial atrial fibrillation. Science 2003; 299:251–254.

167. Chung MK, Martin DO, Sprecher D, Wazni O, Kanderian A, Carnes CA, Bauer JA, Tchou PJ, Niebauer MJ, Natale A, Van Wagoner DR. C-reactive protein elevation in patients with atrial arrhythmias: inflammatory mechanisms and persistence of atrial fibrillation. Circulation 2001; 104:2886–2891.

168. Ortiz J, Niwano S, Abe H, Rudy Y, Johnson NJ, Waldo AL. Mapping the conversion of atrial flutter to atrial fibrillation and atrial fibrillation to atrial flutter. Insights into mechanisms. Circ Res 1994; 74:882–894.

169. Hamer ME, Wilkinson WE, Clair WK, Page PL, McCarthy EA, Pritchett EL. Incidence of symptomatic atrial fibrillation in patients with paroxysmal supraventricular tachycardia. J Am Coll Cardiol 1995; 25:984–988.

170. Chen YJ, Chen SA, Tai CT, Wen ZC, Feng AN, Ding YA, Chang MS. Role of atrial electrophysiology and autonomic nervous system in patients with supraventricular tachycardia and paroxysmal atrial fibrillation. J Am Coll Cardiol 1998; 32:732–738.

171. Janse MJ, Allessie MA. Experimental observations on atrial fibrillation. In:

Falk RH, Podrid PJ, eds. Atrial Fibrillation: Mechanism and Management. 2d ed. New York: Raven Press, 1997:53–73.

172. Allessie MA, Konings K, Kirchhof CJ, Wijffels M. Electrophysiologic mechanisms of perpetuation of atrial fibrillation. Am J Cardiol 1996; 77:10A–23A.

173. Wijffels MC, Kirchhof CJ, Dorland R, Allessie MA. Atrial fibrillation begets atrial fibrillation. A study in awake chronically instrumented goats. Circulation 1995; 92:1954.

174. Wijffels MC, Kirchhof CJ, Dorland R, Power J, Allessie MA. Electrical remodeling due to atrial fibrillation in chronically instrumented conscious goats. Roles of neurohumoral changes, ischemia, atrial stretch, and high rate of electrical activation. Circulation 1997; 96:3710–3720.

175. Fareh S, Villemaire C, Nattel S. Importance of refractoriness heterogeneity in the enhanced vulnerability to atrial fibrillation induction caused by tachycardia-induced atrial electrical remodeling. Circulation 1998; 98:2202–2209.

176. Ramdat Misier AR, Opthof T, Van Hemel N. Increased dispersion of "refractoriness" in patients with idiopathic paroxysmal atrial fibrillation. J Am Coll Cardiol 1992; 19:1531–1535.

177. Roberts DE, Hersch LT, Scher AM. Influence of cardiac fiber orientation on wavefront voltage, conduction velocity and tissue resistivity in the dog. Circ Res 1979; 44:701–712.

178. Spach MS, Miller WT, Dolber PC, et al. The functional role of structural complexities in the propagation of depolarization in the atrium of the dog: cardiac conduction disturbances due to discontinuities of effective atrial resistivity. Circ Res 1982; 50:175–191.

179. Spack MS, Doeber PC. Relating extracellular potentials and their derivatives to anisotropic propagation at a microscopic level in human cardiac muscle: evidence for electrical uncoupling of side-to-side fiber connections with increasing age. Circ Res 1986; 58:356–371.

180. Simpson RJ, Foster JR, Gettes LS. Atrial excitability and conduction in patients with interatrial conduction defects. Am J Cardiol 1982; 50:1331–1337.

181. Simpson RJ, Amara F, Foster JR, et al. Thresholds, refractory periods and conduction times of the normal and diseased human atrium. Am Heart J 1988; 116:1080–1090.

182. Ohe T, Matsuhia M, Kamakura S. Relation between the widening of the fragmental atrial activity zone and atrial fibrillation. Am J Cardiol 1983; 52:1219–1222.

183. Tanigawa M, Fukatani M, Konoe A. Prolonged and fractional right atrial electrograms during sinus rhythm in patients with paroxysmal atrial fibrillation and sick sinus node syndrome. J Am Coll Cardiol 1991; 17:403–408.

184. Moe GK. On the multiple wavelet hypothesis of atrial fibrillation. Arch Int Pharmacodyn Ther 1962; 140:183–188.

185. Allessie MA, Lammers WJEP, Bonke FM. Experimental evaluation of Moe's multiple wavelet hypothesis of atrial fibrillation. In: Zipes DP, Jalife J, eds. Cardiac Arrhythmias. Orlando, FL: Grune & Stratton, 1985:265–276.

186. Danias PG, Caulfield TA, Weigner MJ, Silverman DI, Manning WJ. Likelihood of spontaneous conversion of atrial fibrillation to sinus rhythm. J Am Coll Cardiol 1998; 31:588–592.
187. Tieleman RG, De Langen CDJ, Van Gelder IC, de Kam PJ, Grandjean J, Bel KJ, Wijffels MC, Allessie MA, Crijns HJ. Verapamil reduces tachycardia-induced electrical remodeling of the atria. Circulation 1997; 95:1945–1953.
188. Azuma K, Shinmura H, Shimiza K. Significance of the sinoatrial node on mechanism of occurrence of atrial fibrillation. Br Heart J 1972; 13:84–98.
189. Sani T, Suzaki F, Sato S. Sinus node impulses and atrial fibrillation. Circ Res 1967; 21:507–513.
190. Liu L, Nattel S. Differing sympathetic and vagal effects on atrial fibrillation in dogs: role of refractoriness heterogeneity. Am J Physiol 1997; 273:H805–H816.
191. Tai CT, Chiou CW, Wen ZC, Hsieh MH, Tsai CF, Lin WS, Chen CC, Lin YK, Yu WC, Ding YA, Chang MS, Chen SA. Effect of phenylephrine on focal atrial fibrillation originating in the pulmonary veins and superior vena cava. J Am Coll Cardiol 2000; 36:788–793.
192. Chen SA, Hsieh MH, Tai CT, Tsai CF, Prakash VS, Yu WC, Hsu TL, Ding YA, Chang MS. Initiation of atrial fibrillation by ectopic beats originating from the pulmonary veins: electrophysiological characteristics, pharmacological responses, and effects of radiofrequency ablation. Circulation 1999; 100(18):1879–1886.
193. Haissaguerre M, Jais P, Shah DC, Takahashi A, Hocini M, Quiniou G, Garrigue S, Le Mouroux A, Le Metayer P, Clementy J. Spontaneous initiation of atrial fibrillation by ectopic beats originating in the pulmonary veins. N Engl J Med 1998; 339:659–666.
194. Wit AL, Cranefield PF. Triggered and automatic activity in the canine coronary sinus. Circ Res 1977; 41:434–445.
195. Lewis T, Drury AN, Bulgar HA. Observations upon flutter and fibrillation: Part VII The effect of vagal stimulation. Heart 1921; 8:141–169.
196. Nahum LH, Hoff HE. Production of auricular fibrillation by application of acetyl-beta-methyl-choline chloride to localized region of the auricular surface. Am J Physiol 1990; 129:428–436.
197. Coumel P. Neural aspects of paroxysmal atrial fibrillation. In: Falk RH, Podrid PJ, eds. Atrial Fibrillation: Mechanism and Management. New York: Raven Press, 1992:109–125.
198. Coumel P. Neural aspects of paroxysmal atrial fibrillation in man. Br Heart J 1972; 34:520–525.
199. Coumel P, Leclercq JF. Cardiac arrhythmias and the autonomic nervous system. In: Levy S, Scheinman MM, eds. Cardiac Arrhythmias from Diagnosis to Therapy. Mt Kisco, NY: Futura, 1984:37.

3

Electrophysiological Mechanisms Relating to Pharmacological Therapy of Atrial Fibrillation

Bramah N. Singh
Veterans Affairs Medical Center of West Los Angeles and the David Geffen School of Medicine at UCLA, Los Angeles, California, U.S.A.

As a cardiac arrhythmia, atrial fibrillation (AF) is undoubtedly at the crossroads (1,2). For many decades, it commanded relatively little attention. AF is the most common arrhythmia requiring hospitalization, and its association with significant mortality and morbidity has led to heightened clinician awareness of this important arrhythmia (3–6).

The control of AF either by catheter ablation or the use of implantable devices has been applicable to only a small percentage of patients. Thus, restoration of sinus rhythm by whatever means and its maintenance by pharmacological therapy is still considered a desirable approach to the management of AF (2–4). Effective arrhythmia control presupposes an understanding not only of the precise mechanisms underlying its genesis but also the fundamental mode of action of antifibrillatory compounds that are used (1,4,6).

I. CELLULAR ATRIAL ELECTROPHYSIOLOGY

A great deal of new information is now available on the fundamental mechanisms of atrial fibrillation in the context of expanding knowledge of regional differences of the electrophysiological properties in the atria in health and disease (1). The bulk of the atrial cells are activated by the fast sodium channel associated with rapid conduction velocity. However, from the standpoint of the development of atrial fibrillation and its prevention, the mechanisms underlying atrial repolarization are critical, especially in terms of the ionic currents involved in the action potential duration (APD) and the effective refractory period (ERP). It has become increasingly evident that the electrophysiological properties of atrial cells differ markedly from those in the various regions of the ventricular myocardium (1,8). The important potassium currents in the atrial and ventricular muscle are compared (9) in Figure 1. The time course and the ion channel changes responsible for the inscription of the various phase of the entire atrial action potential are schematically represented in Figure 2.

Atrial repolarization is initiated by the rapid activation and inactivation of the transient outward current, I_{to}, during phase 1 of the action potential (8,9). This phase is followed by the very rapid activation of ultrarapid delayed rectifier current, I_{Kur}, at positive voltage, with very slow inactivation resulting in sustained outward current during phases 1 and 2 of the action potential.

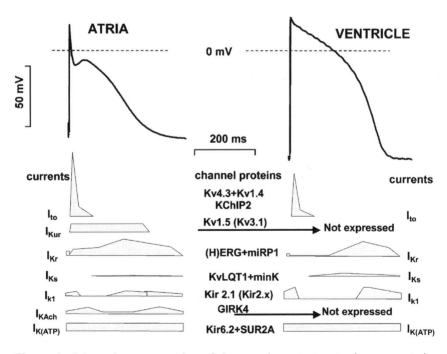

Figure 1 Schematic representation of the most important potassium currents in atrial and ventricular muscle. (From Ref. 9.)

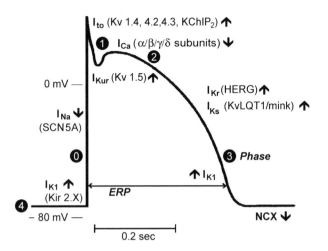

Figure 2 A schematic representation of the atrial action potential with inward current (downward arrows) and outward currents (upward arrows). The molecular basis of each current is indicated in parentheses. The numbers within filled circles indicate the phases of the action potential. (From Ref. 8.)

I_{Kur} is detected only in atrial and not in ventricular cells; phase 3 repolarization is mediated by the rapid (I_{Kr}) and the delayed (I_{Ks}) rectifier currents. The inward rectifier current, I_{K1}, is not only critically important for maintaining the resting membrane potential of cardiac cells, but it also contributes to the final phase of repolarization. Two other K currents have some clinical importance. The first is the ATP-sensitive current, I_{KATP}, which is activated only when the intracellular ATP is markedly decreased, as might occur during myocardial ischemia, resulting in shortening of the APD. The other is the acetylcholine-activated potassium current, I_{KAch}, the activation of which by vagal stimulation leads to shortening of the APD and hyperpolarization of the action potential in the atria. However, this current is not expressed in ventricular cells.

The normal ion-channel characteristics in both the atria and the ventricles are significantly altered in disease in terms of the density of different potassium ion channels. This is especially so in atrial fibrillation and in congestive heart failure, two overlapping syndromes in which changes in the magnitude of the potassium current affect the time course of the action potential and refractoriness as the overall effect of chronic atrial and ventricular remodeling. This is shown in Figure 3. The focus here is on atrial fibrillation. When the arrhythmia has been persistent for a period of time, in addition to the inward calcium current, I_{to} and I_{Kur} are also downregulated (10–12), but I_{K1} is upregulated (10). The overall effect is significant shortening

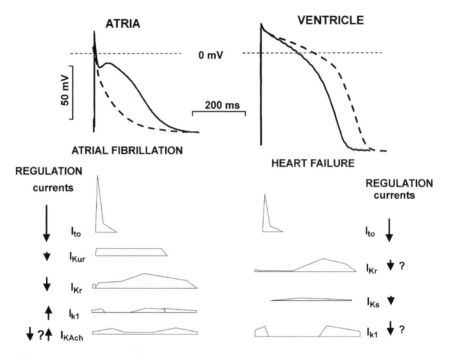

Figure 3 Schematic representation of the down- and upregulation of the most important potassium currents in atrial and ventricular muscle after atrial fibrillation and heart failure. (From Ref. 13.)

of the APD and ERP (13) (Fig. 3), an electrophysiological hallmark of AF associated with loss of rate-dependent APD modulation (Fig. 4). In long-standing atrial fibrillation, the APD or the ERP in atrial muscle does not increase as the frequency of stimulation decreases.

II. MECHANISMS OF ATRIAL FIBRILLATION

There is marked heterogeneity in regional atrial repolarization; this is most likely a significant factor in the genesis of AF (1,6,8). For example, the action potentials in the right atrium vary markedly in certain areas, but of particular importance is the observation that action potentials overall are shorter in the left atrium than those in the right atrium; perhaps they are the shortest in the atrial tissue that extends as a sleeve into the pulmonary veins.

Electrophysiological changes underlying the genesis and perpetuation of AF occur in the setting of anatomic abnormalities that develop as a result

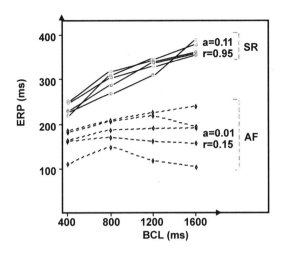

Figure 4   Rate-dependent changes of effective refractory periods (ERP) measured in five different cells at four basic cycle lengths (BCL). The upper part of the panel shows a good adaptation ($r = 0.95$, $a = 0.11$, $p < 0.01$) in a preparation from a patient in sinus rhythm (SR). On the lower part of the panel, lack of adaptation ($r = 0,15$, $a = 0.01$) in a preparation from a patient with atrial fibrillation (AF). Note the shortening and the dispersion of ERP in this last case. (From Ref. 13.)

of the "normal" aging process (14) as well as those that are secondary to such common disorders as hypertension and coronary artery disease. In the case of age, the histopathological changes are characterized by areas of fat deposition in the atrioventricular node and septum as well as in the right atrium; these areas develop hypertrophic and sclerotic changes, followed by atrophy of the smooth layers. In the case of the left atrium, there is endocardial thickening followed by replacement of myocardial fibers with collagen and subsequent loss of myocardial fibers, with diffuse fatty changes and connective tissue infiltration (15,16). In patients with prolonged AF, there is commonly atrial fibrosis, a finding that has been replicated in experimental models (17). For example, in a canine heart failure model, the intense interstitial fibrosis that separates atrial fibers is often associated with significant abnormalities of conduction that can stabilize and perpetuate AF. It has also been shown that, in heart failure, there is upregulation of the Na^+/Ca^{2+} exchanger, which may promote delayed afterdepolarizations, focal atrial ectopy, and rapid triggered activity (18).

For many decades, it was held that AF develops in the wake of repetitive activation of the atria by multiple propagating reentry waves or "wavelets" that rotate around a central obstacle (19). It was recognized that two electrophysiological parameters—conduction velocity and refractory period—were critical for the development of reentry, as their product defined the wavelength of the atrial impulse. It was found that short wavelengths that resulted from short refractory periods (e.g., with thyrotoxicosis, vagal stimulation, or atrial dilatation), and/or slow conduction velocity (e.g., with fibrosis, hypertension, ischemia, heart failure) lead to increases in the number of wavelets that can be accommodated in the atria, which promotes the development of AF. As mentioned above, AF may significantly alter atrial electrophysiology by regulating K^+ ion channels by the process of remodeling, thereby decreasing the atrial ERP and its regional heterogeneity as well as slowing of conduction (20). These overall changes are conducive for the development of multiple-circuit reentry, and its persistence is dependent on the continuous presence of excitable tissue in front of the propagating wavefronts. Drugs or interventions that produce low conduction velocities and short refractory periods will therefore favor multiple-circuit reentry by decreasing minimum circuit size with an increase in the number of circuits. A similar net effect is likely in the case of a large atrium, which can accommodate increased numbers of circuits; moreover, heterogeneity of refractoriness may also favor multicircuit reentry via spatial variability around variably refractory tissue (8). Conversely, drugs and interventions that increase atrial ERP, thereby increasing circuit size, are likely to predictably suppress AF, which provides the rationale for developing drugs that selectively prolong atrial refractoriness.

There is now reasonable consensus that single-circuit reentry is a mechanism for the genesis of AF (21,22). However, clinically, the mechanism is best exemplified in the case of atrial flutter, which is maintained by a single macroreentry circuit. As a reentrant mechanism for AF, a sustained single-circuit reentry critically depends on the wavelength being shorter than the circuit size. There is experimental evidence to suggest that acetylcholine may play a role in the development of single-circuit reentry, and there are data supporting the mechanism of single-circuit macroreentry for AF in the clinical setting (23,24).

It is well established that rapid ectopic activity can also be the basis for the initiation of AF, either as an enhanced, normal phase 4 depolarization that is accelerated to reach the threshold or from triggered activity related to early or delayed afterdepolarizations. In the clinical setting, ectopic foci have been best defined in the ostia of the pulmonary veins (25). Such ectopic foci may trigger single-circuit reentry; by acting as a trigger for induction of reentry and by atrial remodeling, they may also favor multiple-circuit reentry. Moreover, a rapidly firing ectopic beat from a single focus can generate AF if the rate is too fast to conduct 1:1, resulting in fibrillatory conduction when areas of the atria are not able to respond to all the incoming impulses (26). The potential mechanisms are presented in Figure 5. However, as emphasized by

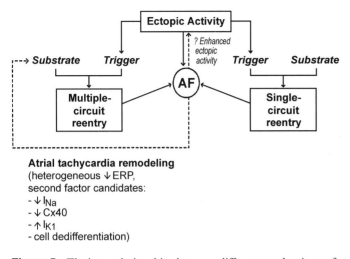

Figure 5 The interrelationships between different mechanisms of atrial fibrillation in a dynamic way. Remodeling due to atrial tachycardia links the potential mechanisms of atrial fibrillation. AF that begins via rapid ectopic activity or single-circuit reentry causes atrial-tachycardia remodeling and tends to move toward multiple circuit reentry. See text for details. (From Ref. 8.)

Nattel (8), while there is compelling evidence indicating differing electrophysiological mechanisms—such as single-circuit reentry, multiple-circuit reentry, and rapid ectopic activity—for the development of atrial fibrillation, they are not discretely independent. Each may play a role in the occurrence of another.

III. ANTIARRHYTHMIC MECHANISMS IN THE CONTROL OF ATRIAL FIBRILLATION

There has recently been concern regarding the clinical wisdom of restoring and maintaining sinus rhythm as a routine practice in most patients with AF (27–29). However, it is known that sustained sinus rhythm in a patient with AF leads to an increase in the left ventricular ejection fraction, with a decrease in left atrial size (30) as well as an increase in maximal exercise capacity and quality of life (31). Thus many patients with AF might benefit from restoration and long-term maintenance of sinus rhythm. Clearly, success in these endeavors depends critically on identifying the precise electrophysiological mechanisms of AF (8) on the one one hand and the fundamental modes of action of antifibrillatory agents on the other (32,33).

Experimental and clinical data have established that the actions of various classes of antiarrhythmic drugs differ significantly with respect to their activity in atrial vs. ventricular muscle (9). As far as the cellular actions of antiarrhythmic drugs are concerned, there are differences in the membrane ion channels that they block in the atrial cells vs. those in the ventricle; there are differences also in selectivity of action with respect to overall lengthening of the APD as well as the magnitude of the differential effects of autonomic transmitters. These differences are relevant in the selection of antifibrillatory agents for the stability of sinus rhythm. The ideal properties of antifibrillatory agents active in atrial tissue have been discussed at length elsewhere (34); they are enumerated briefly below. The ideal antiarrhythmic compound for the control of atrial AF is one that:

> Has a degree of atrial specificity of action with the associated property of blocking atrioventricular (AV) nodal conduction for ventricular rate control if AF recurs during drug therapy
> Has no significant negative inotropic or proarrhythmic action
> Predictably lengthens atrial APD, ERP, and the excitation wavelength
> Exhibits preserved atrial antifibrillatory actions over a wide range of heart rates
> Has a long elimination half-life without significant renally dependent excretion
> Is well tolerated, devoid of organ toxicity, and has no adverse effect on mortality
> Is compatible with most or all mandatory commonly used cardioactive drugs
> Has a high degree of efficacy for maintaining sinus rhythm in patients with AF over prolonged periods of time

A compound with such a range of properties remains to be developed, but lessons learned from experiences with the conventionally available agents and those under development might provide further directions in the search for the ideal agents. However, from the standpoint of effectiveness for maintaining stability of sinus rhythm, the critical features are (1) the prolongation of the excitation wavelength and the APD and ERP and (2) the favorable modulation of the rate-dependent effect on excitation wavelength and APD or refractoriness.

IV. HEART RATE DEPENDENCY OF ANTIARRHYTHMIC ACTIONS

The nature of the rate-dependent effect of the compounds on the atrial APD and ERP appears to be of much significance (7). The patterns of the rate-related effects of various antiarrhythmic agents are shown in Figure 6, and the relationship between rate-related properties relative to other significant electrophysiological parameters are shown in Table 1. The effects of various antiarrhythmic drugs in maintaining sinus rhythm in AF relative to the specific ion channels they block as well as their impact on mortality and their propensity to induce torsades de pointes are shown in Table 2.

There are several distinct consequences in the case of the agents (e.g., dofetilide, quinidine, DL-sotalol, and ibutilide) in which the prolongation of the APD occurs predominantly by blocking the I_{Kr} current; at rapid heart rates, the class III action is attenuated and may variably minimize the effectiveness of antiarrhythmic agents. At less rapid heart rates, these agents are effective in controlling AF. On the other hand, the APD in the ventricular cells increases markedly as the heart is slowed to the extent that there is a tendency for the development of early afterdepolarizations, especially in the

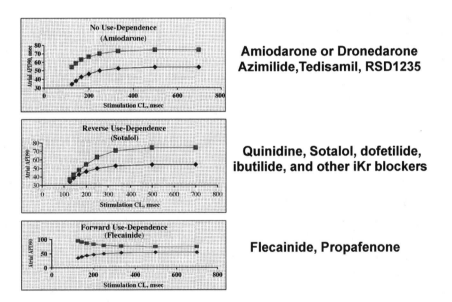

Figure 6 Influence of the changes in stimulation frequency in time course of atrial myocardial repolarization induced by various antiarrhythmic drugs. Three patterns are illustrated: no rate dependence, as in the case of amiodarone (prototype) and azimilide; classical reverse rate and use dependence in which the effect on the APD and ERP shortens as the cardiac frequency increases as typified by sotalol and other I_{Kr} blockers; forward use dependence, as has been demonstrated in the case of flecainide in the atria. These differences may be of much clinical significance as well as important for the development of atrial specific antifibrillatory agents. See text for details. (From Ref. 40.)

Table 1 Potential Mechanisms of Drug Action in Atrial Fibrillation[a]

Antiarrhythmic Drug (class)	Quinidine (Ia)	Flec/Propf (Ic)	Pure Class III (dofetilide)	Sotalol (class III)	Amiodarone Chronic (complex)
β blockade/anti-adrenergic	−	.−	−	+++	++
Conduction velocity	↓↓	↓↓	±	±	↓
Refractoriness	↑↑	↑↑	↑↑	↑↑	↑↑↑
Rate dependence of ERP	Classical reverse	↑ ERP with rate	Classical reverse	Classical reverse	↑ ERP at all frequencies
Wavelength (size)	↑↑→	↑→	↑↑	↑↑	↑↑↑

Key: ↓, reduction; ↑, increase; −, no significant effect; +, magnitude of effect; ERP, effective refractory period; Flec, flecainide; Propf, propafenone.
[a] The magnitude of the drug effects on the parameters indicated is a semiquantitative estimate of the effects gauged from numerous studies. It is cited here merely to provide an estimate of the potential range of differences between various agents.

Purkinje fibers and the M cells of the ventricular myocardium (35–37). Such an effect is now considered to be the basis for the development of proarrhythmic reactions such as torsades de pointes. As emphasized, most such compounds are powerful I_{Kr} blockers, and they are likely to be more effective in terminating atrial flutter than AF when administered acutely. However, there are exceptions. For example, ibutilide is an I_{Kr} blocker, but it also acts by increasing the I_{NAS}; the same may hold for trecetilide, its oral congener. Ersentilide is another I_{Kr} blocker that has class III effects, but it also blocks beta$_1$ receptors in the myocardium. In contrast, azimilide may inhibit I_{Kr} less than it blocks the slow component of the delayed rectifier current (I_{Ks}), while having variable effects on I_{CaL}, and I_{Na}, with a weak depressant action on beta-adrenergic and M2 receptors. It appears to have a different pattern of action on rate dependency (38). It induces a parallel increase in the APD and ERP, as has been demonstrated for amiodarone and dronedarone. Whether this is clinically significant may require a direct comparison of the properties of these compounds with those of other "pure" class III compounds, such as dofetilide. The effectiveness of azimilide in maintaining sinus rhythm is under intense study, as is the drug's proclivity to induce torsades de pointes relative to its QT-prolonging action.

The rate-related effects of amiodarone and dronedarone (Fig. 6) are of clinical importance, being associated with ERP increases in a parallel fashion over a wide range of frequencies (39,40). Of particular theoretical and practical interest are the electropharmacological properties of flecainide and propafenone relative to their rate-related effects on the ERP and APD

Table 2 Effects of I_{Kr} Inhibition on Effectiveness in Sinus Rhythm in AF Patients Relative to the Development of Torsades de Pointes and Total Mortality With and Without Blocking of Other Ionic Currents

Antiarrhythmic Agent	Ionic Currents or Receptors Blocked in Atria	Effectiveness in AF (1 year)	Torsades de pointes	Mortality (Ref. 34)
Amiodarone	I_{Kr}, I_{Ks}, I_{to}, I_{Na}, I_{Ca}, NS anti-adrenergic	60–70%	<0.5%	Neutral or lower
DL-sotalol	I_{Kr}, beta receptor	50%	>2–3%	Neutral
Dofetilide	I_{Kr}	50–60%	>2–3%	Neutral
Azimilide	I_{Kr}, I_{Ks}, I_{Ca}, I_{Na}	50%	?1%	Neutral
Flecainide	I_{to}, I_{Kur}, I_{Kr}, I_{Na}	?50%	—	CAST post-MI mortality increase
Propafenone	I_{to}, I_{Kur}, I_{Kr}, I_{Na}	?50%	—	Increased mortality in cardiac arrest patients
Quinidine	I_{Kr}, I_{K1}, I_{Kur}, I_{to}, I_{Na}	50%	3–5%	1–3% Increased mortality
Dronedarone	I_{Kr}, I_{Kss}, I_{to}, I_{Na}, I_{Ca}, NS anti-adrenergic	?50%	?	Under study
Tedisamil	I_{to}, I_{Kur}, I_{Kr}, I_{Na}, I_{KATP}	IV conversion of AF	?	Not known in a relevant population
RSD1235	I_{to}, I_{Kur}, I_{Na}	IV conversion of AF	?	Not known

in atrial tissue. They are strikingly different from those of most or all other known antiarrhythmic compounds. They prolong the APD and the ERP as a function of rate in so far as greater effects are seen as the stimulation rates are increased—a unique example of class III action selective to the atria in the case of compounds conventionally acting as class I agents in the ventricles. Such a class III action in the atria developing only during fast heart rates (41) is of great value when this action is needed most, as for the control of AF with rapid ventricular response. Such an electrophysiological action can be utilized not only for the maintenance of sinus rhythm but also for the acute conversion of AF and atrial flutter to sinus rhythm. Such electrophysiological properties present in the atria provide a compelling rationale for the development of atrial-specific antifibrillatory compounds that may also be used with impunity in patients with a wide spectrum of ventricular function.

V. EXPERIMENTAL AND CLINICAL CORRELATIONS

It is now established that the electrophysiological parameter that is critical for the pharmacological conversion and maintenance of sinus rhythm in a patient with AF is the acute and chronic lengthening of the atrial ERP (1,4,6,32,33). This is consistent with the notion that the prime determinant for the development of AF is shortening of the atrial APD and refractoriness. Shortening of the APD occurs with vagal stimulation, thyrotoxicosis, and possibly atrial distention from valvular disease or ventricular distention induced by chronic pressure or volume overload.

Many classical class I antiarrhythmic drugs—such as lidocaine, mexiletine, tocainide, and diphenylhydantoin—as well as cardiac glycosides also shorten atrial APD and refractoriness; they appear to have no significant antifibrillatory effects on AF or atrial flutter (42). They may sometimes aggravate AF. Not all class I compounds fall into this category. Dugs such as quinidine, disopyramide, and procainamide not only block I_{Na} but also inhibit I_{Kr} among other ion channels. Thus, their dual electrophysiological properties undoubtedly account for their net actions in the atria (where they prolong repolarization and are antifibrillatory for AF); but their propensity to block I_{Kr} in ventricular cells, especially those in Purkinje fibers and the M cells, accounts for their variable tendency to induce torsades de pointes. It is therefore unlikely that these time-honored compounds will be of much utility in the control of AF unless they are combined with other compounds that tend to offset the latter proclivity.

The quest for antiarrhythmic drugs that combine efficacy with safety has resulted in the synthesis and development of the "pure" class III compounds, including ibutilide, dofetilide, and azimilide, among others. Their ion channel–blocking profiles are shown in Table 3, in which this property is compared to those of the somewhat more complex or multifaceted compounds, such as sotalol and amiodarone, as well as its derivative dronedarone. Included in Table 3 are also two other significant and newer but electrophysiologically discrete compounds, tedisamil and RSD1235.

Dofetilide is an example of the simplest antiarrhythmic drug. It is a highly selective class III antiarrhythmic agent that delays repolarization in the atria, ventricles, and Purkinje fibers by I_{Kr} blockade (43,44). This inhibition of I_{Kr} is the sole identifiable action of the drug in cardiac muscle, in both the atria and ventricles (Table 2). Thus, it confirms the idea that isolated I_{Kr} blockade constitutes an antifibrillatory action in the atria. In controlled clinical trials, this was found to successfully convert 30% of patients, compared with 1.2% on placebo ($p < 0.001$), and it maintained sinus rhythm for 1 year in 62% of patients receiving oral drug. Azimilide also produces a dose-dependent prolongation of the APD via the blockade not only of the I_{Kr} channel but also of the I_{Ks} channel. It is a class III antiarrhythmic agent currently under investigation (45,46).

Table 3 New Antiarrhythmic Drugs for Sinus Rhythm in Atrial Fibrillation[a]

Class III antiarrhythmic drugs without reverse use dependence
  I_{Kr} + I_{Kur} blockers
  I_{Kr} + I_{Na} or I_{CaL} blockers
  I_{Kr} block + I_{Ks} or $I_{K(ATP)}$ activation
Novel mechanisms
  Atrioselective antiarrhythmic drugs
  • I_{Kur} and I_{Ach} blockers
  • Atrioselective Na+ channel blockers
  • Muscarinic M_2-receptor antagonists
  • 5-HT$_4$-receptor antagonists: piboserod RS-1000302
  T-type Ca^{2+} calcium-channel blockers: efonidipine, mibefradil
  Stretch-activated channel blockers: GsMtx-4
  NCX inhibitors: KB-R7943
  K^+-channel agonists
  Modulation of ion-channel expression
    Translational and posttranslational processing of ion-channel subunits
    Overexpression/supression of K^+ channels [HERG, I_{to}, I_{Ks}] and connexins

Key: I_{Na}, inward Na^+ current; I_{CaL}, L-type Ca^{2+} current; I_{KAch}, acetylcholine-activated K^+ current; $I_{K(ATP)}$, ATP-sensitive current; I_{Kr} and I_{Kur}, rapid and slow components of the delayed rectifier K^+ current; I_{to}, transient outward K^+ current; NCX = Na^+/Ca^{2+} exchanger.
[a] *Source*: Modified from Ref. 52.

Of particular interest is the compound RSD1235 [R,2R-hydroxypyr-rolidinyl-1-(3,4dimethylphenethoxy) cyclohexane monohydrochloride] the recent introduction of which marks a new departure in the pharmacological control of atrial fibrillation. Its properties exhibit electrophysiological specificity for atrial tissue (Hesketh and Fedida, unpublished) in therapeutically relevant doses. It acts by blocking repolarizing ion channels (I_{to}, I_{Kur}) and frequency-dependent cardiac I_{Na} channels at high concentrations and is associated with increases in the APD and ERP in atrial myocardium, seemingly independent of cardiac frequency. The drug does not block I_{Kr} in the ventricular tissue; hence there is no increase in the QT interval. It is clearly a prototype of an atrial-specific compound.

In contrast, tedisamil was synthesized as an antianginal agent, but it is a multifaceted compound that exerts potent antifibrillatory effects in converting AF and atrial flutter. This compound is under investigation for its properties for the acute termination of AF and atrial flutter following intravenous injection (47). Of particular interest is the drug's anti-ischemic properties and its bradycardic actions, the nature of which is not understood. Tedisamil inhibits a complex aggregate of repolarizing ion channels with a partial selectivity for the atrial tissue compared to the ventricular myocardial cells, producing modest prolongation of the APD in the ventricle at low drug concentrations while shortening it at high concentrations.

Sotalol and amiodarone (48–51) have recently emerged as atrial antiarrhythmic and antifibrillatory compounds of great therapeutic interest because of the multiplicity of actions that contribute to their efficacy as well as to their side-effect profiles. These two agents have a high degree of effectiveness in maintaining sinus rhythm in patients with persistent AF after the restoration of sinus rhythm. Both drugs prolong repolarization and refractoriness while also having antiadrenergic actions either by competitive receptor blockade (sotalol) or nonspecifically (amiodarone). In the event of relapses to AF during the course of therapy, the ventricular response may remain reasonably well controlled.

Electrophysiologically, there are similarities and differences between the two compounds. Sotalol is a potent nonselective beta-adrenoceptor blocking drug that is also a potent blocker of I_{Kr} (class II and III antiarrhythmic actions) without inhibiting other ion channels in the atria or ventricles. However, the I_{Kr} blockage that the drug produces in the Purkinje fibers or in the M cells of the ventricle may predispose it to inducing early aftedepolarizations, which may lead to the development of torsades de pointes. In contrast, electropharmacologically, amiodarone is an exceedingly complex compound with a multiplicity of actions on cardiac ion channels (Table 2) and autonomic nervous system interactions as well as interactions with organs such as the thyroid gland. The drug blocks sympathetic excitation nonspecifically and selectively, but not by receptor mechanisms; it antagonizes thyroid hormone action in cardiac muscle, with the result that the heart rate is reduced markedly during chronic administration (49,50). Of much interest is the observation that the effect of the drug on I_{Kr} is weak; its inhibitory effect on I_{Ks} and other ion channels is striking (see Table 2). In contrast to sotalol and most other class III compounds, amiodarone tends to shorten the APD in the Purkinje fibers and M cells of the ventricular muscle (37). This is consistent with the findings in large, long-term clinical trials, in which torsades de pointes has not been reported during therapy with amiodarone.

There is now a significant amount of data indicating the superiority of amiodarone over other antiarrhythmic drugs, including sotalol, in the maintenance of sinus rhythm in patients with atrial fibrillation converted to sinus rhythm. However, in a recent placebo-controlled double-blind study, sotalol was as effective as amiodarone in maintaining stability of sinus rhythm in patients having ischemic heart disease with persistent AF converted to normal rhythm (51). In this trial, sotalol and amiodarone were also equipotent in effecting conversions of persistent atrial fibrillation to sinus rhythm. In contrast, amiodarone was four- to six-fold more effective in maintaining sinus rhythm. These observed similarities and differences between sotalol and amiodarone are clearly of great fundamental importance. It appears that the presence of beta-receptor blockade in the context of controlling AF may be of critical importance. Furthermore, the data suggest that the beneficial effects of antifibrillatory drugs may not be predictable solely on the basis of the pattern of ion channels blocked in atrial tissue by an individual pharmacological agent. These considerations may be relevant in the development of newer agents for the conversion and maintenance of sinus rhythm by antifibrillatory compounds.

VI. DEVELOPMENT OF NEWER ANTIARRHYTHMIC COMPOUNDS

As indicated above, the search for the ideal antiarrhythmic drug for the restoration and maintenance of sinus rhythm in patients with AF remains an active investigative scene. It bears emphasis that the focus is still on agents prolonging the APD and the ERP in atrial tissue (39,52). The effects are obtained by blocking I_{Kr} (the rapid component of the delayed rectifier current), I_{Ks} (the slow component of the delayed rectifier current), or I_{to} (the transient outward current). Alternatively, repolarization may be prolonged by slowing the activation of I_{Nas} (the late inward sodium current) or by activating I_{CaL} (the long-lasting L-type calcium current).

Other ionic currents that may affect the APD and ERP in the atria are I_{Kur} and I_{KAch}. The major challenge here has been to develop agents that are antifibrillatory in AF and atrial flutter with lesser effects in ventricular muscle, thus obviating the possibility of a ventricular proarrhythmic reactions. The alternative approach has been the synthesis of the congeners of the most effective agents currently available. This has been particularly applicable to amiodarone, which has now been found to have the most potent antifibrillatory action for maintaining sinus rhythm in patients with AF converted to sinus rhythm (51). Although the unique effectiveness of amiodarone in maintaining sinus rhythm in patients with AF is not known, it has been tested in recent experimental studies. Unlike other antiarrhythmic drugs, amiodarone prevented the electrophysiological and biochemical consequences of adverse remodeling of the atria that may occur with sustained fast heart rates in AF or other supraventricular tachyarrhythmias (53). For this reason, the development of newer derivatives of amiodarone may be of interest. The first of such derivatives has been the compound dronedarone.

Dronedarone is the noniodinated derivative of amiodarone, a compound that was created to reduce the side effect profile of amiodarone without incurring the loss of its complex electrophysiological and pharmacological profile (39,54). The result has been shortening of the elimination half-life to 20 to 30 hr with no effect on thyroid hormone metabolism, but there is a propensity to block M_2 receptors. Thus, despite the significant noncompetitive antiadrenergic actions of dronedarone, the compound has a somewhat lower heart rate–reducing effect than amiodarone.

In other respects, experimental and preliminary clinical studies have shown that the electropharmacological effects of dronedarone and amiodarone are similar (39). In the case of amiodarone and other class III compounds, two properties of dronedarone—QT/QTc interval prolongation and heart rate slowing—are of much importance in the role of the drug as an antifibrillatory agent for the treatment of AF and flutter on the one hand and the ventricular tachycardia and fibrillation on the other. Early clinical trials have suggested a measure of selectivity for the action of dronedarone in atrial vs. ventricular tissue.

VII. THE FUTURE

It is noteworthy that many of the antiarrhythmic drugs in current use for maintaining sinus rhythm in patients with atrial fibrillation were synthesized and developed for the treatment of angina pectoris (amiodarone, sotalol, propranolol and other beta blockers, verapamil) or for the suppression of ventricular tachyarrhythmias (disopyramide, procainamide, flecainide, and propafenone, among others). The effects of many of these compounds—especially those of sotalol, amiodarone, verapamil, and propranolol—were studied in atrial and ventricular tissues relative to changes in APD and ERP many decades ago (55–57). However, recognition of the clinical significance of atrioselectivity in their actions has been relatively recent and has become more marked with continuing increases in the incidence of AF, especially in the elderly. These developments are now reflected in focused strategies for the synthesis and characterization of compounds on the basis of their ability to block certain ion channels relative to rate dependence and atrial selectivity of action, with a minimal proclivity for ventricular proarrhythmia. The potentially important strategies are summarized in Table 3. A detailed discussion of the issues indicated in Table 3 is beyond the scope of this chapter but is available elsewhere (e.g., Ref. 52). A few comments, however, are germane.

Atrial selectivity of action is exemplified by the compound RSD1235, mentioned above. Its major action is on the ultrarapid delayed rectifier potassium current (I_{Kur}), which is expressed in the human atria but not in the ventricle (58). There are data indicating that I_{Kur} blockers may prolong atrial ERP in the remodeled atria and thus prevent recurrences of AF with little or no increases in the QT prolongation in ventricular tissue, carrying low risk of proarrhythmia (59). However, these preliminary findings remain to be confirmed in the larger clinical context.

Of much interest are the effects of flecainide and propafenone, class IC agents that are frequently used in patients with atrial fibrillation and flutter in the setting normal or near-normal ventricular function. They do not increase ventricular repolarization but they do increase the I_{Kur} atrial ERP and reduce atrial ERP dispersion as the rate increases (60). As pointed out above, this unique electrophysiological property is of much clinical importance. This class III effect is manifest only at high heart rates and appears to be due to the delay in Na^+ sodium-channel reactivation and the blockade of a number of K^+ channel such as I_{Kur}, I_{Kr}, I_{Ks}, and I_{KATP}. This may be the basis for the effectiveness of flecainide and propafenone for the acute conversion and long-term maintenance of sinus rhythm in patients with AF.

Clearly a number of practical consequences stem from these observations. First, they raise the possibility of augmenting efficacy for the maintenance of sinus rhythm by combination therapy involving flecainide or propafenone with other antiarrhythmic agents. The net effect might be an additive or a synergistic one. Moreover, the observations raise the possibility of synthesis and development of atrioselective class I antiarrhythmic compounds, as suggested by Tamargo et al. (52).

It is now well documented that the onset and persistence of AF leads to a complex electrophysiological remodeling in atrial tissue that induces a significant decrease in a number of ionic currents such as I_{to}, I_{CaL}, and I_{Kur} (7,61), a finding that raises a number of possibilities, such as the development of K^+ agonists. There is increasing evidence that the arrhythmogenic substrate for AF may be favorably modulated by inhibition of the renin-angiotensin-aldosterone system, certain beta antagonists, tendency for atrial Ca^{2+} overload of whatever origin, oxidative injury, Na^+/H^+ exchange, and selective 5-HT4 blockade (52).

The experimental and clinical data accrued since the concept was first formulated (55–57) support the notion that prolongation of the atrial APD and refractoriness is the mode of action of most or all antiarrhythmic drugs developed to date that have the potential to maintain sinus rhythm in patients in AF; the effect on conduction appears subsidiary but may be desirable. Studies of a range of compounds from the simplest (pure class III, such as dofetilide and azimilide) to the most complex (amiodarone and dronedarone) drugs and those with intermediate complexity (such as dl-sotalol and tedisamil) have provided initial insights into the actions of antiarrhythmic drugs in AF. The properties of flecainide and propafenone have drawn attention to atrial specificity of electrophysiological actions, properties that hold promise for the future. The effects appear to be mediated by the blocking action on one or more of the ionic currents (e.g., I_{Kr}, I_{Ks}, I_{to}, I_{Kur}) or possibly other effects, such as the activation of I_{Nas} or the L-type calcium channel in the atria. Clearly, to further augment the effectiveness of anti-fibrillatory drugs in maintaining sinus rhythm, efforts should also be made to modify the arrhythmogenic substrate, with the goal of a broader strategy for the restoration and long-term maintenance of sinus rhythm in patients with AF.

REFERENCES

1. Nattel S. New ideas about atrial fibrillation 50 years and on. Nature 2002; 415: 219–226.
2. Tsang TS, Gersh BJ. Atrial fibrillation: an old disease, a new epidemic. Am J Med 2002; 113:432–435.
3. Prystowsky EN, Benson DW Jr, Woodrow M, Fuster V, Hart RG, Kay G, Neal MD, Myerburg RJ, Naccarelli GV, Wyse G. Management of patients with atrial fibrillation: a statement for healthcare professionals from the Subcommittee on Electrocardiography and Electrophysiology. American Heart Association. Circulation 1996; 93(6):1262–1286.
4. Singh BN, Mody FV, Lopez B, Sarma JSM. Antiarrhythmic agents for atrial fibrillation: focus on prolonging atrial repolarization. Am J Cardiol 1999; 84: 161–173.
5. Feinberg WM, Blackshear JL, Laupacis A, Kronmal R, Hart RG. Prevalence, age distribution, and gender of patients with atrial fibrillation. Arch Intern Med 1995; 155:469–473.

6. Nattel S, Li D, Yue L. Basic mechanisms of atrial fibrillation. Very new insights into very old ideas. Annu Rev Physiol 2000; 62:51–77.

7. Nattel S, Singh BN. Evolution, Mechanisms, and classification of antiarrhythmic drugs: focus on class III actions. Am J Cardiol 1999; 84(9A):11–19.

8. Nattel S. Atrial electrophysiology and mechanisms of atrial fibrillation. J Cardiovasc Pharmacol Ther 2003; 8(suppl 1):S5–S11.

9. Varro A, Biliczki P, Iost N, Virag L, Hala O, Papp JG. Pharmacology of potassium channel blockers. In: Papp JG, Straub M, Ziegler D, eds. Atrial Fibrillation: New Therapeutic Concepts. Ohmsa, Amsterdam: IOS Press, 2003:27–39.

10. Bosch RF, Zeng JB, Grammer, et al. Ionic mechanisms of electrical modeling in human atrial fibrillation. Cardiovasc Res 1999; 44:121–131.

11. Dovrev, Wettwer, Kortner A, et al. Human inward rectifier potassium channels in chronic and postoperative atrial fibrillation. Cardiovasc Res 2002; 54:397–404.

12. Nattel S, Li D. Ionic remodeling in the heart. Pathophysiological significance and new therapeutic opportunities for atrial fibrillation. Circ Res 2000; 87:440–447.

13. Le Heuzy J-Y, Boutjdir M, Gagey S, Lavergne T, Guize L. Cellular aspects of atrial vulnerability. In: Attuel P, Coumel P, Janse MJ, eds. The Atrium in Health and Disease. Mt Kisco, NY: Futura, 1989:81–94.

14. Lakatta EG. Cardiovascular aging without clinical diagnosis. Dialog Cardiovasc Med 2001; 6:67–80.

15. Davies MJ, Pomerance A. The pathology of atrial fibrillation in man. Br Heart J 1972; 34:520–525.

16. Bharati S, Lev M. Histology of the normal and diseased atrium. In: Falk RH, Podrid PJ, eds. Atrial Fibrillation: Mechanisms and Management. New York: Raven Press, 1992.

17. Li D, Fareh S, Leung TK, Nattel S. Promotion of atrial fibrillation by heart failure in dogs—atrial remodelling of a different kind. Circulation 1999; 100:87–95.

18. Li D, Menyk P, Feng J, et al. Effects of experimental heart failure on atrial cellular and ionic electrophysiogy. Circulation 1999; 101:2631–2638.

19. Moe GK. On the multiple wavelet hypothesis of atrial fibrillation. Arch Int Pharmacodyn Ther 1962; 140:183–188.

20. Schram G, Pourier M, Melnyk P, Nattel S. Differential distribution of cardiac ion-channel expression as a basis for regional specialization in electrical function. Circ Res 2002; 90:939–950.

21. Schuessler RB, Grayson TM, Bromberg BI, Cox JL, Boineau JP. Cholinergically mediated tachyarrhythmias induced by a single extrastimulus in the isolated canine right atrium. Circ Res 1992; 71:1254–1267.

22. Mandapati R, Skanes A, Chen J, Berenfeld O, Jalife J. Stable microreentrant sources as a mechanism of atrial fibrillation in the isolated sheep heart. Circulation 2000; 90:194–1999.

23. Katrisis D, Iliodromitis E, Fragakis N, Adamopoulos S, Kremastinos D.

Ablation therapy of type I atrial flutter may eradicate paroxysmal atrial fibrillation. Am J Cardiol 1996; 78:345–347.

24. Liu TY, Tai CT, Chen SA. Treatment of atrial fibrillation by catheter ablation of conduction gaps in the crista terminalis and cavotricuspid isthmus of the right atrium. J Cardiovasc Electrophysiol 2002; 13:1044–1046.

25. Haissaguerre M, Jais P, Shah DC, Takahashi A, Hocini M, Quiniou G, Garrigue S, Mouroux AL, Metayer PL, Clementy J. Spontaneous initiation of atrial fibrillation by ectopic beats originating in the pulmonary veins. N Engl J Med 1998; 339:659–666.

26. Berenfeld O, Zaitsev AV, Mironov SF, Pertsov AM, Jalife J. Frequency-dependent breakdown of wave propagation into fibrillatory conduction across the pectinate muscle network in the isolated sheep right atrium. Circ Res 2002; 90:1173–1180.

27. Atrial Fibrillation Follow-up Investigation of Rhythm Management (AFFIRM) Investigators. A comparison of rate control and rhythm control in patients with atrial fibrillation. N Engl J Med 2002; 34:1825–1833.

28. Van Gelder IC, Hagens VE, Bosker HA, Kingma JH, et al. for The Rate Control versus Electrical Conversion for Persistent Atrial Fibrillation Study Group. A comparison of rate control and rhythm control in patients with recurrent persistent atrial fibrillation. N Engl J Med 2002; 347:1834–1840.

29. Hohnloser SH, Kuck KH, Lilienthal J, for the PIAF Investigators. Rhythm versus rate control in atrial fibrillation—pharmacological intervention in atrial fibrillation (PIAF): a randomized trial. Lancet 2000; 356:1789–1794.

30. Manning W, Leeman DE, Gotch PJ, Come PC. Pulsed Doppler evaluation of atrial mechanical function after electrical cardioversion of atrial fibrillation. J Am Coll Cardiol 1989; 13:617–623.

31. Van Gelder IC, Crijns HJGM, Blanksma PK, et al. Time course of hemodynamic changes and improvement of exercise tolerance after cardioversion of chronic atrial fibrillation unassociated with cardiac valve disease. Am J Cardiol 1993; 72:560–566.

32. Singh BN. Current antiarrhythmic drugs: An overview of mechanisms of action and potential clinical utility. J Cardiovasc Electrophysiol 1999; 10:283–301.

33. Singh BN. Atrial fibrillation: epidemiologic considerations and rationale for Conversion and maintenance of sinus rhythm. J Cardiovasc Pharmacol Ther 2003; 8(suppl 1):S11–S26.

34. Singh BN, Sarma JSM. Mechanisms of antiarrhythmic actions in the maintenance of sinus rhythm in patients with atrial fibrillation: clinical and experimental correlations. In: Papp JG, Straub M, Ziegler D, eds. Atrial Fibrillation: New Therapeutic Concepts. Ohmsa, Amsterdam: IOS Press, 2003: 41–55.

35. Antzelevitch C, Sicouri S. Clinical relevance of cardiac arrhythmias generated by afterdepolarizations. Role of M cells in the generation of U waves, triggered activity and torsades de pointes. J Am Coll Cardiol 1994; 23:259–277.

36. Papp J, Gy, Nemeth M, Krassoi I, Mester L, Hala O, Varro A. Differential electrophysiologic effects of chronically administered amiodarone on canine Pur-

kinje fibers versus ventricular muscle. J Cardiovasc Pharmacol Ther 1996; 1(4): 187–196.

37. Sicouri S, Moro S, Litovsky S, Elizari M, Antzelevitch C. Chronic amiodarone reduces transmural dispersion of repolarization in the canine heart. J Cardiovasc Electrophysiol 1997; 8:1269–1279.
38. Salata JJ, Brooks RR. Pharmacology of azimilide dihydrochloride (NE-10064), a class III antiarrhythmic agent. Cardiovasc Drug Rev 1997; 15:137–156.
39. Sun W, Sarma JSM, Singh BN. Chronic and acute effects of dronedarone on the action potential of rabbit atrial muscle preparations: comparison with amiodarone. J Cardiovasc Pharmacol 2002; 39:677–684.
40. Singh BN, Wadhani N, Sarma JSM. Rate dependence of antiarrhythmic action. J Cardiovasc Pharmacol Ther 2002; 7:203–206.
41. Wang Z, Pelletier LC, Talajic M, Nattel S. Effects of flecainide and quinidine on human atrial potentials: role of rate dependence and comparison with guinea pig, rabbit and dog tissues. Circulation 1990; 82:274–283.
42. Singh BN. Antiarrhythmic drugs: a re-orientation in light of recent developments in the control of disorders of rhythm. Am J Cardiol 1998; 81(6A):3D–13D.
43. Torp-Pedersen C, Moller C, Bloch Thomsen PE, Kober L, Sandoe E, Egstrup K, et al. Dofetilide in patients in congestive heart failure and left ventricular dysfunction. Danish Investigators of Arrhythmia and Mortality on Dofetilide Study Group. N Engl J Med 1999; 341:857–865.
44. Singh SN, Berk M, Yellen L, Zoble R, Haley JA, Abrahamson D, et al. Efficacy and safety of oral dofetilide in maintaining sinus rhythm: 12 months follow-up results of the SAFFIRE-D. Circulation 1999; 100:1–501.
45. Camm AJ, Karam R, Pratt CM. The azimilide post-infarct survival evaluation (ALIVE) trial. Am J Cardiol 1998; 81:35D–39D.
46. Pritchett E, Page R, Connolly S, Marcello S. Azimilide treatment of atrial fibrillation. Circulation 1998; 98(17):1:633.
47. Wallace AA, Stupienski RF, Baskin EP, et al. Cardiac electrophysiology and antiarrhythmic actions of tedisamil. J Phamacol Exp Therapeut 1995; 273:168–175.
48. Singh BN. Sotalol: Current status and expanding indications. J Cardiovasc Pharmacol Therapeut 1999; 4(1):49–65.
49. Singh BN. Antiarrhythmic actions of amiodarone: A profile of a paradoxical agent. Am J Cardiol 1996; 78:41–53.
50. Singh BN. Antiarrhythmic drugs: A re-orientation in light of recent developments in the control of disorders of rhythm. Am J Cardiol 1998; 81(6A):3D–13D.
51. Singh BN, Singh SN, Reda DJ, Tang XC, Lopez B, Harris CL, Fletcher RD, Sharma SC, Atwood JE, Jacobson AK, Lewis HD Jr., Ezekowitz MD, and SAFE-Investigators. Antiarrhythmic Therapy in Maintaining Stability of Sinus Rhythm in Atrial Fibrillation—Sotalol Amiodarone Atrial Fibrillation Efficacy Trial (SAFE-T). A Veterans Affairs Cooperative Study 2004. Submitted.
52. Tamargo J, Caballero R, Delpon E. New mechanistic targets for the treatment

of atrial fibrillation. In: Papp JG, Straub M, Ziegler D, eds. Atrial Fibrillation: New Therapeutic Concepts. Ohmsa, Amsterdam: IOS Press, 2003:133–155.

53. Shinagawa K, Shiroishita A, Schram G, Nattel S. Effects of antiarrhythmic drugs on fibrillation in the remodeled atrium. Insights into the mechanism of the superior efficacy of amiodarone. Circulation 2003; 107:1440–1446.

54. Guillemare E, Martion A, Nisato D, et al. Acute effects of dronedarone and amiodarone on I_{K1}, I_{Kr}, and I_{Ks} in guinea pig ventricular myocytes. Fund Clin Pharmacol 1999; 13:389–395.

55. Singh BN, Vaughan Williams EM. A third class of antiarrhythmic action. Effects on atrial and ventricular intracellular potentials, and other pharmacological actions on cardiac muscle, of MJ 1999 and AH 3474. Br J Pharmacol 1970; 39:675–687.

56. Singh BN, Vaughan Williams EM. The effect of amiodarone, a new antianginal drug, on cardiac muscle. Br J Pharmacol 1970; 39:657–667.

57. Hauswirth O, Singh BN. Ionic mechanisms in heart muscle in relation to the genesis and the pharmacological control of cardiac arrhythmias. Pharmacol Rev 1979; 30:5–63.

58. Yue L, Feng J, Li GR, et al. Characterization of an ultrarapid delayed rectifier potassium channel involved in canine atrial repolarization. J Physiol 1996; 496(pt 3):647–662.

59. Yamahshita T, Murakawa Y, Hayami N, et al. Short-term effects of rapid pacing on MRNA level of voltage K^+– dependent channels in rat atrium. Electrical remodeling in paroxysmal atrial tachycardia. Circ Res 2000; 101:2007-2014

60. Wang J, Bourne GW, Wang Z, et al. Comparative mechanisms of antiarrhythmic drug action in experimental atrial fibrillation: importance of use-dependent effects on refractoriness. Circulation 1993; 88:1030–1044.

61. van Wagoner DR, Nerbonne JM. Molecular basis of electrical remodeling in atrial fibrillation. J Mol Cell Cardiol 2000; 32:1101–1117.

4

Preclinical Models: What Clinical Lessons Have We Learned?

Yuri Blaauw, Ulrich Schotten, and Maurits A. Allessie
*Cardiovascular Research Institute Maastricht, Maastricht University,
Maastricht, The Netherlands*

I. INTRODUCTION

Atrial fibrillation (AF) is a common arrhythmia responsible for a substantial morbidity (1) and mortality (2) in the general population. It affects mainly the elderly, with a prevalence of 0.5% in patients aged 50 to 59 years, incrementing to almost 9% in men aged over 80 years (3). Atrial fibrillation sometimes occurs in individuals without cardiac abnormalities (lone atrial fibrillation) (4). More often it is associated with an underlying heart disease such as hypertension, valvular disorders, coronary artery disease, and/or congestive heart failure (3).

In the last century, several animal models of atrial fibrillation were developed. This has led to a considerable improvement in our understanding of the mechanisms of the arrhythmia. The aim of the current chapter is to review the various animal models of atrial fibrillation and assess what they have taught us about the treatment of AF.

II. AF IS DUE TO MULTIPLE MECHANISMS

Atrial fibrillation can easily be diagnosed on the basis of the characteristic features of the surface electrocardiogram. However, this does not provide much information on the many possible causes and mechanisms of the arrhythmia in individual patients. Experimental and clinical studies have revealed that AF has several different etiologies and that the mechanisms by which AF sustains itself are diverse. Atrial fibrillation can be perpetuated by either a single source or by multiple sources. In Figure 1, different mechanisms of AF are presented schematically. Some of them are still hypothetical; others have been demonstrated experimentally or clinically.

A. Single-Source AF

An important characteristic of AF "driven" by a single source is that the arrhythmia should terminate after elimination of the rapid source.

1. Automatic Focus

In this type of AF, an automatic focus is present, which fires so rapidly that the atria cannot follow 1:1 (fibrillatory conduction). Clinical studies have shown that the vast majority of these atrial ectopic foci are located in the myocardial "sleeves" of the pulmonary veins (5).

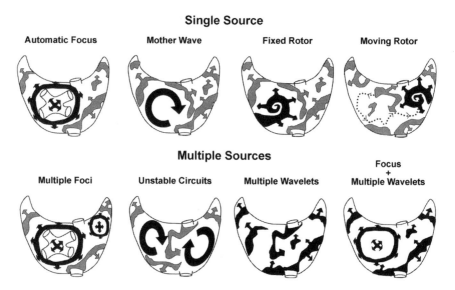

Figure 1 Schematic representation of the different mechanisms that can give rise to AF. See text for details.

2. Mother Wave

This is a single stable macro–reentrant circuit with a short cycle length and a fixed anatomically or functionally determined pathway. The high frequency of the reentrant circuit leads to fibrillatory conduction in the rest of the atria. Interruption of the circulating mother wave should terminate AF.

3. Fixed Rotor

AF can also be "driven" by a stable, fixed micro–reentrant circuit with a high frequency.

4. Moving Rotor

This is AF driven by a stable micro–reentrant circuit drifting through the atria. AF results because the rest of the atrium cannot follow the high frequency in a 1:1 fashion. Rotors may have preferential locations determined by anatomical and functional properties of the atria.

B. Multiple-Source AF

1. Multiple Foci

Foci due to enhanced automaticity can be present at multiple sites. In this case the successful elimination of one of these foci will not restore sinus rhythm.

2. Multiple Circuits

Multiple reentrant circuits may coexist in the atria. Their circular pathways can be anatomically or functionally determined. Because they are multiple, the circuits do not have to be stable in order to perpetuate AF.

3. Multiple Wavelets

The atria are activated with a high frequency by multiple wavelets wandering simultaneously through the atrial myocardium. The pathways of the wavelets are determined by the anatomical and functional properties of the atrial wall. While traveling through the atria, the wavelets often reenter the tail of refractoriness of other waves (random reentry). Incidentally, they can also reenter their own refractory tail. However, stable rotors are not observed during this type of AF. The stability of AF depends on the number of wavelets that "fit" on the atrial surface. The shorter the wavelength of the atrial impulse, the more wavelets will coexist and the less likely AF will terminate.

Prolongation of the wavelength by class III drugs reduces the number of wavelets and terminates AF.

4. Focus and Multiple Wavelets

It is not unlikely that different mechanisms of AF can be operative at the same time. If a rapid focus exists together with randomly reentering multiple wavelets, atrial fibrillation will be highly persistent or even permanent.

III. ACONITINE-INDUCED AF

Already in 1907, Winterberg (6) proposed that AF can originate from a single automatic focus. Experiments by Scherf et al. (7) confirmed this hypothesis. Local application of aconitine on canine atria induced a rapidly firing focus that, depending on the frequency, created either atrial flutter or fibrillation. When the focus was eliminated by clamping off the site of aconitine application, the arrhythmia stopped. This is illustrated in Figure 2a. In this experiment performed by Moe and Abildskov (8), AF was induced by injecting aconitine in the tip of the atrial appendage. To investigate whether the focal discharge was responsible for perpetuation of AF, the focus was isolated from the rest of the atrium by clamping the atrial appendage. Indeed, after electrical isolation of the appendage, the arrhythmia was promptly terminated.

In a recent clinical study, Haissaguerre and coworkers (5) demonstrated that in patients with paroxysmal AF, AF was initiated by a rapidly firing focus in the pulmonary veins. Selective ablation of these foci strongly reduced the number of AF episodes; in many patients, antiarrhythmic drugs could be discontinued. The ionic electrophysiological mechanism underlying the rapid focal activity is not clear. It is also not understood whether these foci act solely as the trigger to start AF or whether they also act as a "driver" that perpetuates the arrhythmia. So far, only anecdotal reports have shown that chronic AF can be terminated by focal ablation inside the pulmonary veins (9). Circumferential radiofrequency ablation of the pulmonary veins has been reported to cardiovert long-lasting chronic AF in some patients (10). However, it is important to note that this rather extensive ablation procedure will not only isolate the trigger within the pulmonary veins but also affect the substrate of AF by markedly reducing the atrial tissue mass of the diseased left atrium (debulking). Although the clinical outcome of pulmonary vein ablation is often beneficial, complete and permanent electrical isolation of the veins is seldom accomplished (11). This raises the question of whether alternative mechanisms like a reduction of atrial mass, autonomic denerva-

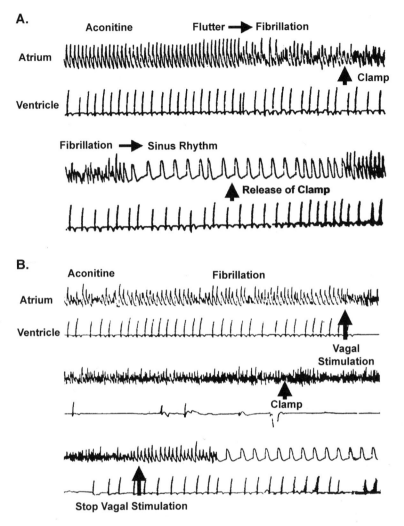

Figure 2 A. Demonstration of AF "driven" by a rapidly firing focus. Shown are electrograms recorded from the right atrium and ventricle. Injection of aconitine into the atrial myocardium resulted in the degeneration of atrial flutter into fibrillation. Isolation of the site of injection from the rest of the atrium by clamping the atrial appendage caused the arrhythmia to terminate. When the clamp was released, atrial fibrillation restarted. B. Illustration of the effect of vagal stimulation on the stability of AF. Shown are the same tracings as in 2A. Aconitine injection into the right atrial appendage resulted in AF. When the vagal nerve was stimulated, the rate of fibrillation accelerated. Isolation of the aconitine focus by clamping at this point did not terminate the arrhythmia. When vagal stimulation was stopped, atrial fibrillation slowed down and sinus rhythm resumed. (From Ref. 8.)

tion, or interruption of critical reentry crossroads may explain the clinical efficacy of pulmonary vein ablation.

IV. VAGAL AF

The autonomic nervous system, in particular the vagal nerves, has been recognized to play an important role in the initiation and perpetuation of atrial fibrillation. Already in 1897, Knoll (12) observed that AF often occurred during vagal stimulation in rabbits and dogs. In 1915, Rothberger and Winterberg (13) showed that AF could easily be induced during vagal stimulation in normal canine atria. Figure 2B demonstrates the importance of the vagal nerves for the stability of AF. When the driver of AF (aconitine) was eliminated by clamping the atrial appendage, AF persisted when the vagal nerves were stimulated. To demonstrate that vagal stimulation was responsible for the maintenance of AF, vagal stimulation was stopped (see arrow in Fig. 2B). This led to prompt termination of AF.

Induction of AF by vagal stimulation, either by direct stimulation of the vagal nerve or by intravenous infusion of cholinergic agents, is an established way to induce AF. The main underlying electrophysiological mechanism is a shortening of the atrial refractory period and possibly an increase in the spatial dispersion of refractoriness (14). When a premature impulse encounters an area of prolonged refractoriness, the wavefront will be blocked locally, while in other directions (with shorter refractory periods) it will be propagated. When the time required for the impulse to travel around the area of block exceeds the refractory period of the cells proximal to the area of block, these cells will be reexcited by the returning wavefront and a reentrant arrhythmia will be initiated. Not only the induction but also the persistence of fibrillation is facilitated by vagal stimulation. When the refractory period shortens, the length of the fibrillation waves will decrease and AF may become sustained, because more wavelets can now circulate simultaneously in the atria. The multiple-wavelet hypothesis of Moe (8) was experimentally confirmed by Allessie et al. (15) in isolated canine atria perfused with acetylcholine. Using a multichannel mapping system, they recorded the electrical activity from several hundred atrial sites. It was found that a critical number of four to six wavelets was required to sustain AF. The experiments by Wang et al. (16) are in line with this observation. In a canine model of vagal AF, they demonstrated that class IC drugs terminated AF by decreasing the number of wavelets. In 1992, Schuessler et al. (17) demonstrated that, at high dosages of acetylcholine, a single rotor with a very short cycle length of ~ 40 ms caused fibrillatory conduction in the rest of the atria. The small functionally determined reentry circuit was either stationary or drifted slowly through the atrial wall. In addition, these authors demonstrated that, in specific regions, activation of the epicardium was discordant from the endocardial surface (18). The role of anatomical heterogeneities for the pattern of atrial activation during AF was further supported by Wu et al. (19). In isolated canine atria, they found that pectinate muscles were involved in lines of conduction block, thus allowing stationary reentry. Also, in isolated perfused sheep heart, Skanes et al. (20) demonstrated that in the presence of acetyl-choline, single sources of microreentry of very rapid rates caused loss of 1:1 conduction in other parts of the atria. Mandapati et al. (21) demonstrated that these "rotors" were predominantly located in the posterior left atrium. However, evidence that such a mechanism is responsible for clinical AF is as yet lacking.

Although the above-mentioned experiments have contributed significantly to our understanding of the mechanism of AF, one must be cautious in extrapolating these observations to clinical arrhythmias. First of all, it is important to note that contrary to most clinical cases of AF, no structural abnormalities are present in the atria in most animal studies. It is also questionable whether the extreme shortening of atrial refractoriness by vagal stimulation is encountered in patients. After the first description of vagal AF by Coumel et al. (22), several studies addressed this issue. In most studies, the neurohumoral activity was evaluated by analysis of heart rate variability. No consistent picture regarding the onset of AF can be derived from these studies. While in some studies vagal tone was found to be increased (23,24), other studies demonstrated a predominance of sympathetic activity (25,26). Also, the circadian pattern of onset of paroxysmal AF does not support the concept of vagally induced AF. Since vagal tone is higher during the night, one would expect most episodes of AF to occur during the night. In contrast, Irwin et al. (27) and Kupari et al. (28) found that most paroxysms of AF actually occurred during the day.

V. AF-INDUCED ATRIAL REMODELING

Clinical studies have shown that atrial fibrillation is progressive in nature. In many patients with paroxysmal AF, the arrhythmia tends to become persistent with time (29). In 1995, two studies helped to explain these clinical observations (30,31). Morillo et al. (30) subjected dogs to 6 weeks of continuous rapid atrial pacing (400 bpm) and observed a shortening of the atrial refractory period by about 15%. In chronically instrumented goats, Wijffels et al. (31) maintained AF by a fibrillation pacemaker that automatically delivered bursts of stimuli (1 sec, 50 Hz) as soon as sinus rhythm was detected (Fig. 3). Using this method, AF could be maintained 24 hr a day, 7

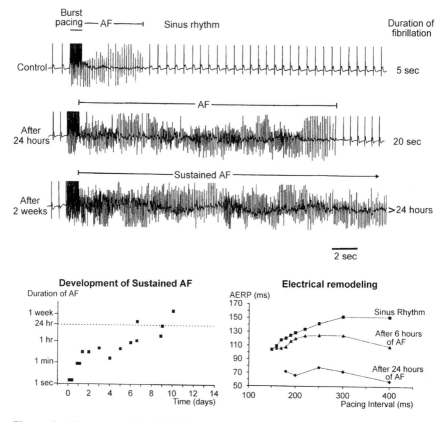

Figure 3 The goat model of AF. Upper panel: Induction of AF by burst pacing. An atrial bipolar electrogram was continuously analyzed by a custom-made fibrillation pacemaker. As soon as sinus rhythm occurred, a burst of stimuli was given to reinduce AF. In this way AF could be maintained 24 hr a day, 7 days a week. Left lower panel: Time course of the development of sustained AF. In the example shown, AF became persistent (>24 hr) after 7 to 10 days of artificially maintained AF. Lower right panel: AF-induced atrial electrical remodeling. After 6 to 24 hr of AF, the refractory period had shortened and the physiological rate adaptation was lost. (From Ref. 58.)

days a week. After 2 to 4 days of AF, the atrial refractory period had shortened from ∼ 150 to ∼ 80 ms (−45%). In addition, the normal physiological rate dependency of the refractory period was lost. Restoration of sinus rhythm completely restored the normal refractory period within 2 to 3 days (reverse electrical remodeling). In both studies, the rapid atrial rate led to a progressive increase in the duration of AF paroxysms. After 6 weeks of rapid atrial pacing in the dog, 82% of the paroxysms of AF lasted longer than 15 min. In the goat model, as a result of 2 to 3 weeks of repetitive induction of AF, 90% of the animals developed persistent AF (31). Both in the dog model of Morillo et al. (30) and the goat model of Wijffels et al. (31) it was hypothesized that the mechanism of increased susceptibility for AF was based on a shortening of atrial refractoriness and wavelength. Morillo et al. (30) observed a significantly shorter atrial fibrillation cycle length in the left atrium compared to the right. Cryoablation of the area with the highest dominant frequency terminated AF in 9 of 11 dogs.

The ionic mechanisms underlying AF-induced electrical remodeling have been extensively studied. (32) Yue et al. (33) were the first to demonstrate that the L-type Ca^{2+} current (I_{CaL}) was reduced in cardiomycytes of electrically remodeled atria (Fig. 4). Inhibition of I_{CaL} by nifedipine produced a shortening of the action potential, comparable to the changes caused by prolonged atrial tachycardia. On the other hand, an increase of the L-type Ca^{2+} current by BayK 8644 could partly reverse the shortening of the action potential by rapid atrial pacing. These data strongly suggest that a reduction of I_{CaL} underlies the tachycardia-induced shortening of the refractory period. In additional studies it was shown that AF also reduces the transient outward current (I_{to}) and the ultrarapid delayed rectifier current (I_{Kur}) (33,34). The

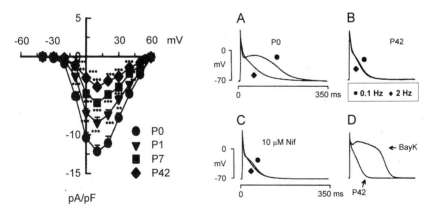

Figure 4 Left panel: Voltage current relationships of I_{CaL} during control (P0) and after 1, 7, and 42 days of rapid atrial pacing in the dog. The density of I_{CaL} was progressively reduced with the duration of rapid pacing. Right panel: Action potentials recorded at 0.1 (●) and 2 Hz (♦) in control atrial cells (P0) and after 42 days of rapid atrial pacing (P42). Addition of nifedipine (C) mimicked the effects of electrical remodeling, whereas the Ca agonist BayK 8644 restored the plateau phase of the action potential (D). (From Ref. 33.)

ionic remodeling resulting from prolonged high atrial rates or atrial fibrillation are reviewed by Bosch and Nattel (32).

Electrical remodeling of the atria also occurs in humans. As far back as 1982, Attuel et al. (35) observed a shortening and abnormal rate adaptation of atrial refractoriness in patients with AF. In 1986, Boutjdir et al. (36) found that atrial action potentials were shorter in patients with AF compared to those with normal sinus rhythm. Franz et al. (37) demonstrated that, after electrical cardioversion of atrial flutter or fibrillation, the human atrial action potential was shortened. The time course of reverse electrical remodeling was studied by Yu et al. (38). In 19 patients, the change in atrial refractoriness was monitored daily after electrical cardioversion of chronic AF. It was found that the shortening of the refractory period was completely reversible within 3 to 4 days of sinus rhythm. After the initial description of the AF-induced shortening of atrial refractoriness, several studies have tried to prevent tachycardia-induced electrical remodeling. First, it was reported that administration of the L-type Ca^{2+} antagonist verapamil could delay the AF-induced shortening of refractoriness (39,40). In other studies, initially a protective effect was described for angiotensin II antagonists (41), Na^+/H^+ exchanger inhibitors (42), antioxidants (ascorbate) (43), mibefadril (T-type Ca^{2+} channel blocker) (44), and amiodarone (45). However, most of these studies addressed the short-term effects (hours) of atrial tachycardia. When the atria were paced for longer periods of time (days), most drugs failed to prevent electrical remodeling (46,47). Only mibefadril (44) and amiodarone (45) retained their protective effects during 7 days of rapid pacing and could prevent the development of persistent AF in dogs. Recently, it was found that the class III action of I_{Kr} blockers like d-sotalol, ibutilide, and dofetilide was strongly reduced after 48 hr of AF (48,49). In contrast, the class III effect of AVE 0118, a substance blocking early activated K^+ currents (I_{Kur} and I_{to}), was *enhanced* after electrical remodeling (49). If these observations are reproduced in humans, such "early" class III drugs may become very useful in the cardioversion and prevention of AF.

From clinical studies, it is known that the atrial contractile function is impaired after successful cardioversion of AF (50). The degree of contractile dysfunction seems to be related to the duration of AF. In patients with lone AF, Sanfillippo et al. (51) observed an increase in atrial volume of ~40% after 20.6 months of AF. After restoration of sinus rhythm, atrial contractile function can recover, although this may take several months (52). Schotten et al. (53) hypothesized that the reduction in I_{CaL} during AF-induced electrical remodeling may also underlie atrial contractile dysfunction. To test this hypothesis, they chronically instrumented goats with pairs of piezoelectric crystals on both atria and a pressure catheter in the cavity of the right atrium (Fig. 5). With the atrial volume-pressure loops obtained in this way, the

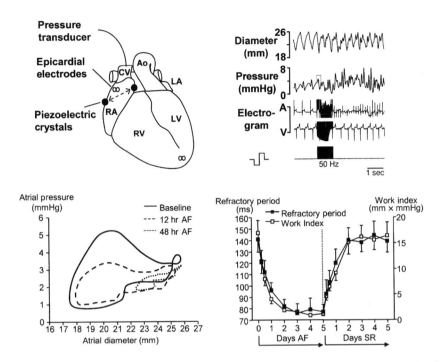

Figure 5 Contractile remodeling during the first 5 days of AF. Upper left: A pair of piezoelectric crystals sutured on the right atrium. Right atrial pressure was measured by an implanted pressure transducer. LA, left atrium; RA, right atrium; CV, superior caval vein; Ao, aorta. Upper right: Simultaneous recording of right atrial diameter and pressure. AF was induced by 1 sec (50 Hz) of burst pacing. Lower left: Right atrial pressure-volume loops recorded at baseline and after 12 and 48 hr of AF. Lower right: Time course of electrical and contractile remodeling and their reversibility in seven goats. (From Ref. 53.)

external work performed by the right atrium could be measured chronically. During the first 5 days of AF, the strength of the atrial contractions markedly declined. After 2 days the pressure-volume loop already showed that atrial contractile function was almost completely abolished. The atrial work index decreased from 16 to 2 mm × mmHg. The time course of electrical and contractile remodeling was the same. Also, during reverse remodeling, the time course of restoration of the refractory period and atrial contractile function were the same; after 2 days of sinus rhythm, the pressure-diameter loop returned to control values. These findings indicate that during the first 5 days of AF, electrical and contractile remodeling are closely linked. They are probably both the result of the same mechanism—i.e., a downregulation of the L-type Ca^{2+} current.

Apart from inducing electrical and contractile remodeling, AF also changes the structure of the atrium. The first experimental study in which this was demonstrated was done by Morillo et al. (30). Dogs subjected to 6 weeks of rapid atrial pacing revealed a marked disarray of atrial myofilaments, increased number and size of mitochondria, and disruption of the sarcoplasmic reticulum. Ausma et al. (54) found similar changes in the atria of goats in which AF was maintained for 9 to 23 weeks. The atrial myocytes were markedly increased in size, and changes in cellular structure were characterized by loss of myofibrils, accumulation of glycogen, reduction in connexin 40, changes in mitochondrial shape and size, fragmentation of sarcoplasmic reticulum, and dispersion of nuclear chromatin (Fig. 6). It was suggested that these ultrastructural alterations closely resembled the changes observed in ventricular myocardium due to low-flow ischemia, termed "hibernation."

Myolysis
Sinus rhythm   Atrial fibrillation

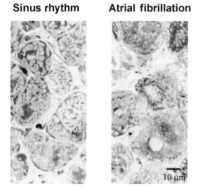

Connexin 40

Figure 6 Structural remodeling of caprine atria by 4 months of AF. Top: Light microscopy shows enlarged atrial cells with severe myolysis and accumulation of glycogen. Bottom: Immunolabeling of Cx40 showing a clear reduction in Cx40 expression. (From Refs. 54 and 90.)

Hibernating atrial myocytes were heterogeneously distributed, with some cells strongly affected and neighboring cells virtually normal.

In two recent studies, the reversibility of structural atrial remodeling was evaluated. Everett et al. (55) found no recovery of structural remodeling 2 weeks after restoration of sinus rhythm in dogs subjected to 2 months of AF. Ausma et al. (56) investigated the reversibility of structural changes in the atria of goats that had been in AF for 4 months. Four months after restoration of sinus rhythm, structural abnormalities were still present. Although by that time cell size, connexin 40, and myocytes with severe myolysis were normal again, 25% of atrial myocytes still showed a moderate degree of myolysis. Also, the duration of induced AF episodes was still prolonged.

VI. ATRIAL DILATATION

The impact of atrial dilatation on the propensity for AF is being studied in several experimental models. In most models, the *acute* effects of atrial dilatation were studied. In the Langendorf perfused rabbit heart, Ravelli et al. (57) found that acute atrial stretch was associated with a shortening of the atrial action potential and refractory period. In contrast, other studies have reported no change (58) or a prolongation of atrial refractoriness (59) after acute volume overload. In a recent study, Eijsbouts et al. (60) evaluated the effects of acute atrial dilatation on atrial conduction. As a result of dilatation, atrial conduction slowed and the number of areas with local conduction delays increased significantly. In combination with a short atrial wavelength, such stretch-induced lines of intra-atrial conduction block may serve as sites of wavebreak, which can initiate AF.

Although the models of acute dilation have provided important information about the electrophysiological effects of acute atrial stretch, atrial dilatation develops more gradually in patients. As early as 1981, Boyden et al. (61) evaluated the effects of *chronic* atrial dilatation on atrial electrophysiology in dogs. Right atrial dilatation was created by cutting the chordae tendineae of the septal cusps of the tricuspid valves and partly occluding the pulmonary artery. After a mean follow-up of 93 days, the right atrial volume had increased by 39%. The propensity for atrial arrhythmias had clearly increased and the incidence of AF episodes lasting >10 min was significantly higher. However, in vitro recorded atrial action potentials did not differ in duration from action potentials recorded from nondilated atria (62). An increased trabeculation of the right atrium was observed and atrial histology was characterized by hypertrophy and fibrosis. Cox et al. (63) developed a canine model of chronic mitral regurgitation by cutting the chordae tendineae of the mitral valve. After 3 months of regurgitation, AF could easily be induced by burst pacing. Multisite mapping revealed multiple activation patterns, "ranging from the simplest pattern, in which a single reentrant circuit was present, to the most complex cases, in which no consistent pattern of activation could be identified." Of note, animals with sustained AF demonstrated the highest degree of dilatation. The most complex AF activation patterns were observed in these animals. Similar observations were made by Verheule et al. (64). In dogs with 1 month of mitral regurgitation, the inducibility of AF was strongly increased. Atrial conduction did not change, but atrial refractory periods in the right and left atria were prolonged. Structural alterations in the atrial myocardium were confined to the left atrium and consisted of increased glycogen accumulation and interstitial fibrosis.

Recently Neuberger et al. (65) investigated the relation between the time course of atrial dilatation and the stability of AF in goats with chronic atrioventricular (AV) block. Endocardial screw-in leads with sonomicrometer ultrasound crystals were chronically implanted in the right atrium. In this way, atrial electrophysiology and atrial size could be monitored simultaneously. After His bundle ablation, a progressive increase in atrial size was observed; after 4 weeks, atrial diameter had increased by 12%. Before the creation of this AV block, episodes of AF induced by burst pacing were generally brief (lasting seconds). After 4 weeks of AV block, the duration of AF paroxysms gradually increased. In goats with the largest degree of dilatation, AF now lasted longer than 1 hr (Fig. 7). As in the study of Boyden

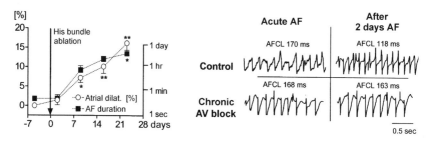

Figure 7 Effects of atrial dilatation on the electrophysiological properties of the atria in six goats with chronic AV block. Left: Relative changes in atrial diameter and duration of induced AF episodes during 4 weeks of complete AV block. Right: Representative examples of unipolar endocardial atrial electrograms. Under control conditions (upper panels), the median AF interval shortened within the first 2 days of AF from 170 to 118 ms. After chronic AV block (lower panels), 2 days of AF still shortened the atrial refractoriness (not shown) but no longer shortened the AF cycle length. (From Ref. 91.)

et al. (62), no changes in atrial refractoriness were observed. Detailed mapping of the right and left atria revealed an increased heterogeneity in conduction.

Whereas maintenance of AF still resulted in shortening of the atrial refractory period, the AF cycle length did not shorten accordingly. This suggests that, in this model of atrial dilatation, structural conduction defects are involved in the reentrant process.

Clinical data on the effects of chronic atrial stretch on atrial electrophysiology are scarce. Sparks et al. (66,67) evaluated the effects of chronic VVI and DDD pacing on atrial size and electrophysiology in patients requiring permanent pacing. In this prospective randomized study, it was found that VVI pacing increased atrial dimension (66) and that this was associated with a prolongation of the atrial refractory period (AERP) (67). No changes, either in atrial size or electrophysiological properties, were observed after DDD pacing. Although a prolongation of atrial refractoriness can be expected to prevent arrhythmias by prolonging the atrial wavelength, VVI pacing clearly increased the propensity for AF compared to DDD pacing. The underlying mechanisms are unknown, but it is likely that changes in atrial conduction due to an increase in connective tissue play a role in the genesis of AF in patients with dilated atria.

VII. INFLAMMATION

In 1986, the group of Waldo developed a new canine model of atrial flutter (68). After a thoracotomy, both atria were dusted with sterile talc and a gauze dressing was left on them. Electrodes were sutured to the atria and the chest was closed. During the first week after surgery, susceptibility for atrial arrhythmias was evaluated daily. In more than 90% of the animals, atrial flutter could be induced by programmed electrical stimulation on at least one of the first four postoperative days. With time, the susceptibility for arrhythmias declined; 1 week after surgery, flutter could be induced in only one of four animals. The mechanism of this temporarily high atrial vulnerability is still unclear. Atrial refractoriness and conduction velocity were not different in susceptible or nonsusceptible dogs. In subsequent studies also, atrial fibrillation was induced. Extensive mapping of electrical activation showed that one to four unstable reentrant circuits of short cycle length were responsible for the maintenance of AF (69). Reentrant circuits involved the septum, right atrial free wall, pulmonary veins, and inferior and superior caval veins. Importantly, Bachmann's bundle was involved in most of these reentrant circuits. Radiofrequency catheter ablation of this "critical crossroad" completely abolished AF in this model. It is of interest to note that the time course of inducibility of atrial flutter and fibrillation observed in the model shows striking similarities with the incidence of postoperative AF in patients. Atrial AF/atrial flutter occurs in 70% of patients during the first 4 days after surgery (70). The canine model of sterile pericarditis can thus be useful in elucidating the mechanisms of postoperative atrial arrhythmias in humans. In a recent study, Waldo's group evaluated the antiarrhythmic effects of steroids in the canine model of pericarditis (71). Administration of oral prednisone completely prevented atrial arrhythmias during the first 4 days after surgery. Histological examination revealed that the degree of inflammation was clearly reduced in steroid-treated animals. In an earlier clinical study, Yared et al. (72) showed that, in patients undergoing elective coronary or valvular heart surgery, administration of a single dose of dexamethasone reduced the incidence of postoperative AF from 32.3 to 18.9%. These studies clearly indicate a link between postoperative AF and inflammatory responses.

VIII. CONGESTIVE HEART FAILURE

In clinical practice, it is well known that heart failure often leads to AF (73). On the other hand, AF can also worsen ventricular function. Not surprisingly, AF and heart failure coexist in many patients. To elucidate how heart failure increases the vulnerability for AF, Nattel and coworkers (74) subjected dogs to rapid ventricular pacing (220 to 240 bpm) for a period of 3 weeks. The animals progressively developed clinical and hemodynamical signs of heart failure. In 10 of 18 dogs, sustained AF could be induced. AF was characterized by long AF cycle lengths and a relatively low degree of polymorphism of the fibrillation electrograms. Atrial mapping suggested that AF was maintained by a small number of reentrant waves. Unlike the case in the rapid atrial pacing model, the increased stability of AF was not based on a shortening of the atrial wavelength. No changes in refractoriness, conduction velocity, or wavelength were noted. However, when the local conduction properties were studied in more detail, discrete regions of slow conduction were found. Histological analysis revealed a marked increase in fibrous tissue, which was held responsible for the local disturbances in atrial conduction (Fig. 8). Characterization of the cellular electrophysiological changes showed a decrease in I_{to}, I_{Ca}, and I_{Ks} and an increase in the Na^+/Ca^{2+} exchange current (75). Thus, in the setting of congestive heart failure (CHF) an increase in atrial fibrosis and tissue anisotropy may promote AF by facilitating microreentry. Of note, the structural abnormalities showed striking similarities with the histological findings observed in atrial myocardia of the elderly (76) and in patients with rheumatic heart disease (77).

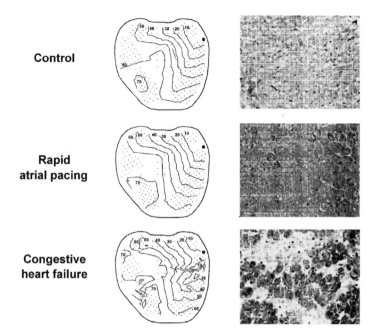

Control

Rapid
atrial pacing

Congestive
heart failure

Figure 8 Different kinds of atrial remodeling in canine atria. Left: Crowding of isochrones was observed only in dogs with congestive heart failure, indicating local slowing of conduction. Right: Histological examination revealed severe atrial fibrosis in dogs with congestive heart failure, whereas prolonged rapid atrial pacing had no significant effect on the amount of connective tissue. (Modified from Ref. 74.)

Sanders et al. (78) recently investigated the atrial electrophysiological properties in patients with CHF. Using electroanatomic mapping, they found that right atrial conduction velocity was markedly slowed and that the number of electrograms with fractionated potentials was increased. Although no clear difference in the inducibility of AF was observed, the duration of induced AF paroxysms was clearly prolonged.

Since the renin-angiotensin system is thought to play a pivotal role in the development of cardiac fibrosis, Li et al. (79) investigated whether the angiotensin converting enzyme (ACE) inhibitor enalapril could prevent AF in the canine CHF model. After 5 weeks of rapid ventricular pacing, drug-treated animals showed a lower level of angiotensin II in the atrial wall. At the same time, the duration of induced AF episodes was significantly shorter than in the placebo group. ACE inhibition attenuated the development of inter-stitial fibrosis and could partly prevent the development of intra-atrial conduction abnormalities. Recent clinical data suggest that ACE inhibitors may have beneficial effects in patients with atrial fibrillation. In the TRACE study (80), it was found that trandolapril reduced the incidence of AF during a 2- to 4-year follow-up in patients with reduced left ventricular function. Similar results were obtained in the SOLVD trial (81). Recurrences of atrial fibrillation after electrical cardioversion were significantly less in patients treated with amiodarone and irbesartan (an angiotensin II type 1 blocker) vs. patients treated with amiodarone alone (82). However, it remains to be determined whether the observed antiarrhythmic action of ACE inhibition is based on an antifibrotic effect. Other effects, such as lowering of the atrial pressure, might also explain a reduction in susceptibility for AF.

IX. ISCHEMIA

Myocardial infarction is an independent risk factor for the development of AF (3). Up to 21% of patients admitted with an acute myocardial infarction suffer from atrial fibrillation/flutter during their hospital stay (83). The pathophysiological mechanisms of ischemia related AF are not well understood. Most of our knowledge of the arrhythmogenic mechanisms of ischemia has been acquired in the ventricles. Both a marked heterogeneity in refractoriness and areas of slow and discontinuous conduction may lead to a substrate of reentrant arrhythmias. It is unclear whether the same electrophysiological effects also occur in ischemic atria. Only recently, the effects of coronary occlusion on atrial arrhythmias have been studied. In a dog model, Jayachandran et al. (42) observed an acute shortening of the atrial refractory period after occlusion of the proximal right coronary artery. In a study of Sinno et al. (84), no effects on atrial refractoriness were observed during the first hours after ligation of a branch of the right coronary artery (right intermediate atrial artery). In ischemic atrial tissue, the pacing threshold was increased, conduction was slowed, and the duration of induced AF episodes increased significantly. Miyauchi et al. (85) investigated the long-term effects on the susceptibility of the atria for AF of occlusion of the left descending artery below the first diagonal branch in dogs. After 8 weeks of occlusion, atrial electrophysiological measurements were performed. Both the induction and stability of AF were increased after myocardial infarction; in the control group, the duration of induced AF lasted for only 3 sec; after myocardial infarction, AF lasted for an average of 41 days. Mapping of atrial activation during application of premature stimulation showed epicardial wavebreaks degenerating into AF. No differences in the duration of atrial action potentials or refractoriness were found after myocardial infarction. However, at fast pacing rates, a higher spatial dispersion in the duration of monophasic action potentials was found. The slope of the restitution curve was also steeper. Immunocytochemical staining of sympathetic nerves showed an increased density and marked heterogeneities in different parts of the atria. The amount of connexin 40 was reduced and it was also more heterogeneously distributed (86). No signs of atrial ischemia or fibrosis could be found. Thus it appears that ventricular infarction *itself* leads to the creation of a substrate for AF, possibly due to nerve sprouting, atrial stretch, or modulation of the autonomic nervous system.

X. COMPUTER MODELS OF AF

In the early 1960s, Moe and coworkers (87) developed the first computer model of AF, consisting of a two-dimensional matrix of 992 units. Each unit could have five different states of excitability, ranging from fully excitable to absolutely refractory (Fig. 9, left panel). Spatial dispersion in refractoriness was simulated by varying the duration of the lowest excitable state in different units. The "turbulent activity" within the matrix was sustained by multiple wandering wavelets varying in both number and size (Fig. 9, right panel). When the refractory period was increased or the surface area reduced, the activity was terminated. The creation of internal obstacles resulted in a circus movement flutter. The growing knowledge of cellular electrophysiology led to the design of more sophisticated computer models implementing various ionic currents and concentrations, subcellular compartments, membrane capacity, and cell-to-cell coupling. One example is the model recently developed by Zou et al. (88). These authors simulated cell grids of varying

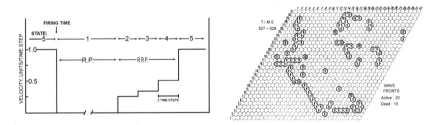

Figure 9 The early computer model of AF by Moe and Abildskov. Left: Each unit of a 992-unit matrix was assigned one of five states of excitability. State 1: absolutely refractory. State 2 to 4: relatively refractory with decreased conduction velocity in case of activation. State 5: fully recovered excitability. Right: Several simultaneously propagating wavefronts differing in size and direction of propagation. Arrows indicate progress of wavefronts. (From Ref. 87.)

size in the presence of spatially different acetylcholine concentrations, causing different patterns of spatial dispersion of refractoriness. In almost all cases, AF was sustained by a single spiral wave rotating around an area of low acetylcholine concentration. When the grid became too small, AF was not sustained. Since, above this critical size, the behavior of AF was qualitatively the same in an 11-fold increase in atrial grid size, these authors stated that the emphasis on tissue mass as an important determinant of AF stability may have been overstated (88). Virag et al. (89) developed a model of AF based on the anatomy of human atria. An ion-based membrane model was implemented in an anatomical structure derived from segmented magnetic resonance images. However, anisotropy and differences in wall thickness were not implemented in this model, in which burst pacing induced atrial fibrillation even when the membrane properties were uniform. As expected, shortening of the refractory period increased the duration of AF.

REFERENCES

1. Wolf PA, Abbott RD, Kannel WB. Atrial fibrillation as an independent risk factor for stroke: the Framingham study. Stroke 1991; 22:983–988.
2. Benjamin EJ, Wolf PA, D'Agostino RB, Silbershatz H, Kannel WB, Levy D. Impact of atrial fibrillation on the risk of death: the Framingham Heart Study. Circulation 1998; 98:946–952.
3. Benjamin EJ, Levy D, Vaziri SM, D'Agostino RB, Belanger AJ, Wolf PA. Independent risk factors for atrial fibrillation in a population-based cohort. The Framingham Heart Study. JAMA 1994; 271:840–844.
4. Kopecky SL, Gersh BJ, McGoon MD, Whisnant JP, Holmes DR Jr, Ilstrup DM, Frye RL. The natural history of lone atrial fibrillation. A population-based study over three decades. N Engl J Med 1987; 317:669–674.
5. Haissaguerre M, Jais P, Shah DC, Takahashi A, Hocini M, Quiniou G, Garrigue S, Le Mouroux A, Le Metayer P, Clementy J. Spontaneous initiation of atrial fibrillation by ectopic beats originating in the pulmonary veins. N Engl J Med 1998; 339:659–666.
6. Winterberg H. Studien über Herzflimmern. 1. Uber die Wirkung des N Vagus und Accelerans auf das Flimmern des Herzens. Pflugers Arch Physiol 1907; 117: 223–256.
7. Scherf D. Studies on auricular tachycardia caused by aconitine administration. Proc Soc Exp Biol Med 1947; 64:233.
8. Moe GK, Abildskov JA. Atrial fibrillation as a self-sustaining arrhythmia independent of focal discharge. Am Heart J 1959; 58:59–70.
9. Herweg B, Kowalski M, Steinberg JS. Termination of persistent atrial fibrillation resistant to cardioversion by a single radiofrequency application. Pacing Clin Electrophysiol 2003; 26:1420–1423.

10. Pappone C, Rosanio S, Oreto G, Tocchi M, Gugliotta F, Vicedomini G, Salvati A, Dicandia C, Mazzone P, Santinelli V, Gulletta S, Chierchia S. Circumferential radiofrequency ablation of pulmonary vein ostia: a new anatomic approach for curing atrial fibrillation. Circulation 2000; 102:2619–2628.

11. Cappato R, Negroni S, Pecora D, Bentivegna S, Lupo PP, Carolei A, Esposito C, Furlanello F, De Ambroggi L. Prospective assessment of late conduction recurrence across radiofrequency lesions producing electrical disconnection at the pulmonary vein ostium in patients with atrial fibrillation. Circulation 2003; 108:1599–1604.

12. Knoll P. Über die Wirkungen des Herzvagus bei Warmblutern. Archiv Ges Physiol 1897; 67:587–614.

13. Rothberger C, Winterberg H. Uber Vorhofflimmern und vorhofflattern. Arch Ges Physiol 1914; 160:42–91.

14. Alessi R, Nusynowitz M, Abildskov J, Moe G. Nonuniform distribution of vagal effects on the atrial refractory period. Am J Physiol 1958; 194:406–410.

15. Allessie M, Lammers WJ, Bonke FI, Hollen J. Experimental evaluation of Moe's multiple wavelet hypothesis of atrial fibrillation. In: Zipes DP, ed. Cardiac Electrophysiology and Arrhythmias. Orlando, FL: Grune & Stratton, 1985.

16. Wang Z, Page P, Nattel S. Mechanism of flecainide's antiarrhythmic action in experimental atrial fibrillation. Circ Res 1992; 71:271–287.

17. Schuessler RB, Grayson TM, Bromberg BI, Cox JL, Boineau JP. Cholinergically mediated tachyarrhythmias induced by a single extrastimulus in the isolated canine right atrium. Circ Res 1992; 71:1254–1267.

18. Schuessler RB, Kawamoto T, Hand DE, Mitsuno M, Bromberg BI, Cox JL, Boineau JP. Simultaneous epicardial and endocardial activation sequence mapping in the isolated canine right atrium. Circulation 1993; 88:250–263.

19. Wu TJ, Yashima M, Xie F, Athill CA, Kim YH, Fishbein MC, Qu Z, Garfinkel A, Weiss JN, Karagueuzian HS, Chen PS. Role of pectinate muscle bundles in the generation and maintenance of intra-atrial reentry: potential implications for the mechanism of conversion between atrial fibrillation and atrial flutter. Circ Res 1998; 83:448–462.

20. Skanes AC, Mandapati R, Berenfeld O, Davidenko JM, Jalife J. Spatiotemporal periodicity during atrial fibrillation in the isolated sheep heart. Circulation 1998; 98:1236–1248.

21. Mandapati R, Skanes A, Chen J, Berenfeld O, Jalife J. Stable microreentrant sources as a mechanism of atrial fibrillation in the isolated sheep heart. Circulation 2000; 101:194–199.

22. Coumel P, Attuel P, Lavallee J, Flammang D, Leclercq JF, Slama R. The atrial arrhythmia syndrome of vagal origin. Arch Mal Coeur Vaiss 1978; 71:645–656.

23. Herweg B, Dalal P, Nagy B, Schweitzer P. Power spectral analysis of heart period variability of preceding sinus rhythm before initiation of paroxysmal atrial fibrillation. Am J Cardiol 1998; 82:869–874.

24. Bettoni M, Zimmermann M. Autonomic tone variations before the onset of paroxysmal atrial fibrillation. Circulation 2002; 105:2753–2759.

25. Dimmer C, Tavernier R, Gjorgov N, Van Nooten G, Clement DL, Jordaens L. Variations of autonomic tone preceding onset of atrial fibrillation after coronary artery bypass grafting. Am J Cardiol 1998; 82:22–25.

26. Wen ZC, Chen SA, Tai CT, Huang JL, Chang MS. Role of autonomic tone in facilitating spontaneous onset of typical atrial flutter. J Am Coll Cardiol 1998; 31:602–607.

27. Irwin JM, McCarthy EA, Wilkinson WE, Pritchett EL. Circadian occurrence of symptomatic paroxysmal supraventricular tachycardia in untreated patients. Circulation 1988; 77:298–300.

28. Kupari M, Koskinen P, Leinonen H. Double-peaking circadian variation in the occurrence of sustained supraventricular tachyarrhythmias. Am Heart J 1990; 120:1364–1369.

29. Godtfredsen J. Atrial fibrillation: a review of course and prognosis. In: Kulbertus HE, Olsson SB, Schlepper M, eds. Atrial Fibrillation. Molndal, Sweden: Lindgren and Soner, 1982:134–145.

30. Morillo CA, Klein GJ, Jones DL, Guiraudon CM. Chronic rapid atrial pacing. Structural, functional, and electrophysiological characteristics of a new model of sustained atrial fibrillation. Circulation 1995; 91:1588–1595.

31. Wijffels MC, Kirchhof CJ, Dorland R, Allessie MA. Atrial fibrillation begets atrial fibrillation. A study in awake chronically instrumented goats. Circulation 1995; 92:1954–1968.

32. Bosch RF, Nattel S. Cellular electrophysiology of atrial fibrillation. Cardiovasc Res 2002; 54:259–269.

33. Yue L, Feng J, Gaspo R, Li GR, Wang Z, Nattel S. Ionic remodeling underlying action potential changes in a canine model of atrial fibrillation. Circ Res 1997; 81:512–525.

34. Van Wagoner DR, Pond AL, McCarthy PM, Trimmer JS, Nerbonne JM. Outward K+ current densities and Kv1.5 expression are reduced in chronic human atrial fibrillation. Circ Res 1997; 80:772–781.

35. Attuel P, Childers R, Cauchemez B, Poveda J, Mugica J, Coumel P. Failure in the rate adaptation of the atrial refractory period: its relationship to vulnerability. Int J Cardiol 1982; 2:179–197.

36. Boutjdir M, Le Heuzey JY, Lavergne T, Chauvaud S, Guize L, Carpentier A, Peronneau P. Inhomogeneity of cellular refractoriness in human atrium: factor of arrhythmia? Pacing Clin Electrophysiol 1986; 9:1095–1100.

37. Franz MR, Karasik PL, Li C, Moubarak J, Chavez M. Electrical remodeling of the human atrium: similar effects in patients with chronic atrial fibrillation and atrial flutter. J Am Coll Cardiol 1997; 30:1785–1792.

38. Yu WC, Lee SH, Tai CT, Tsai CF, Hsieh MH, Chen CC, Ding YA, Chang MS, Chen SA. Reversal of atrial electrical remodeling following cardioversion of long-standing atrial fibrillation in man. Cardiovasc Res 1999; 42:470–476.

39. Tieleman RG, De Langen C, Van Gelder IC, de Kam PJ, Grandjean J, Bel KJ, Wijffels MC, Allessie MA, Crijns HJ. Verapamil reduces tachycardia-induced electrical remodeling of the atria. Circulation 1997; 95:1945–1953.

40. Goette A, Honeycutt C, Langberg JJ. Electrical remodeling in atrial fibrillation. Time course and mechanisms. Circulation 1996; 94:2968–2974.

41. Nakashima H, Kumagai K, Urata H, Gondo N, Ideishi M, Arakawa K. Angiotensin II antagonist prevents electrical remodeling in atrial fibrillation. Circulation 2000; 101:2612–2617.

42. Jayachandran JV, Zipes DP, Weksler J, Olgin JE. Role of the Na^+/H^+ exchanger in short-term atrial electrophysiological remodeling. Circulation 2000; 101:1861–1866.

43. Carnes CA, Chung MK, Nakayama T, Nakayama H, Baliga RS, Piao S, Kanderian A, Pavia S, Hamlin RL, McCarthy PM, Bauer JA, Van Wagoner DR. Ascorbate attenuates atrial pacing-induced peroxynitrite formation and electrical remodeling and decreases the incidence of postoperative atrial fibrillation. Circ Res 2001; 89:E32–E38.

44. Fareh S, Benardeau A, Thibault B, Nattel S. The T-type Ca^{2+} channel blocker mibefradil prevents the development of a substrate for atrial fibrillation by tachycardia-induced atrial remodeling in dogs. Circulation 1999; 100:2191–2197.

45. Shinagawa K, Shiroshita-Takeshita A, Schram G, Nattel S. Effects of antiarrhythmic drugs on fibrillation in the remodeled atrium: insights into the mechanism of the superior efficacy of amiodarone. Circulation 2003; 107:1440–1446.

46. Lee SH, Yu WC, Cheng JJ, Hung CR, Ding YA, Chang MS, Chen SA. Effect of verapamil on long-term tachycardia-induced atrial electrical remodeling. Circulation 2000; 101:200–206.

47. Shinagawa K, Mitamura H, Ogawa S, Nattel S. Effects of inhibiting Na^+/H^+-exchange or angiotensin converting enzyme on atrial tachycardia-induced remodeling. Cardiovasc Res 2002; 54:438–446.

48. Duytschaever M, Wijffels MCEF, Allessie MA. Effect of AF induced remodeling on class IC and III drug action: loss of class III effect by atrial fibrillation [abstr]. Pacing Clin Electrophysiol 2000; 23:564.

49. Blaauw Y, Gögelein H, Tieleman RG, van Hunnink A, Schotten U, Allessie MA. Early class III drugs for the treatment of atrial fibrillation: efficacy and atrial selectivity of AVE0118 in remodeled atria of the goat. Circulation 2004. In Press.

50. Logan W, Rowlands D, Howitt G, Holmes A. Left atrial activity following cardioversion. Lancet 1965; 2:471–473.

51. Sanfilippo AJ, Abascal VM, Sheehan M, Oertel LB, Harrigan P, Hughes RA, Weyman AE. Atrial enlargement as a consequence of atrial fibrillation. A prospective echocardiographic study. Circulation 1990; 82:792–797.

52. Manning WJ, Silverman DI, Katz SE, Riley MF, Doherty RM, Munson JT, Douglas PS. Temporal dependence of the return of atrial mechanical function on the mode of cardioversion of atrial fibrillation to sinus rhythm. Am J Cardiol 1995; 75:624–626.

53. Schotten U, Duytschaever M, Ausma J, Eijsbouts S, Neuberger HR, Allessie M. Electrical and contractile remodeling during the first days of atrial fibrillation go hand in hand. Circulation 2003; 107:1433–1439.

54. Ausma J, Wijffels M, Thone F, Wouters L, Allessie M, Borgers M. Structural changes of atrial myocardium due to sustained atrial fibrillation in the goat. Circulation 1997; 96:3157–3163.

55. Everett THT, Li H, Mangrum JM, McRury ID, Mitchell MA, Redick JA, Haines DE. Electrical, morphological, and ultrastructural remodeling and reverse remodeling in a canine model of chronic atrial fibrillation. Circulation 2000; 102:1454–1460.

56. Ausma J, van der Velden HM, Lenders MH, van Ankeren EP, Jongsma HJ, Ramaekers FC, Borgers M, Allessie MA. Reverse structural and gap-junctional remodeling after prolonged atrial fibrillation in the goat. Circulation 2003; 107:2051–2058.

57. Ravelli F, Allessie M. Effects of atrial dilatation on refractory period and vulnerability to atrial fibrillation in the isolated Langendorff-perfused rabbit heart. Circulation 1997; 96:1686–1695.

58. Wijffels MC, Kirchhof CJ, Dorland R, Power J, Allessie MA. Electrical remodeling due to atrial fibrillation in chronically instrumented conscious goats: roles of neurohumoral changes, ischemia, atrial stretch, and high rate of electrical activation. Circulation 1997; 96:3710–3720.

59. Satoh T, Zipes DP. Unequal atrial stretch in dogs increases dispersion of refractoriness conducive to developing atrial fibrillation. J Cardiovasc Electrophysiol 1996; 7:833–842.

60. Eijsbouts SC, Majidi M, van Zandvoort M, Allessie MA. Effects of acute atrial dilation on heterogeneity in conduction in the isolated rabbit heart. J Cardiovasc Electrophysiol 2003; 14:269–278.

61. Boyden PA, Hoffman BF. The effects on atrial electrophysiology and structure of surgically induced right atrial enlargement in dogs. Circ Res 1981; 49:1319–1331.

62. Boyden PA, Tilley LP, Pham TD, Liu SK, Fenoglic JJ Jr, Wit AL. Effects of left atrial enlargement on atrial transmembrane potentials and structure in dogs with mitral valve fibrosis. Am J Cardiol 1982; 49:1896–1908.

63. Cox JL, Canavan TE, Schuessler RB, Cain ME, Lindsay BD, Stone C, Smith PK, Corr PB, Boineau JP. The surgical treatment of atrial fibrillation: II Intraoperative electrophysiologic mapping and description of the electrophysiologic basis of atrial flutter and atrial fibrillation. J Thorac Cardiovasc Surg 1991; 101:406–426.

64. Verheule S, Wilson E, Everett TT, Shanbhag S, Golden C, Olgin J. Alterations in atrial electrophysiology and tissue structure in a canine model of chronic atrial dilatation due to mitral regurgitation. Circulation 2003; 107:2615–2622.

65. Neuberger HR, Schotten U, Ausma J, Blaauw Y, Eijsbouts S, Hunnik van A, Allessie MA. Atrial remodeling in the goat due to chronic complete atrioventricular block [abstr]. Eur Heart J 2002; 23:813.

66. Sparks PB, Mond HG, Vohra JK, Yapanis AG, Grigg LE, Kalman JM. Mechanical remodeling of the left atrium after loss of atrioventricular synchrony. A long-term study in humans. Circulation 1999; 100:1714–1721.

67. Sparks PB, Mond HG, Vohra JK, Jayaprakash S, Kalman JM. Electrical remodeling of the atria following loss of atrioventricular synchrony: a long-term study in humans. Circulation 1999; 100:1894–1900.

68. Page PL, Plumb VJ, Okumura K, Waldo AL. A new animal model of atrial flutter. J Am Coll Cardiol 1986; 8:872–879.

69. Kumagai K, Khrestian C, Waldo AL. Simultaneous multisite mapping studies during induced atrial fibrillation in the sterile pericarditis model. Insights into the mechanism of its maintenance. Circulation 1997; 95:511–521.
70. Aranki SF, Shaw DP, Adams DH, Rizzo RJ, Couper GS, VanderVliet M, Collins JJ Jr, Cohn LH, Burstin HR. Predictors of atrial fibrillation after coronary artery surgery. Current trends and impact on hospital resources. Circulation 1996; 94:390–397.
71. Goldstein RN, Khrestian CM, Ryu K, Van Wagoner DR, Stambler BS, Waldo AL. Prevention of postoperative atrial fibrillation and flutter using steroids [abstr]. Pacing Clin Electrophysiol 2003; 26:1068.
72. Yared JP, Starr NJ, Torres FK, Bashour CA, Bourdakos G, Piedmonte M, Michener JA, Davis JA, Rosenberger TE. Effects of single dose, postinduction dexamethasone on recovery after cardiac surgery. Ann Thorac Surg 2000; 69:1420–1424.
73. Stevenson WG, Stevenson LW. Atrial fibrillation in heart failure. N Engl J Med 1999; 341:910–911.
74. Li D, Fareh S, Leung TK, Nattel S. Promotion of atrial fibrillation by heart failure in dogs: atrial remodeling of a different sort. Circulation 1999; 100:87–95.
75. Li D, Melnyk P, Feng J, Wang Z, Petrecca K, Shrier A, Nattel S. Effects of experimental heart failure on atrial cellular and ionic electrophysiology. Circulation 2000; 101:2631–2638.
76. Lie JT, Hammond PI. Pathology of the senescent heart: anatomic observations on 237 autopsy studies of patients 90 to 105 years old. Mayo Clin Proc 1988; 63:552–564.
77. Pham TD, Fenoglio JJ Jr. Right atrial ultrastructural in chronic rheumatic heart disease. Int J Cardiol 1982; 1:289–304.
78. Sanders P, Morton JB, Davidson NC, Spence SJ, Vohra JK, Sparks PB, Kalman JM. Electrical remodeling of the atria in congestive heart failure. Electrophysiological and electroanatomic mapping in humans. Circulation 2003; 108: 1461–1468.
79. Li D, Shinagawa K, Pang L, Leung TK, Cardin S, Wang Z, Nattel S. Effects of angiotensin-converting enzyme inhibition on the development of the atrial fibrillation substrate in dogs with ventricular tachypacing-induced congestive heart failure. Circulation 2001; 104:2608–2614.
80. Pedersen OD, Bagger H, Kober L, Torp-Pedersen C. Trandolapril reduces the incidence of atrial fibrillation after acute myocardial infarction in patients with left ventricular dysfunction. Circulation 1999; 100:376–380.
81. Vermes E, Tardif JC, Bourassa MG, Racine N, Levesque S, White M, Guerra PG, Ducharme A. Enalapril decreases the incidence of atrial fibrillation in patients with left ventricular dysfunction: insight from the Studies Of Left Ventricular Dysfunction (SOLVD) trials. Circulation 2003; 107:2926–2931.
82. Madrid AH, Bueno MG, Rebollo JM, Marin I, Pena G, Bernal E, Rodriguez A, Cano L, Cano JM, Cabeza P, Moro C. Use of irbesartan to maintain sinus rhythm in patients with long-lasting persistent atrial fibrillation: a prospective and randomized study. Circulation 2002; 106:331–336.

83. Pedersen OD, Bagger H, Kober L, Torp-Pedersen C. The occurrence and prognostic significance of atrial fibrillation/flutter following acute myocardial infarction. TRACE Study group. TRAndolapril Cardiac Evaluation. Eur Heart J 1999; 20:748–754.

84. Sinno H, Derakhchan K, Libersan D, Merhi Y, Leung TK, Nattel S. Atrial ischemia promotes atrial fibrillation in dogs. Circulation 2003; 107:1930–1936.

85. Miyauchi Y, Zhou S, Okuyama Y, Miyauchi M, Hayashi H, Hamabe A, Fishbein MC, Mandel WJ, Chen LS, Chen PS, Karagueuzian HS. Altered atrial electrical restitution and heterogeneous sympathetic hyperinnervation in hearts with chronic left ventricular myocardial infarction. Implications for atrial fibrillation. Circulation 2003; 108:360–366.

86. Ohara K, Miyauchi Y, Ohara T, Fishbein MC, Zhou S, Lee MH, Mandel WJ, Chen PS, Karagueuzian HS. Downregulation of immunodetectable atrial connexin40 in a canine model of chronic left ventricular myocardial infarction: implications to atrial fibrillation. J Cardiovasc Pharmacol Ther 2002; 7:89–94.

87. Moe GK, Rheinboldt WC, Abildskov JA. A computer model of atrial fibrillation. Am Heart J 1964; 67:200–220.

88. Zou R, Kneller J, Leon LJ, Nattel S. Development of a computer algorithm for the detection of phase singularities and initial application to analyze simulations of atrial fibrillation. Chaos 2002; 12:764–778.

89. Virag N, Jacquemet V, Henriquez CS, Zozor S, Blanc O, Vesin JM, Pruvot E, Kappenberger L. Study of atrial arrhythmias in a computer model based on magnetic resonance images of human atria. Chaos 2002; 12:754–763.

90. van der Velden HM, van Kempen MJ, Wijffels MC, van Zijverden M, Groenewegen WA, Allessie MA, Jongsma HJ. Altered pattern of connexin40 distribution in persistent atrial fibrillation in the goat. J Cardiovasc Electrophysiol 1998; 9:596–607.

91. Schotten U, Neuberger HR, Allessie MA. The role of atrial dilatation in the domestication of atrial fibrillation. Prog Biophys Mol Biol 2003; 82:151–162.

5
Rate Control Versus Maintenance of Sinus Rhythm

D. George Wyse
University of Calgary and Calgary Health Region, Calgary, Alberta, Canada

I. INTRODUCTION: BACKGROUND TO THE QUESTION OF RHYTHM VS. RATE

Atrial fibrillation (AF) is a very common cardiac arrhythmia associated with a number of clinical outcomes, including death, thromboembolism (primarily stroke), congestive heart failure (CHF), and other morbidity; it also causes symptoms. However, association between AF and these consequences does not prove that AF is the cause of these problems. Much of the research about rhythm management for AF during the last two decades has ignored or forgotten this principle. An apparently widely held view was that when AF is abolished, the problems associated with it are also abolished. Accordingly, many studies of therapy for AF have used maintenance of sinus rhythm itself as their endpoint. Such research ignores the possibility—indeed, the probability—that the morbidity associated with AF is at least partly caused by the disease process that is the background for AF, not the AF itself.

Furthermore, such research negates the fact that adverse effects of the therapy for AF may be contribute to the clinical outcomes associated with it. For example, the association of AF with increased mortality may be partly explained by the potentially fatal adverse effects of antiarrhythmic drugs used to treat it. Finally, the approach of using sinus rhythm as the endpoint for arrhythmia management research is based on the mistaken notion that there are methods that reliably measure the absence of AF. Thus, trials of therapy for AF need to focus on clinical endpoints rather than the presence or absence of AF itself (1). In the trials of rhythm control vs. rate control discussed in this chapter, such endpoints have been used much more extensively than they have been in previous studies of rhythm management for AF, with somewhat surprising results.

Before reviewing the trials themselves, it is worthwhile to examine briefly the basis for the research that seeks to compare the rhythm-control strategy to the rate control strategy for the management of AF. The background observations on which this research question is based were made in the late 1980s and early 1990s. During and before that time, drug therapy was (and still is) the mainstay of rhythm management for AF. However, the drugs available had relatively poor efficacy for the maintenance of sinus rhythm (2). They also had serious adverse effects, including death, particularly in those with underlying cardiac disease such as CHF (3). For these reasons there was general dissatisfaction with and apprehension of antiarrhythmic drug therapy for maintenance of sinus rhythm. Indeed, much research effort is now being directed at alternative, nonpharmacological therapies for rhythm management in patients with AF. During this same period of time, the remarkable efficacy of oral anticoagulants for stroke prevention was clearly demonstrated (4). The inefficacy and adverse effects of the antiarrhythmic drugs along with the efficacy of oral anticoagulants caused many to wonder if it might not be preferable to treat many patients who have AF with anticoagulation and the rate-control strategy rather than continuing efforts to restore and to maintain sinus rhythm. Beginning about 1995, a number of randomized clinical trials were undertaken to examine this question. The results of these trials are summarized in this chapter.

II. OVERVIEW OF THE COMPLETED TRIALS: SOME SIMILARITIES AND SOME DIFFERENCES

Five randomized trials comparing the rate-control strategy to the rhythm-control strategy in management of AF have been completed and published (5–9). The total number of patients studied in these five trials is greater than 5000. The basic comparison is the same in all five trials: the strategy of restoring and maintaining sinus rhythm is compared to the strategy of controlling the heart rate without making any specific effort to achieve sinus rhythm. Both strategies in all trials used anticoagulation with oral anticoagulants, although slightly differently within each strategy. There are some differences between the trials. In the discussion that follows, the trials are compared and contrasted under a series of headings; a summary of the characteristics of each trial is presented in Table 1.

A. Patient Selection

In these five trials, primarily elderly patients were recruited, reflecting the preponderance of older patients among those afflicted with AF in Europe and North America, where the trials took place (10). The Pharmacologic Intervention in Atrial Fibrillations (PIAF) trial, The Strategies of Treatment of Atrial Fibrillation (STAF) trial and The Rate Control versus Electrical Cardioversion for Persistent Atrial Fibrillation (RACE) trial selected only patients with persistent AF. In the case of RACE, all patients had been previously cardioverted and AF had returned. The Paroxysmal Atrial Fibrillation 2 (PAF 2) trial studied patients highly symptomatic from paroxysmal AF who were having implantation of a DDDR pacemaker and radiofrequency ablation of the atrioventricular junction. The patients in the Atrial Fibrillation Follow-up Investigation of Rhythm Management (AFFIRM) trial had a mixture of the persistent and paroxysmal (predominantly persistent) forms of AF as their qualifying episodes.

B. Therapies Used

The therapies used in either strategy were predominantly pharmacological in all five trials. In PIAF, amiodarone was the antiarrhythmic drug used. The other trials used a variety of antiarrhythmic drugs including amiodarone, sotalol, and class I antiarrhythmic drugs, although amiodarone was the drug most frequently used in all cases. Electrical cardioversion was used in the rhythm-control strategy in all trials except PAF 2. In RACE, there was a prescribed sequence for electrical cardioversion and change of antiarrhythmic drug therapy that was dependent on the time from the last cardioversion to recurrence of atrial fibrillation. As mentioned above, all patients in PAF 2 had a DDDR pacemaker and radiofrequency ablation of the atrioventricular junction. Patients were then randomized to receive antiarrhythmic drug or no antiarrhythmic drug. That is, antiarrhythmic drug therapy was added to a background of nonpharmacological heart rate control (atrioventricular junction ablation and a pacemaker). In the other trials, beta blockers, diltiazem, verapamil, and digitalis—alone or in combination—were used to achieve rate control. Only a small number of patients in the trials other than PAF 2 had a pacemaker and radiofrequency ablation of the atrioventricular junction. All the trials extensively used anticoagulation with oral anticoagulants, according to published guidelines. In PIAF, which had the shortest follow-up, anticoagulation was supposed to be continued in all patients throughout the study unless a contraindication to its use developed. In the other trials, discontinuation of oral anticoagulants was allowed according to published guidelines for antithrombotic therapy in atrial fibrillation. In

Table 1 An Overview of Published Randomized Trials of Rhythm Control *vs.* Heart Rate Control in the Management of Atrial Fibrillation

	PIAF	PAF2	AFFIRM	RACE	STAF
Name of trial	Pharmacological Intervention in Atrial Fibrillation	Paroxysmal Atrial Fibrillation 2	Atrial Fibrillation Follow-up Investigation of Rhythm Management	Rate Control vs. Electrical Cardioversion for Persistent Atrial Fibrillation	Strategies of Treatment of Atrial Fibrillation
Number of subjects enrolled	252	141	4060	522	200
Duration of follow-up	1.0 years	1.3 years	3.5 years	2.3 years	1.7 years
Patients' characteristics	60 years old; 92% male; 50% hypertension and 23% coronary artery disease; 16% no heart disease; few CHF	68 years old; 42% male; 30% hypertension and 16% coronary artery disease; 35% no heart disease; few CHF	70 years old; 61% male; 71% hypertension and 38% coronary artery disease; 13% no heart disease; 9% CHF	68 years old; 63% male; 49% hypertension and 27% coronary artery disease; 21% no heart disease; half CHF	65 years old; 64% male; 63% hypertension and 44% coronary artery disease; 11% no heart disease; 46% CHF
Characteristics of AF	Persistent 7 days to 1 year	Paroxysmal; severely symptomatic	Persistent ($\geq$69%) & paroxysmal	Persistent; median 32 days; recurrent after ECV	Persistent > 4 weeks
Rhythm-control therapies used	Amiodarone; ECV	Amiodarone; propafenone, flecainide; sotalol; ECV not allowed	Amiodarone; sotalol; propafenone; other class I; ECV; few non-pharmacological	Sotalol; flecainide/ propafenone, amiodarone; ECV (prescribed sequence)	Amiodarone; propafenone; flecainide; ECV

Rate control therapies used	Diltiazem; beta blockers; digitalis; AV junction RF ablation	AV junction RF ablation	Beta blockers; diltiazem; verapamil; digitalis; AV junction RF ablation	Beta blockers; diltiazem; verapamil; digitalis; AV junction RF ablation	Beta blockers; diltiazem; verapamil; digitalis; AV junction RF ablation
Oral anticoagulant use	Continued for duration of study	Discontinuation for SR permitted by guidelines	Discontinuation for SR permitted by guidelines	Discontinuation for SR permitted by guidelines	Discontinuation for SR permitted by guidelines
Primary endpoints	Proportion symptomatically improved	Development of permanent AF	Death	Composite of clinical events	Composite of clinical events
Other endpoints	QoL; functional capacity; hospitalization; adverse drug effects; bleeding	QoL; echo measurements; worsening CHF; hospitalization; bleeding	Composite of clinical events; QoL; functional capacity; bleeding; hospitalization; adverse drug effects; cost	Individual components of the composite; QoL; bleeding; cost	Individual components of the composite; QoL; echo measurements; worsening heart failure; bleeding
Summary of results	No difference in primary endpoint and QoL; rhythm = slightly better functional capacity; rate = fewer hospitalizations and adverse drug effects	Rhythm = less permanent AF; no difference in QoL & echo; rate = less worsening CHF and fewer hospitalizations	No difference in primary endpoint (trend favors rate) and QoL; rate = fewer hospitalizations and adverse drug effects; rhythm = slightly better functional capacity	Rate not inferior on primary endpoint; no difference in QoL; rate = fewer hospitalizations and adverse drug effects	No difference in primary endpoint and all secondary endpoints; rate = fewer hospitalizations

Key: AF, Atrial fibrillation; AV, atrioventricular; CHF, congestive heart failure (New York Heart Association class ≥II); ECV, electrical cardioversion; QoL, quality of life perceived by patient (questionnaire); RF, radiofrequency; SR, sinus rhythm.

aggregate, however, anticoagulation was used less in the rhythm-control strategy in all of these trials.

C. Mortality Results

The five trials varied considerably in size (number of subjects randomized) and the length of time over which the patients were followed (Table 1). Careful consideration of the duration of follow-up is needed in discussing some endpoints. For example, the average follow-up of the 4060 patients in the AFFIRM trial was 3.5 years. The number of patients enrolled in the other trials was considerably smaller, and the duration of follow-up was shorter. This difference in duration of follow-up is important, for example, in pooling events such as death, because in AFFIRM, the difference in mortality between the two strategies did not begin to emerge until almost 2 years after randomization (Fig. 1) (7). Thus the other trials, with average follow-up of less than 2 years, probably contribute very little to an understanding of the impact of the two strategies on mortality. Nevertheless, the result of pooling the data on mortality from all four trials enrolling similar patients is illustrated in Figure 2, which is a meta-analysis of the combined nominal (nonactuarial) mortality from the four trials that recruited a similar type of patient. In this analysis, it can be seen that the trials other than AFFIRM

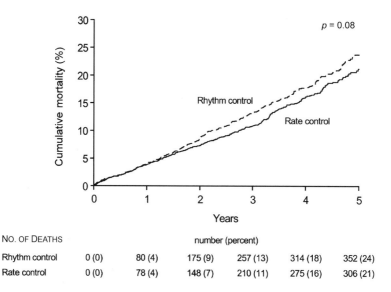

NO. OF DEATHS			number (percent)			
Rhythm control	0 (0)	80 (4)	175 (9)	257 (13)	314 (18)	352 (24)
Rate control	0 (0)	78 (4)	148 (7)	210 (11)	275 (16)	306 (21)

Figure 1   Total mortality in the AFFIRM trial by intention to treat. (From Ref. 7.)

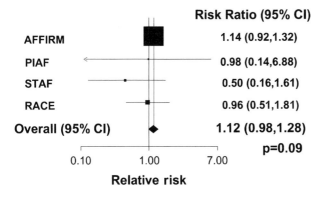

Figure 2 Meta-analysis of the nominal mortality rate in the four trials enrolling primarily elderly patients with persistent AF. The squares illustrate the point estimate of the hazard ratios for the individual trials and their size reflects the number of subjects in each trial. The horizontal lines depict the 95% confidence intervals of each point estimate. The diamond is the overall point estimate and its 95% confidence interval for the hazard ratio calculated by pooling the data.

contribute little to this endpoint (total mortality), partly because of their smaller size but also partly because of their shorter follow-up (see Fig. 1). Long-term follow-up is important in trials of management in AF because this arrhythmia is often treated for years and even decades.

D. Other Results

None of these five trials with perhaps one exception demonstrated any clear superiority of the rhythm-control strategy (Table 1). With respect to most results, no significant difference was noted between the two treatment strategies. In the PIAF trial, it was noted that patients in the rhythm-control group could walk further on a 6-min walk test (5). However, the difference was about a 10% change. In AFFIRM, the other trial that did 6-min walk tests, there was a similar small increase in the distance walked by patients assigned to the rhythm-control strategy (11). Thus, the rhythm-control strategy may offer superior physical functional capability. It might be expected that such an effect on functional capacity might be even greater in those with disabling symptoms, who were underrepresented in most of these trials. The rate-control approach is superior to the rhythm-control approach with respect to need for subsequent hospitalization and adverse drug effects. Hospitalization has important implications with respect to cost. Several of the trials measured patient-perceived quality of life, and in all cases there was no difference between the two strategies, although quality of life improved over time in both strategies. It is interesting that improvement in quality of life over time was greatest in the PAF 2 trial (6). That trial is different from the other four trials because it enrolled severely symptomatic patients. It is noteworthy in PAF 2 that attempting to control rhythm with antiarrhythmic drugs did not improve patient-perceived quality of life over that obtained with rate control alone (pacemaker and atrioventricular junction ablation). However, in PAF 2, the attempt to control rhythm with antiarrhythmic drugs was not very successful, as judged by the actuarial proportion of patients who developed permanent AF (6).

Figure 3 presents the pooled nominal incidence of thrombotic stroke in the four remaining trials after excluding the PAF 2 patients. After death, the next most frequent major clinical endpoint was thrombotic stroke; this event was more frequent with the rhythm-control approach. This event (thrombotic stroke) occurred at about one-third the rate of death itself. The absolute difference was small (3.4 vs. 4.1%, rate vs. rhythm) and the hazard ratio was not significant, although it (1.63; $p = 0.20$) was the largest point estimate seen among hazard ratios for the major clinical events. Major hemorrhage occurred at about the same nominal frequency as thrombotic stroke and was more frequent in the rate-control approach (4.9 vs. 4.5%, rate vs. rhythm; HR 0.92, 95% CI 0.72 to 1.18). To some degree these findings reflect the differential use of oral anticoagulants in the two treatment strategies (Table 1),

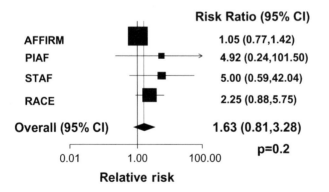

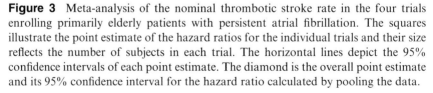

Figure 3 Meta-analysis of the nominal thrombotic stroke rate in the four trials enrolling primarily elderly patients with persistent atrial fibrillation. The squares illustrate the point estimate of the hazard ratios for the individual trials and their size reflects the number of subjects in each trial. The horizontal lines depict the 95% confidence intervals of each point estimate. The diamond is the overall point estimate and its 95% confidence interval for the hazard ratio calculated by pooling the data.

where oral anticoagulants was discontinued more frequently in the rhythm-control strategy (7–9). Major bleeding complications occurred mainly when the International Normalized Ratio (INR) exceeded 3.0 (7,8). Accordingly, it could be argued that an antithrombotic therapy that is safer and easier to use than oral anticoagulants would negate the counterbalanced risk of thrombotic stroke (favors rate control) and risk of major hemorrhage (favors rhythm control) that was observed. If there were a safe and convenient antithrombotic therapy, it would have been equally within the two strategies.

The least frequent major clinical events were intracerebral hemorrhage (0.9 vs. 0.8%, rate vs. rhythm) and systemic embolus (0.5% in each group). The event rates for intracerebral hemorrhage and systemic embolus are too low to say much and point estimates of the risk ratios are not presented here.

III. BRIEF SUMMARY OF UNPUBLISHED TRIALS AND TRIALS IN PROGRESS

One other trial comparing the strategy of rhythm control to the strategy of rate control in the management of AF has been published as an abstract (11). That trial is different from the others because it included an entirely different type of patient. Specifically, the patients in that trial had rheumatic heart disease and most had had a mitral valve procedure. The study population was much younger, and it included a higher proportion of women. It was done primarily in New Delhi. There were three treatment groups in this trial: rate control with open-label diltiazem, rhythm control with amiodarone and electrical cardioversion, and a placebo matching amiodarone with electrical cardioversion. There were only 48 patients in each of the three groups. It is not possible to comment on the results of this trial without further information, partly because the authors chose to combine the last two groups and compare them to the diltiazem-treated patients (12).

Another large trial [the Atrial Fibrillation and Congestive Heart Failure (AF-CHF) Trial] is currently being conducted (13), comparing the two strategies (rate vs. rhythm) in patients with reduced systolic function (left ventricular ejection fraction < 0.35) and a history of CHF. In many ways, AF-CHF is similar to the AFFIRM trial, but only amiodarone, dofetilide, and sotalol, in a very restricted way, are being used for rhythm control and warfarin is not discontinued unless a contraindication develops. The primary endpoint of the AF-CHF trial is cardiovascular mortality, but total mortality is a secondary endpoint. The trial aims to enroll 1450 patients and an average follow-up of over 3 years is planned. The results of AF-CHF will not be available until 2006. A second large trial has just begun in Japan, where some physicians believe pathophysiology of AF to be different (more vagally mediated AF), and the drugs used are different than they are in North America and Europe (personal communication, Professor S. Ogawa).

IV. CLINICAL IMPLICATIONS OF THE PUBLISHED TRIALS

The integration of the information from this recent spate of randomized clinical trials into the overall management of AF is challenging and important. Although the trial results are remarkable consistent, they can be over-interpreted. The basic conclusion from these trials is that the rate-control strategy is a perfectly acceptable primary therapy for the types of patients enrolled in these trials. Until now, the rate-control approach has been considered a "second best," or alternative, to rhythm control when the latter approach has been unsuccessful. However, it should not now be concluded that all such patients should be started with the rate-control approach, any more than it was previously thought by many that all patients should start with the rhythm-control approach. It is still necessary to individualize initial therapy for each patient. It can be concluded, however, that the trials support the concept that the primary purpose of rhythm-management therapy in such patients is relief of symptoms (anticoagulation cannot be stopped). Therefore one potential approach for patients such as those enrolled in these trials is to start with rate control and then reassess for symptoms and adverse drug effects. When symptoms persist, an attempt at rhythm control should be made. In the latter case, there is continued need for better and safer rhythm-control therapies, either pharmacological or nonpharmacological. When a physician and patient choose to start with the rhythm-control strategy, there should be no hesitation to switch to the rate-control strategy when the former is not going well. Finally, when long-term therapy is needed the increased mortality after 2 years of therapy in the AFFIRM trial mandates careful monitoring for adverse drug effects in patients being treated with the rhythm-control approach.

In making clinical decisions using these trial results, it is also important to consider the generalizability of the trials with respect to two aspects of the trials: the types of patients who are underrepresented in them and the therapies used. For example, in the case of patients underrepresented in the trials, there are few younger patients with little or no heart disease in these trials and not very many with CHF and poor ventricular systolic function. The results of the completed trials should not be generalized to subsets of patients who were not included or included in only small numbers. Second, the results should not be generalized to therapies, pharmacological or nonpharmacological, that were not used or infrequently used in the completed trials. This preclusion about generalizability includes drugs other than amiodarone, sotalol, and propafenone and newer nonpharmacological therapies, such as pulmonary vein isolation. If a highly effective therapy with no adverse effects were available, the results of these trials might have been quite different. Finally, the importance of continuous antithrombotic therapy, regardless of the rhythm-management approach, is emphasized by these trials. Effective and simple alternatives to oral anticoagulants would be welcome.

Some of the next areas for research in the management of atrial fibrillation include extension of the comparison of the rate-control strategy to the rhythm-control strategy to other populations not studied thus far. As mentioned above, this is already under way. Furthermore, now that rate control has been elevated to a primary therapy, more information is needed on how to accomplish it effectively. More research is also need on alternatives to warfarin for antithrombotic therapy and on development of more effective and safer therapies, both pharmacological and nonpharmacological, for rhythm control.

V. CONCLUSIONS

A more coherent picture of the role of the rate-control strategy vs. the rhythm-control strategy in the management of AF is beginning to emerge with the recent completion of five published trials that examined this issue. In aggregate, these trials have failed to confirm the expected superiority of the rhythm-control approach. Instead, they have demonstrated that rate control is an underappreciated primary therapy for AF in many patients. The trials have also underscored the importance of continued anticoagulation in high-risk patients, even when it is felt that rhythm control has been achieved. More research is needed to build on these concepts.

REFERENCES

1. Wyse DG. Selection of endpoints in atrial fibrillation studies. J Cardiovasc Electrophysiol 2002; 13(suppl):S47–S52.
2. Miller MR, McNamara RL, Segal JB, Kim N, Robinson KA, Goodman SN, Powe NR, Bass EP. Efficacy of agents for pharmacological conversion of atrial fibrillation and subsequent maintenance of sinus rhythm: a meta-analysis of clinical trials. J Fam Pract 2000; 49:1033–1046.
3. Flaker GC, Blackshear JL, McBride R, Kronmal RA, Halperin JL, Hart RG. Antiarrhythmic drug therapy and cardiac mortality in atrial fibrillation. J Am Coll Cardiol 1992; 20:527–532.

4. Connolly SC. Preventing stroke in patients with atrial fibrillation: current treatments and new concepts. Am Heart J 2003; 145:430–437.

5. Hohnloser SH, Kuck K-H, Lilienthal J, for the PIAF Investigators. Rhythm or rate control in atrial fibrillation—Pharmacologic Intervention in Atrial Fibrillation (PIAF): a randomized trial. Lancet 2000; 356:1789–1794.

6. Brignole M, Menozzi C, Gasparini M, Bongiorni MG, Botto GL, Ometto R, Alboni P, Bruna C, Vincenti A, Verlato R, for the PAF 2 investigators. An evaluation of the strategy of maintenance of sinus rhythm by antiarrhythmic drug therapy after ablation and pacing therapy in patients with paroxysmal atrial fibrillation. Eur Heart J 2002; 23:892–900.

7. The AFFIRM investigators. A comparison of rate control and rhythm control in patients with atrial fibrillation. N Engl J Med 2002; 347:1825–1833.

8. Van Gelder IC, Hagens VE, Bosker HA, Kingma JH, Camp O, Kingma T, Said SA, Darmanata JI, Timmermans AJ, Tijessen JG, Crijns HJ, for the RACE investigators. A comparison of rate control and rhythm control in patients with recurrent persistent atrial fibrillation. New Engl J Med 2002; 347:1834–1840.

9. Carlsson L, Miketic S, Windeler J, Cuneo A, Haun S, Micus S, Walter S, Tebbe U, for the STAF investigators. Randomized trial of rate-control versus rhythm-control in persistent atrial fibrillation: the Strategies of Treatment of Atrial Fibrillation (STAF) trial. J Am Coll Cardiol 2003; 41:1690–1696.

10. Go AS, Hylek EM, Phillips KA, Chang Y, Henault LE, Selby JV, Singer DE. Prevalence of diagnosed atrial fibrillation in adults. National implications for rhythm management and stroke prevention: the AnTicoagulation and Risk Factors In Atrial Fibrillation (ATRIA) study. JAMA 2001; 285:2370–2375.

11. Chung Mk, Sherman D, Shemanski D, for the AFFIRM Investigators. Effect of rate versus rhythm control strategies on the functional status of patients in the Atrial Fibrillation Follow-up Investigation of Rhythm Management (AFFIRM) study. Submitted.

12. Vora AM, Goyal VS, Naik AM, Lokhandwala YY, Gupta A, Karnad DR, Kulkarni HL, Singh B. Maintenance of sinus rhythm by amiodarone is superior to ventricular rate control in rheumatic atrial fibrillation: a blinded placebo-controlled study [abstr]. Pacing Clin Electrophysiol 2001; 24:546.

13. The AF-CHF Investigators. Rationale and design of a study assessing treatment strategies of atrial fibrillation in patients with heart failure: the Atrial Fibrillation and Congestive Heart Failure (AF-CHF) trial. Am Heart J 2002; 144:597–607.

6
Strategies for Rate Control

Andrew E. Epstein
The University of Alabama at Birmingham, Birmingham, Alabama, U.S.A.

Atrial fibrillation (AF) can be managed by either a rate-control or a rhythm-control strategy. For patients at risk for stroke, anticoagulation with warfarin is clearly indicated. The rationale for using a rate-control strategy as first-line therapy has been confirmed by the concordant results of the Pharmacologic Intervention in Atrial Fibrillation (PIAF) trial (1), the Strategies of Treatment of Atrial Fibrillation (STAF) trial (2), the Rate Control versus Electrical Cardioversion (RACE) trial (3), and the Atrial Fibrillation Follow-up Investigation of Rhythm Management (AFFIRM) trial (4). For patients with minimal or asymptomatic atrial fibrillation, a rate-control strategy is eminently reasonable.

I. RATIONALE FOR A RATE-CONTROL STRATEGY (TABLE 1)

In the PIAF trial, 252 patients with recent-onset AF (7 to 360 days, average 110 days) were randomly assigned to a rate-control strategy with diltiazem or a rhythm-control strategy with amiodarone plus electrical cardioversion as necessary (1). At 1 year follow-up, 56% of patients receiving amiodarone were in sinus rhythm vs. 10% of controls ($p < 0.001$). Rate- and rhythm-control management strategies produced similar improvements in symptoms and quality of life. Patients in the rhythm-control group performed better on 6 min walk tests. Hospitalizations and adverse events occurred more frequently in patients receiving amiodarone.

The STAF trial was a pilot study to determine whether a larger trial might show that a rhythm-control strategy would improve outcome of a

Table 1 Overview of Randomized Clinical Trials Comparing Rate-Control and Rhythm-Control Strategies to Manage Atrial Fibrillation

Trial	Hypothesis/Objective	Entry criteria	Treatments	Outcomes	Conclusions
AFFIRM (4)	Compare survival with rate-control and rhythm-control strategies for managing AF.	65 years of age, or <65 years of age with a risk factor for stroke or death.	Rate control with beta-blockers, calcium channel blockers, digoxin, and combinations. Rhythm control with class I and III antiarrhythmic drugs.	Similar survival in rate-control and rhythm-control arms.	1. A rhythm-control strategy offers no survival advantage over a rate-control strategy. 2. Anticoagulation should be continued in high-risk patients such as those in the AFFIRM trial with a high risk for stroke, since the majority of strokes occurred after warfarin had been stopped or when anticoagulation was subtherapeutic.
PIAF (1)	Compare outcomes with rate- and rhythm-control strategies for managing AF.	AF 7–360 days in duration.	Rate control with diltiazem vs. rhythm control with amiodarone plus electrical cardioversion if necessary.	Better 6-min walk but higher hospitalization and adverse event rates in rhythm-control group. Quality of life same for both groups.	1. Rate- and rhythm-control strategies provide similar improvement is symptoms and quality of life. 2. Rhythm control improves exercise capacity at a cost of need for cardioversion, adverse effects, and more frequent hospitalization.

Study	Objective	Inclusion criteria	Intervention	Results	Conclusions
RACE (3)	Ventricular rate control is not inferior to maintenance of sinus rhythm for the treatment of AF as assessed by composite endpoint of death from cardiovascular causes, heart failure, thromboembolic complications, bleeding, pacemaker implantation, and serious adverse antiarrhythmic drug events.	Persistent AF after a previous electrical cardioversion; anticoagulation not contraindicated.	Rate control vs. electrical cardioversion as needed in setting of therapy with class IC or III antiarrhythmic drugs.	No difference in composite primary endpoint.	1. Rate control is not inferior to rhythm control for the prevention of death and morbidity from cardiovascular causes. 2. Rate control may be appropriate therapy with persistent AF after electrical cardioversion.
STAF (2)	Compare composite endpoint of death, cerebrovascular events, systemic embolism, and cardiopulmonary resuscitation in patients with AF treated with a rate- vs. rhythm-control strategy.	AF >4 weeks, left atrial size >45 mm, CHF NYHA class >II, LVEF <45%, >1 prior cardioversion with AF recurrence.[a]	Rate control with AV-node blocking agents. Rhythm control with cardioversion followed by antiarrhythmic drug therapy.	No difference in composite primary endpoint.	1. No difference in primary endpoint. 2. Maintenance of sinus rhythm was low, 23% after 3 years, despite repeated cardioversions and antiarrhythmic therapy. 3. Almost all events occurred in AF.

[a] Inclusion criteria in Carlsson J, Neuzner J, Rosenberg YD. Therapy for atrial fibrillation: rhythm control versus rate control. PACE 2000; 23:891–902.
Key: AF, atrial fibrillation; AFFIRM, Atrial Fibrillation Follow-up Investigation of Rhythm Management study; PIAF, Pharmacologic Intervention in Atrial Fibrillation study; RACE, Rate control versus Electrical Cardioversion for Persistent Atrial Fibrillation study; STAF, Strategies of Treatment of Atrial Fibrillation pilot study.

primary composite endpoint including death, cerebrovascular events, systemic embolism, and cardiopulmonary resuscitation compared to a rate-control strategy in patients with AF (2). Patients with AF were randomized to either a rhythm-control (cardioversion followed by antiarrhythmic drug therapy) or rate-control strategy. At 1- and 3-year follow-up, only 40 and 23% of patients assigned to the rhythm-control strategy were in sinus rhythm. There was no difference in achievement of the primary endpoint in the two groups.

The RACE trial was designed to determine whether a rate-control strategy to manage persistent AF after a previous electrical cardioversion was not inferior to a rhythm-control strategy (3). Patients in the rhythm-control group underwent serial cardioversions and received antiarrhythmic drugs and anticoagulation. The goal for rate control was a resting heart rate <100 beats per minute (bpm). Over 90% of patients in both groups had a risk factor for stroke. At a mean follow-up of 2.3 years, 39% of patients in the rhythm-control group and 10% of the patients in the rate-control group were in sinus rhythm. The frequency of the composite primary endpoint (cardiovascular death, heart failure, thromboembolic complications, bleeding, pacemaker implantation, and severe adverse antiarrhythmic drug effects) was 17% in the rate-control and 23% in the rhythm-control groups, respectively ($p = $ NS).

The AFFIRM trial involved 4060 patients with AF and a high risk for stroke (4). These individuals were either >65 years in age or had a risk factor for stroke including diabetes, hypertension, left ventricular hypertrophy, heart failure, a prior transient ischemic attack (TIA) or stroke, or left atrial enlargement. Patients were randomized to a rhythm-control or a rate-control strategy. Rhythm control to maintain sinus rhythm was attempted with at least two class I and/or III antiarrhythmic drugs. Amiodarone was used in 63% of patients in the rhythm-control arm at some point during the study. Rate control used standard drugs—including digoxin, beta-blockers, and calcium channel blockers—to slow the ventricular response. The goal was to have a heart rate of ≤80 bpm at rest and ≤110 bpm on a 6-min walk test. Warfarin was used for anticoagulation in both groups, and discontinuation was allowed in the rhythm-control group if sinus rhythm was maintained for at least 4 and preferably 12 consecutive weeks with antiarrhythmic drug therapy. At the 5-year follow-up, 63 and 35% of patients in their rhythm- and rate-control groups, respectively, were in sinus rhythm. Mortality rates at 5 years were 24 and 21%, respectively ($p = $ NS). The annual rate of ischemic stroke was approximately 1% in both groups, although it was slightly higher in the rhythm-control group. Most strokes occurred in patients who had either stopped warfarin or had sub-therapeutic International Normalized Ratios (INRs).

The PIAF, STAF, RACE, and AFFIRM trials showed that a rate-control strategy is an acceptable first alternative to the management of AF in patients with minimal or asymptomatic AF (1–4). Furthermore, attempts to maintain sinus rhythm were far from successful in the long term in any of the trials. The higher thromboembolic event rates in the rhythm-control arms of the RACE and AFFIRM trials attest to the importance of maintaining anticoagulation indefinitely (3,4). It is likely that either asymptomatic recurrences of AF or other factors are responsible for strokes in these patient, regardless of whether or not sinus rhythm is maintained.

II. FURTHER REASONS TO CONSIDER A RATE-CONTROL STRATEGY

There is evidence—as presented above—that survival, quality of life, and exercise tolerance are similar with rate- and rhythm-control strategies for patients with asymptomatic and minimally symptomatic AF; there is also a rationale for the avoidance antiarrhythmic drugs if possible (5–7). Specifically, antiarrhythmic drugs are associated with toxicities and expense that can be avoided if rate-control agents are used alone. Class IA antiarrhythmic drugs (quinidine, procainamide, and disopyramide) and class IC antiarrhythmic drugs (flecainide and propafenone) can all increase mortality, especially in patients with coronary artery disease (6,7). Both class IA and class III drugs (sotalol and dofetilide) can cause torsades de pointes ventricular tachycardia. As noted above, most of these agents are expensive.

III. METHODS OF RATE CONTROL

Primary methods for rate control include drug therapy, maintenance of sinus rhythm (discussed elsewhere, including antiarrhythmic drug therapy and the surgical or catheter-based Maze procedure), and ablation (Table 2). Atrioventricular (AV) junction ablation with pacemaker implantation can also achieve this goal. Drug therapy has the broadest application.

Beta-blockers and calcium channel blockers are accepted as front-line therapy for ventricular rate control in AF (8,9). These agents are effective for the management of new-onset and chronic AF as well as AF with an acute exacerbation and a rapid ventricular response.

For years, digitalis has been the drug of choice for managing AF, especially with rapid ventricular responses (10–12). Unfortunately, digitalis is ineffective in controlling the ventricular rate in the majority of active patients, because the primary mechanism of the drug effect is by the enhancement

Table 2 Outcomes of Therapy

	Rhythm control with antiarrhythmic drug therapy	Rate control				Catheter-Based maze procedure	Surgical maze procedure
		Digoxin	Beta-blockers	Calcium channel blockers	AV Junction ablation		
Symptom relief	Moderate	Moderate to neutral		Moderate	Yes	Yes	Yes
Chronotropic competence	Moderate	No		No	Moderate with rate responsive pacemaker	Yes	Yes
AV synchrony	Yes	No		No	No	Yes	Yes
Emboli prevented	No	No		No	No	Unknown	Yes
Survival	Equal to rate control	Neutral to detrimental		Equal to rhythm control	Probably neutral	Unknown	Good

of parasympathetic tone (12). Indeed, digitalis is most useful in patients with heart failure who are minimally active (9). On the other hand, beta-adrenergic blockers and calcium channel blockers are more effective in blunting the ventricular response during exercise (9,13,14). In addition, verapamil has been shown to prevent atrial remodeling and may thereby help maintain sinus rhythm in patients with paroxysmal AF (15).

Falk et al. have reviewed the use of digitalis in AF (12). These authors point out that, in the absence of congestive heart failure, digitalis preparations are not antirrrhythmic. Although digitalis affects both atrial tissue and the AV node, its predominant effect is indirect, mediated via the autonomic nervous system through vagal influences on the atrium and AV node. Although the effect of vagal stimulation in the atrium is to shorten refractoriness and increase the dispersion of refractoriness, digoxin's direct effect is to prolong atrial refractoriness and decrease the vulnerable zone for repetitive atrial depolarizations. The apparent paradox that digoxin has no effect on controlling the ventricular response in paroxysmal AF but controls the heart rate in chronic AF, especially in patients with heart failure, is explained by the high sympathetic tone that is incurred at the onset of AF. In contrast, beta-adrenergic blockers and calcium channel blockers blunt these adrenergic effects during a paroxysm.

A number of studies support the use of beta-adrenergic blockade and calcium channel blockade in managing AF (10,13,14). David et al. studied 28 patients with chronic AF (10). In these individuals, digoxin failed to prevent excessively rapid heart rates with exertion. However, the addition of timolol to digoxin therapy resulted in attenuation of the rapid ventricular response both at rest and during exercise. Compared to treatment with digoxin alone, the resting heart rate was reduced by timolol from 98 to 67 bpm at rest, and from 139 to 92 bpm during exercise. Lang et al. showed that verapamil (240 mg a day), with or without digoxin, in 52 patients with chronic AF decreased the heart rate at rest and during all levels of exercise. This effect was sustained for months. Furthermore, there was a marked improvement in the maximal effort capacity when compared to that during treatment with digoxin alone (13).

The above findings were confirmed by Farshi et al. (14). In this investigation, 12 patients with chronic AF and five standardized daily regimens—including digoxin 0.25 mg a day, diltiazem CD 240 mg a day, atenolol 50 mg a day, digoxin with diltiazem, and digoxin with atenolol—were tested. Not only were the baseline heart rates decreased in the diltiazem and atenolol groups, either with or without digoxin, but the maximal heart rates reached during exercise were similarly blunted. The study showed that digoxin and diltiazem as single agents were least effective in controlling the ventricular response in atrial fibrillation during daily activity. In contrast, the combination of digoxin with atenolol was most effective in controlling the heart rate both at rest and during exercise.

IV. OTHER DRUG THERAPIES FOR CONTROLLING THE VENTRICULAR RESPONSE

Not all patients can tolerate a beta-blocker due to pulmonary disease, heart failure, or bradycardia during sinus rhythm ("sick sinus syndrome"). Other agents can be tried as alternatives to diltiazem or beta-blockers, although blunting of the heart rate in sinus rhythm can also be problematic. Clonidine is one such agent (16,17). Roth et al. studied 18 stable patients with AF and a rapid ventricular response (16) who were randomized to receive either no antiarrhythmic therapy or clonidine 0.075 mg orally at baseline and after 2 hr if the heart rate did not decrease by at least 20%. Compared to patients in the control group, 8 of 9 patients receiving clonidine had heart rate decreases to below 100 bpm after clonidine, in contrast to 2 of 9 patients in the control group. The authors concluded that low-dose clonidine was an easy and effective treatment for patients with AF and a rapid ventricular response who were hemodynamically stable.

Simpson et al. confirmed these results (17). Forty patients with new-onset stable AF with a rapid ventricular response were randomized to receive digoxin, verapamil, or clonidine. The mean reduction in heart rate over 6 hr was 52 bpm in the digoxin group, 42 bpm in the verapamil group, and 44 bpm in the clonidine group. The authors concluded that clonidine was as effective as verapamil or digoxin in the management of acute atrial fibrillation.

Although not traditionally though of as rate-control agents, amiodarone and propafenone have been used to slow the ventricular response in atrial fibrillation (8,9). Both intravenous and oral amiodarone are efficacious for this indication (8,9). In intensive care unit settings, intravenous amiodarone may be especially useful for acute rate control and to achieve rapid loading in the event that the drug is to be used long-term (18). Peripheral administration should be avoided due to a high incidence of cellulitis. Propafenone has been used in part because of its beta-adrenergic blockade component.

V. ASSESSMENT OF RATE CONTROL

If a rate-control strategy is chosen for the management of AF, demonstration of the adequacy of drug therapy is important (19). A controlled ventricular response is maintained not only for symptom control but also to prevent tachycardia-mediated cardiomyopathy. Both Holter monitoring and exercise testing are alternatives for efficacy analysis. A 24-hr Holter monitor is ideal, since it allows patients to perform their usual activities and have their heart rate observed. Similarly, for patients who perform vigorous exercise and do not wish to wear a Holter monitor, an exercise test can be used to judge the ventricular response during exertion.

In clinical trials, the efficacy of rate control has been judged using 6-min walk tests. In the AFFIRM trial, the goal was to achieve a resting heart rate not higher than 80 bpm at rest and not over 110 bpm during a 6-min walk (4).

VI. SPECIAL DISEASE STATES

A number of conditions warrant special consideration for rate-control strategies. AF following open-heart surgery is common, occurring in up to 30% of patients. Perioperative AF and atrial flutter are associated with an increased risk of stroke as well as other morbidity and mortality (20,21). Although most perioperative AF and atrial flutter episodes are self-limited, others require aggressive management to either control the ventricular response or restore sinus rhythm. Anticoagulation has been recognized as an important component of therapy because of the risk of perioperative stroke.

Because hyperadrenergic tone is present in the perioperative period, beta-adrenergic blockers and calcium channel blockers are accepted as the mainstays of therapy for this condition (21). In general, either drug class is effective in controlling the rate. In one study, esmolol was shown to be as effective as diltiazem for controlling the ventricular response at 24 hr in patients who did not convert to sinus rhythm (22). Class IV drugs (diltiazem and verapamil) have also been shown to be effective in controlling the ventricular response in AF following open-heart surgery. As discussed above, both propafenone and amiodarone have also been used in the perioperative period, with similar results (21).

AF in patients with hypertrophic cardiomyopathy can be particularly devastating (23). In these individuals, ventricular hypertrophy and diastolic dysfunction limit ventricular filling in the absence of atrial transport. For many of these individuals, maintenance of sinus rhythm is imperative. On the other hand, for others, by simply controlling the rate and allowing more time for diastolic filling, symptoms can be markedly improved. Either beta-adrenergic blockers or calcium channel antagonists can be extremely effective.

AF that occurs in patients with hyperthyroidism is often particularly difficult to manage. The hyperadrenergic tone leads to extremely rapid ventricular responses, especially in young individuals. Because of the adrenergic component of the disease as well as concomitant heart failure and the potential salutary effects of beta-blockers on ventricular remodeling, beta-blockers are considered a mainstay of treatment (24).

Finally, mitral stenosis is a less common condition in modern medicine. As in patients with hypertrophic cardiomyopathy, intact atrial transport function is extremely important (25). Furthermore, because of limitations of transmitral flow, shortened diastole markedly impairs cardiac output. Thus, rate control is extremely important in these individuals. Digoxin, verapamil, and metoprolol have all been shown to be beneficial (25,26).

VII. NONPHARMACOLOGICAL OPTIONS FOR RATE CONTROL

A subset of patients cannot achieve rate control with pharmacological therapy. For these individuals, several options are available. First, ablation of the AV junction followed by pacemaker implantation has been shown to be extremely effective in decreasing symptoms (27). Furthermore, for patients with depressed left ventricular function, the ejection fraction improves with rate control (28). The latter is probably related to reversal of tachycardia-mediated cardiomyopathy (15,29). Although patients are rendered pacemaker-dependent with AV junction ablation, the improved quality of life and improvement of left ventricular function in many instances outweigh the cost of this therapy, both financially and physiologically.

For younger patients with AF that is extremely symptomatic and difficult to control and in whom AV junction ablation and pacemaker therapy is deemed undesirable, either the catheter-based or surgical Maze procedure are alternatives (30). The catheter management of AF is discussed elsewhere. In brief, either compartmentalization of the left atrium by the construction of linear ablation lines and/or isolation of the pulmonary veins can be effective. Similar physiological effects can be achieved with a surgical Maze procedure. Although time-tested and having greater efficacy than the catheter-based approach, the surgical method entails open heart surgery, entailing greater morbidity. In short, for young patients, especially those in whom rate control is problematic, a catheter-based approach to AF is reasonable.

Sinus node dysfunction may be considered an associated disease state. When it occurs in the setting of AF, the condition is described as the "brady-tachy syndrome." In these individuals, rate control may not be achievable without providing rate support with a pacemaker. Although dual-chamber pacing may decrease the risk of AF, the risk of stroke is unchanged (31,32).

Finally, and despite the results of the clinical trials reviewed, since patients with significant heart failure were not well represented, it is unknown whether a rhythm-control strategy may have special benefit for patients with congestive heart failure. Thus, the Atrial Fibrillation and Congestive Heart Failure (AF-CHF) trial has been initiated to address this large and ill population (33).

VIII. WHEN IS A RATE-CONTROL STRATEGY NOT DESIRABLE?

Patients with extremely symptomatic AF, especially if the rate cannot be controlled, are not candidates for continued rate-control management. In these individuals, the options are (1) restoration of sinus rhythm, (2) performance of a definitive procedure such as AV junction ablation with pacemaker implantation, or (3) a catheter-based or surgical Maze procedure. Although no clinical trial data are available, young patients with "lone AF" may also be better candidates for a rhythm-rather than a rate-control strategy. With continued paroxysms of AF, atrial remodeling may occur, both electrically and pathologically (15,29). In these individuals, maintenance of sinus rhythm with an antiarrhythmic drug may provide time to allow for either further progress in AF ablation technology to become more refined or continued drug therapy if that is acceptable to the patient.

IX. SUMMARY

Recent clinical trial data show that for a large proportion of patients with AF who either asymptomatic or minimally symptomatic, a rate-control strategy is acceptable. This approach leads to similar survival, quality of life, and exercise tolerance as does one directed at the restoration and maintenance of sinus rhythm. On the other hand, some patients do not tolerate AF well and are not candidates for a rate-control strategy. In these individuals, restoration and maintenance of sinus rhythm is desirable, either with antiarrhythmic drug therapy, surgical therapy, catheter-based therapy, or AV junctional ablation and pacemaker implantation. Regardless of the approach, in patients who have AF and a risk for thromboembolic events, warfarin should be continued indefinitely.

REFERENCES

1. Hohnloser SH, Kuck KH, Lilienthal J. Rhythm or rate control in atrial fibrillation—Pharmacological Intervention in Atrial Fibrillation (PIAF): a randomised trial. Lancet 2000; 356:1789–1794.

2. Carlsson J. Mortality and stroke rates in a trial of rhythm control versus rate control in atrial fibrillation: results from the STAF pilot phase (Strategies of Treatment of Atrial Fibrillation). J Am Coll Cardiol 2001; 38:603.

3. van Gelder IC, Hagens VE, Bosker HA, Kingma JH, Kamp O, Kingma T, Said SA, Darmanata JI, Timmermans AJM, Tijssen JGP, Crijns HJGM, for the Rate Control versus Electrical Cardioversion for Persistent Atrial Fibrillation Study Group. A comparison of rate control and rhythm control in patients with recurrent persistent atrial fibrillation. N Engl J Med 2002; 347:1834–1840.

4. The Atrial Fibrillation Follow-Up Investigation of Rhythm Management (AFFIRM) investigators. A comparison of rate control and rhythm control in patients with atrial fibrillation. N Engl J Med 2002; 347:1825–1833.

5. Flaker GC, Blackshear JL, McBride R, Kronmal RA, Halperin JL, Hart RG, on behalf of the Stroke Prevention in Atrial Fibrillation investigators. Antiarrhythmic drug therapy and cardiac mortality in atrial fibrillation. J Am Coll Cardiol 1992; 20:527–532.

6. Echt DS, Liebson PR, Mitchell LB, Peters RW, Obias-Manno D, Barker AH, Arensberg D, Baker A, Friedman L, Green HL, Huther ML, Richardson DW, and the CAST Investigators. Mortality and morbidity in patients receiving encainide, flecainide, or placebo: the Cardiac Arrhythmia Suppression Trial. N Engl J Med 1991; 324:781–788.

7. Epstein AE, Hallstrom AP, Rogers WJ, Liebson PR, Seals AA, Anderson JL, Cohen JD, Capone RJ, Wyse DG, for the CAST investigators. Mortality following ventricular arrhythmia suppression by encainide, flecainide, and moricizine after myocardial infarction: the original design concept of the Cardiac Arrhythmia Suppression Trial (CAST). JAMA 1993; 270:2451–2455.

8. Fuster V, Rydén LE, Asinger RW, Cannom DS, Crijns HJ, Frye RL, Halperin JL, Kay GN, Klein WW, Lévy S, McNamara RL, Prystowsky EN, Wann LS, Wyse DG. ACC/AHA/ESC guidelines for the management of patients with atrial fibrillation: executive summary: a report of the American College of Cardiology/American Heart Association Task Force on Practice Guidelines and the European Society of Cardiology Committee for Practice Guidelines and Policy Conferences (Committee to Develop Guidelines for the Management of Patients With Atrial Fibrillation). Circulation 2001; 104:2118–2150.

9. Segal JB, McNamara RL, Miller MR, Kim N, Goodman SN, Powe NR, Robinson K, Yu D, Bass EB. The evidence regarding the drugs used for ventricular rate control. J Fam Pract 2000; 49:47–59.

10. David D, Di Segni E, Klein HO, Kaplinsky E. Inefficacy of digitalis in the control of heart rate in patients with chronic atrial fibrillation: beneficial effect of an added beta-adrenergic blocking agent. Am J Cardiol 1979; 44:1378–1382.

11. Falk RH, Knowlton AA, Bernard SA, Gotlieb NE, Battinelli NJ. Digoxin for converting recent onset atrial fibrillation to sinus rhythm: a randomized, double-blinded trial. Ann Intern Med 1987; 106:503–506.

12. Falk RH, Leavitt JI. Digoxin for atrial fibrillation: a drug whose time has gone? Ann Intern Med 1991; 114:573–575.

13. Lang R, Klein HO, Weiss E, David D, Sareli P, Levy A, Guerrero J, Di Segni E,

Kaplinsky E. Superiority of oral verapamil therapy to digoxin in treatment of chronic atrial fibrillation. Chest 1983; 83:491–499.

14. Farshi R, Kistner D, Sarma JSM, Longmate JA, Singh BN. Ventricular rate control in chronic atrial fibrillation during daily activity and programmed exercise: a crossover open-label study of five drug regimens. J Am Coll Cardiol 1999; 33:304–310.

15. Gallagher MM, Obel OA, Camm AJ. Tachycardia-induced atrial myopathy: an important mechanism in the pathophysiology of atrial fibrillation? J Cardiovasc Electrophysiol 1997; 8:1065–1074.

16. Roth A, Kaluski E, Felner S, Heller K, Laniado S. Clonidine for patients with rapid atrial fibrillation. Ann Intern Med 1992; 116:388–390.

17. Simpson CS, Ghali WA, Sanfilippo AJ, Moritz S, Abdollah H. Clinical assessment of clonidine in the treatment of new-onset rapid atrial fibrillation: a prospective, randomized clinical trial. Am Heart J 2001; 142:e3.

18. Clemo HF, Wood MA, Gilligan DM, Ellenbogen KA. Intravenous amiodarone for acute heart rate control in the critically ill patient with atrial tachyar-rhythmias. Am J Cardiol 1998; 81:594–598.

19. Prystowsky EN. Management of atrial fibrillation: therapeutic operations and clinical decisions. Am J Cardiol ; 85:3D–11D.

20. Hogue CW, Hyder ML. Atrial fibrillation after cardiac operation: risks, mechanisms, and treatment. Ann Thorac Surg 2000; 69:300–306.

21. Maisel WH, Rawn JD, Stevenson WG. Atrial fibrillation after cardiac surgery. Ann Intern Med 2001; 135:1061–1073.

22. Mooss AN, Wurdeman RL, Mohiuddin SM, Reyes AP, Sugimoto JT, Scott W, Hilleman DE, Seyedroudbari A. Esmolol versus diltiazem in the treatment of postoperative atrial fibrillation/atrial flutter after open heart surgery. Am Heart J 2000; 140:176–180.

23. Spirto P, Seidman CD, McKenna WJ, Maron BJ. The management of hypertrophic cardiomyopathy. N Engl J Med 1997; 336:775–785.

24. Toft AD, Forfar JC. Atrial fibrillation in hyperthyroidism. Pathogenesis, incidence, and management. Intern Med 1982; 3:35–39.

25. Meisner JS, Keren G, Pajaro OE, Mani A, Strom JA, Frater RWM, Laniado S, Yellin EL. Atrial contribution to ventricular filling in mitral stenosis. Circulation 1991; 84:1469–1480.

26. Ahuja RC, Sinha N, Saran RK, Jain AK, Hasan M. Digoxin or verapamil or metoprolol for heart rate control in patients with mitral stenosis—a randomized cross-over study. Int J Cardiol 1989; 25:325–332.

27. Wood MA, Brown-Mahoney C, Kay GN, Ellenbogen KA. Clinical outcomes after ablation and pacing therapy for atrial fibrillation. a meta-analysis. Circulation 2000; 101:1138–1144.

28. Kay GN, Ellenbogen KA, Giudici M, Redfield MM, Jenkins LS, Mianulli M, Wilkoff B, and the APT Investigators. The Ablate and Pace Trial: a prospective study of catheter ablation of the AV conduction system and permanent pacemaker implantation for treatment of atrial fibrillation. J Intervent Cardiac Electrophysiol 1998; 2:121–135.

29. Wijffels MCEF, Kirchhof CJHJ, Dorland R, Power J, Allessie MA. Electrical remodeling due to atrial fibrillation in chronically instrumented conscious goats. Roles of neurohumoral changes, ischemia, atrial stretch, and high rate of electrical activation. Circulation 1997; 96:3710–3720.

30. Cannom DS. Atrial fibrillation: nonpharmacologic approaches. Am J Cardiol 2000; 85:25D–35D.

31. Lamas GA, Lee KL, Sweeney MO, Silverman R, Leon A, Yee R, Marinchak RA, Flaker G, Schron E, Orav EJ, Hellkamp AS, Goldman L, for the Mode Selection Trial in Sinus-Node Dysfunction. Ventricular pacing or dual-chamber pacing for sinus-node dysfunction. N Engl J Med 2002; 346:1854–1862.

32. Connolly SJ, Kerr CR, Gent M, Roberts RS, Yusuf S, Gillis AM, Sami MH, Talajic M, Tang ASL, Klein GJ, Lau C, Newman DM, for the Canadian Trial of Physiologic Pacing Investigators. Effects of physiologic pacing versus ventricular pacing on the risk of stroke and death due to cardiovascular causes. N Engl J Med 2000; 342:1385–1391.

33. The AF-CHF Investigators. Rationale and design of a study assessing treatment strategies of atrial fibrillation in patients with heart failure: the Atrial Fibrillation and Congestive Heart Failure (AF-CHF) trial. Am Heart J 2002; 144:597–607.

7

Atrial Fibrillation and Anticoagulation

Greg C. Flaker and Mohammed Murtaza
University of Missouri, Columbia, Missouri, U.S.A.

I. INTRODUCTION

Anticoagulation plays an important role in the management of patients with atrial fibrillation (AF). In this chapter we review studies that have emphasized the importance of this form of therapy and introduce new therapies for the future.

The association of stroke with AF has been known for years, particularly in patients with mitral stenosis. In the Framingham Heart Study, the risk of stroke in patients with AF and rheumatic heart disease was 18 times higher than in patients without AF and without rheumatic heart disease (1). Several autopsy studies in patients with rheumatic heart disease and stroke frequently revealed an intracardiac thrombus (2,3). Clinicians understood that thrombus could form in the left atrium or left ventricle, dislodge, and cause distal embolization. A number of retrospective studies published between 1952 and 1974, mainly in patients who had experienced stroke, demonstrated a reduction in stroke and systemic embolism with warfarin derivatives (4–8). Thus, although not conclusively proven, the use of warfarin for patients with rheumatic valvular heart disease and AF was generally accepted in the 1980s (9).

The use of warfarin for stroke prevention in AF without rheumatic heart disease was more controversial. Again, the Framingham study demonstrated that patients with nonvalvular atrial fibrillation had a stroke risk of approximately 5% per year, which was nearly five times the risk of patients matched for age and sex without AF (1). Although several retrospective studies demonstrated a reduction in stroke risk with warfarin in AF with a wide range of heart diseases (10,11), the use of warfarin for stroke prevention in AF without associated mitral stenosis was low in the 1980s.

II. RANDOMIZED CLINICAL TRIALS

From 1989 to 1999, a total of 16 randomized clinical trials involving nearly 10,000 patients with nonvalvular or, more accurately, nonrheumatic AF demonstrated the unequivocal efficacy of warfarin in preventing stroke when compared with placebo (relative risk reduction 62%) or compared with aspirin (relative risk reduction 36%). Aspirin was more effective than placebo (relative risk reduction 22%). Low-dose warfarin was less effective in stroke prevention (12). It is instructive to review the major findings of these randomized clinical trials.

A. The Copenhagen Atrial Fibrillation Aspirin Anticoagulation (AFASAK) Study

AFASAK (13) randomized 1007 patients into one of three treatment groups: (1) oral anticoagulation with warfarin; (2) aspirin at 75 mg per day; or (3) placebo. Patients were followed for up to 2 years. The aspirin and placebo arms were double-blinded; the warfarin treatment arm was unblinded. During this study, warfarin anticoagulation was monitored by a prothrombin time ratio. The goal for this ratio was 1.5 to 2, which is roughly translated into an International Normalized Ratio (INR) of 2.8 to 4.2 today. Only 42% of patients were maintained in this range throughout the study. Levels below an estimated INR of 2.4 were obtained 26% of the time. In addition, 38% of the warfarin-treated patients withdrew from this study.

Despite the high dropout rate and the frequent subtherapeutic level of anticoagulation, the risk of stroke, transient ischemic attack, or systemic embolism was 2% in the warfarin-treated patients (95% CI 0.6 to 4.8%) vs. 5.5% in both the aspirin- and placebo-treated patients (95% CI 2.9 to 9.4%, $p < 0.05$). The 5.5% risk per year of events in the placebo-treated patients was similar to the stroke rate of 5% per year in the Framingham study.

Bleeding was more common in the warfarin-treated patients, with 6% of these patients having a bleeding-related side effect, as compared to only 1% in the aspirin group and none in the placebo-treated patients.

The AFASAK study was the first prospective study to demonstrate the beneficial effects of chronic warfarin therapy. It also suggested that anti-platelet therapy at a dose of 75 mg per day was not effective for stroke prevention.

B. The Stroke Prevention in Atrial Fibrillation I (SPAF I) Study

The second major multicenter trial was SPAF I, a randomized study comparing warfarin or aspirin to placebo for the prevention of stroke or systemic embolism in patients with nonrheumatic AF (14,15). Eligible patients were categorized as being warfarin-eligible (group 1) or warfarin-ineligible (group 2). Patients with gastrointestinal or intracranial bleeding were randomized in group 2, as were patients who were unwilling to receive warfarin. During the initial phase of this study, patients over the age of 75 were automatically excluded from group 1. Later, this age restriction was eliminated. A variety of other reasons were given for assignment to the warfarin-ineligible (group 2) arm. These included patient or physician refusal of warfarin therapy and inability to obtain adequate follow-up for anti-coagulation monitoring.

Group 1 patients were randomized to receive warfarin, aspirin, or placebo. Warfarin doses were adjusted to achieve a prothrombin time of between 1.3 and 1.8 times control values which translated into an INR of 2 to 4.5. The aspirin dose was 325 mg per day.

After follow-up of 1330 randomized patients for a period of 1.3 years, the study was interrupted by the Data and Safety Monitoring Board because of a significant benefit of active therapy (warfarin or aspirin) over placebo. The rate of ischemic stroke and systemic embolism was substantially reduced with warfarin (2.3% per year) compared with placebo (7.4% per year). The risk reduction was 67%, (95% CI 27 to 85%, $p = 0.01$). The rate of ischemic stroke and systemic embolism was also reduced in the group 1 and 2 patients treated with aspirin (3.6% per year) compared with placebo (6.3% per year, $p = 0.02$). The risk reduction was 42%, (95% CI 9 to 63%, $p = 0.02$). Major bleeding complications occurred in 1.5% of warfarin-treated patients and 1.4% of aspirin-treated patients. Between 1.6 and 1.9% of placebo treated patients had major bleeding.

In SPAF, an events committee classified the type of stroke as presumed cardioembolic or noncardioembolic based on published guidelines. Members of the committee were blinded to the type of therapy received. Sixty percent of strokes in the placebo group were cardioembolic, lending support to the idea that a cardiac source in patients with AF was plausible. Interestingly, aspirin seemed to be more effective for strokes classified as noncardioembolic than for strokes considered to be cardioembolic (16).

Too few events occurred in the warfarin-versus-aspirin-treated arm of group 1, and the relative benefits of aspirin or warfarin could not be addressed by the SPAF I study, but this was the subject of a subsequent randomized trial, the SPAF II study (17).

C. SPAF II

The SPAF II study randomized 1100 patients with nonrheumatic AF to aspirin, 325 mg per day, or warfarin, with an INR maintained between 2 and 4.5. Patients were also stratified by age (<75 years in one group, ≥75 years in another group). The average follow-up was 3 years. Patients in SPAF I who were assigned to aspirin or warfarin were allowed to continue into SPAF II. A number of anticoagulation-eligible patients assigned to placebo or patients originally considered to be anticoagulation ineligible (assigned to either aspirin or placebo in SPAF I) were rerandomized to either aspirin or warfarin. These rerandomized patients composed 24% of the SPAF II population.

The findings of the SPAF II study were controversial. In patients under 75 years of age, the risk of ischemic stroke or systemic embolism was 1.9% per year with aspirin (95% CI 1.3 to 3.0) and 1.3% per year with warfarin (95% CI 0.8 to 2.2, $p = 0.24$). The risk of major bleeding was 0.9% with aspirin and 1.7% with warfarin ($p = 0.17$).

In contrast, patients 75 years of age or older had a higher event rate. Warfarin-treated patients had an event rate of stroke or systemic embolism of 3.6% per year (95% CI 2.1 to 6.0) compared with an event rate of 4.8% per year (95% CI 3.0 to 7.6, $p = 0.39$) on aspirin. Bleeding was more common in these older patients and was more common with warfarin than with aspirin. Major bleeding occurred in 1.6% of aspirin treated patients and in 4.2% of warfarin treated patients ($p = 0.04$). A high rate (1.8% per year) of intracranial bleeding occurred in SPAF II.

The SPAF II study concluded that warfarin was only modestly more effective than aspirin in stroke prevention in AF. A number of patients with AF could be identified who had an intrinsically low risk for stroke or systemic embolism, and these patients could be treated with aspirin The risk of ischemic stroke was higher in older patients, and risk of bleeding, particularly intracranial bleeding, was also higher. Increasing age, the number of pre-scribed medications (an index for increased comorbid conditions), and the intensity of anticoagulation were associated with increased bleeding (18).

D. The Boston Area Anticoagulation Trial for Atrial Fibrillation (BAATAF)

After SPAF II, additional studies supported the efficacy of warfarin in stroke prevention in AF. BAATAF (19) was a small trial involving 420 patients with nonrheumatic atrial fibrillation. Patients were randomized to receive warfarin or placebo, although the placebo-treated patients could receive aspirin on the advice of their personal physician. The use of aspirin was not randomized, but it was monitored. After a mean follow-up of 2.2 years, there were 13 strokes in the placebo arm (2.98% per year) and only 2 strokes in the warfarin group (0.41% per year). The risk reduction was 86%, (95% CI 51 to 96%, $p =$ 0.0022). Patients who received no aspirin and no warfarin had a yearly risk of stroke of 1.8%. Those who took less than 7 aspirin per week had a yearly risk of 2.8% and those who took at least 7 aspirin per week had a yearly risk of 4.1%. The efficacy of aspirin was not demonstrated in this nonrandomized assessment (20).

E. The Veterans Affairs Stroke Prevention in Nonrheumatic Atrial Fibrillation (SPINAF) Study, Canadian Atrial Fibrillation Anticoagulation (CAFA) Trial, and European Atrial Fibrillation Trial (EAFT)

Three other multicenter studies supported the use of warfarin in stroke prevention. The SPINAF study demonstrated a 79% risk reduction with warfarin compared to placebo ($p = 0.001$) after a follow-up of 1.75 years (21). The CAFA trial noted a relative risk reduction of 37% in warfarin-treated patients compared to placebo-treated patients (22). The study was stopped prematurely because of the positive findings of the previous studies. The relative risk reduction was similar to that of the other studies, and the lack of statistical significance ($p = 0.17$) was likely due to the premature termination of the study, with only 60% of the anticipated recruitment and 50% of the planned follow-up completed. Finally, the EAFT divided 1007 patients with nonrheumatic atrial fibrillation who had a recent transient ischemic attack (TIA) or minor ischemic stroke into two groups, those eligible for anti-coagulation and those not eligible for anticoagulation (23). After a mean follow-up of 2.3 years, the yearly risk of any stroke was 4% in warfarin-treated patients, 10% in all patients receiving aspirin, and 12% in any patient receiving placebo. Compared to placebo, warfarin was highly effective at preventing stroke (HR 0.34, 95% CI 0.20 to 0.57, $p < 0.001$). Aspirin was not effective at preventing stroke in these patients (HR 0.86, 95% CI 0.64 to 1.15, $p = 0.31$). Most strokes occurred with subtherapeutic INR values (24).

F. SPAF III

The SPAF I and SPAF II studies recognized the disutility of using warfarin. Anticoagulation with warfarin increases the risk of bleeding, especially in elderly patients. Aspirin was thought to be effective in stroke prevention in certain patients but not others. Four clinical and echocardiographic features were identied from the SPAF I and II studies that were helpful in identifying high-risk patients. These risk factors included being female and over 75 years of age, a history of a previous stroke, blood pressure greater than 160 mmHg, and a history of congestive heart failure or an echocardiographic fractional shortening of ≤25% (25). In these patients, the risk of stroke was greater than 5% per year, and this could justify placing them on warfarin, with an expected 2% per year risk of major hemorrhage. In SPAF III, these aspirin nonresponders were randomized to receive either standard or adjusted-dose warfarin with an INR of 2 to 3 or low-dose warfarin plus aspirin. The latter therapy recognized the benefit of aspirin in stroke prevention but also provided the hoped for added protection of warfarin, although at a low dose, which did not require monthly monitoring. In patients without these risk factors, the expected event rate was less than 2% per year. Based on an estimated 2% yearly risk of major bleeding on warfarin, these patients were offered aspirin.

The results of the SPAF III study did confirm that patients could be identified who have a low risk of stroke on aspirin. In these nonrandomized patients, the risk of stroke or systemic embolism was 1.1% per year in those without a history of hypertension. In patients with a history of hypertension, the yearly event rate was 3.6%, emphasizing the importance of hypertension management for stroke prevention in atrial fibrillation (26).

The randomized portion of the trial was stopped at an interim analysis after a mean follow-up of 1.1 years because of the favorable response to adjusted-dose warfarin. The risk of stroke or systemic embolism was 7.9% per year (95% CI 5.9 to 10.6%) in those on the combination therapy, compared with an event rate of 1.9% per year (95% CI 1.0 to 3.4%, $p < 0.0001$) in patients treated with adjusted-dose warfarin. This study reaffirmed the efficacy of adjusted-dose warfarin. Since most strokes in this study occurred with an INR of less than 2, it was recommended that if warfarin was used, an INR of 2 to 3 be used for stroke prevention. Aspirin was not effective in these high-risk patients, even when combined with low-dose warfarin.

III. HIGH-RISK GROUPS

The investigators of five randomized controlled trials (AFASAK, SPAF, BAATAF, CAFA, and SPINAF) analyzed the pooled data to identify patient features predictive of high or low risk and assessed the efficacy and risks of antithrombotic therapy. These Atrial Fibrillation Investigators reported that the best predictors of risk for ischemic stroke were increasing age, a previous stroke or TIA, diabetes, and a history of hypertension. Patients with a previous stroke or TIA had a stroke risk of approximately 12% per year (27). The risk of stroke in patients with diabetes was 8 to 9% per year. In patients with hypertension, the risk of stroke was 5 to 6% per year. In patients with heart failure, the risk of stroke was 6 to 7% per year. They confirmed that warfarin therapy was associated with a dramatic reduction in stroke, with a relative risk reduction of 68%. The efficacy of aspirin was less, with a relative risk reduction of 23%.

Currently there are several published guidelines for the identification of high-risk patients (28,29). The American College of Cardiology, the American Heart Association, and the European Society of Cardiology in conjunction with the North American Society for Pacing and Electrophysiology created a committee of experts to develop guidelines for the management of

Table 1 American College of Cardiology/American Heart Association/ European Society of Cardiology Recommendation for Stroke Prevention in Atrial Fibrillation

Age < 60, no heart disease, (lone AF)	ASA (325 mg) or no therapy
Age < 60, heart disease, no risk factors	ASA (325 mg)
Age ≥ 60, no risk factors	ASA (325 mg)
Age ≥ 60 with diabetes or CAD	Oral anticoagulation (INR 2–3), optional ASA (81–162 mg)
Age ≥ 75, especially women	Oral anticoagulation (INR 2–3)
Heart failure	Oral anticoagulation (INR 2–3)
LVEF ≤ 35%	Oral anticoagulation (INR 2–3)
Thyrotoxicosis	Oral anticoagulation (INR 2–3)
Hypertension	Oral anticoagulation (INR 2–3)
Rheumatic heart disease (MS)	Oral anticoagulation (INR 2.5–3.5 or higher may be appropriate)
Prosthetic heart valve	Oral anticoagulation (INR 2.5–3.5 or higher may be appropriate)
Prior thromboembolism	Oral anticoagulation (INR 2.5–3.5 or higher may be appropriate)
Atrial thrombus (TEE)	Oral anticoagulation (INR 2.5–3.5 or higher may be appropriate)

High Risk	Moderate Risk
Prior stroke, TIA	Age 65–75 years
Systemic embolism	Diabetes
Hypertension	Coronary artery disease
Poor LV function	
Age > 75 years	
Rheumatic mitral disease	
Prosthetic heart valves	

Key: CAD, coronary artery disease; ASA, aspirin; INR, International Normalized Ratio; LVEF, left ventricular ejection fraction; MS, multiple sclerosis; TEE, transesophageal echocardiography; TIA, transient ischemic attack.

Table 2 Guidelines of the American College of Chest Physicians for Stroke Prevention

Risk factors	Therapy
Any high-risk factor or > 1 moderate	Oral anticoagulation
One moderate risk factor	Oral anticoagulation or ASA
No high-risk, no moderate risk factor	ASA

patients with AF and have made specific recommendations for anticoagulation strategies. Similarly, the American College of Chest Physicians has regularly convened a consensus conference to evaluate antithrombotic therapy. Patients with AF at high or moderate risk for stroke are identified on the basis of risk factors (Table 1) and appropriate antithrombotic therapy is suggested (Table 2). Both of these expert panels have focused predominantly on clinical risk factors in the identification of patients at high, moderate, or low risk of stroke.

Transthoracic echocardiographic (TTE) studies can be helpful in refining the risk for stroke (30). Patients with global left ventricular dysfunction had a stroke risk of over 12% per year. Patients with an enlarged left atrium had a stroke risk of 5 to 9% per year. Patients without clinical risk factors rarely (3%) had echocardiographic evidence of left ventricular dysfunction. However, when left atrial enlargement was considered as a risk factor, 38% of patients originally classified as low-risk on clinical criteria were reclassified as high-risk, emphasizing the importance of echocardiography in risk stratification.

Transesophageal echo may be even more helpful in identifying high-risk patients. Atrial abnormalities associated with stroke were spontaneous echo contrast, atrial septal aneurysm and other septal abnormalities, a patent foramen ovale, and left atrial thrombus. Patients with nonvalvular AF who undergo TEE have a 10 to 15% chance of a left atrial thrombus, which occurs primarily in the left atrial appendage (31–33). There appears to be a correlation between left atrial thrombus and dense spontaneous echo contrast, supporting the concept that stasis in the left atrium plays an important role in clot formation. The risk of stroke is increased threefold with a left atrial thrombus (34). Sequential TEE studies indicate that short-term warfarin therapy may dissolve left atrial thombi (35).

IV. LOW-RISK GROUPS

Patients at low risk of stroke may be considered for aspirin therapy or no therapy. The Atrial Fibrillation Investigators (27) noted that approximately

14% of patients in the pooled studies had none of the features associated with high risk, and the incidence of stroke among them was only 1% per year. Chronic anticoagulation is not warranted in these low-risk patients, given the risk of major bleeding with warfarin. The identification of a population of patients with AF at low risk for stroke extended the findings from previous studies that patients under the age of 60 years with AF and no identifiable heart disease ("lone AF") have a very low risk of thromboembolism over a period of observation of up to 25 years. Rates of thromboembolic events as low as 0.55% per year were reported (36). The stroke risk of patients with lone AF was higher in the Framingham Heart Study. In this study, patients had AF without preexisting or coexisting coronary artery disease, congestive heart failure, rheumatic heart disease, or hypertensive cardiovascular disease. The stroke risk in these patients was 2.6% per year. Of note was that 56% of these patients were above age 70 and 32% had a history of controlled or treated hypertension (37). These factors illustrate the importance of age and hypertension in the development of stroke in AF.

V. CARDIOVERSION

The risk of clinical thromboembolism following cardioversion to sinus rhythm in patients with AF varies from 5 to 7% (38–40), depending upon the underlying risk factors (35–37). The use of anticoagulation with warfarin for several weeks before cardioversion is associated with a reduction in cardioversion-related thromboembolism to 0 to 1.6% (38–40). It is generally believed that anticoagulant therapy stabilizes thrombus in the atrium by allowing enhanced organization and adherence to the atrial wall (39,41,42). However, Collins and colleagues have shown that dissolution of atrial thrombi may be the predominant mechanism of benefit of warfarin therapy in this setting (35). Using serial TEE, they studied 14 patients with nonrheumatic AF who had atrial thrombi and found resolution of 89% of thrombi after a median of 4 weeks of warfarin therapy.

The current recommendations suggest that warfarin be given to achieve an INR of 2.0 to 3.0 for at least 3 weeks before elective cardioversion in patients with AF lasting for longer than 48 hr. Patients with AF lasting less than 48 hours have a low likelihood of cardioversion-related thromboembolism, and cardioversion can be performed without anticoagulation in these patients (28,43).

After successful cardioversion, thromboembolic events may occur even when atrial thrombus has been excluded before cardioversion. It has become apparent that, although atrial electrical activity may be restored by cardioversion, normal mechanical atrial function may take longer to recover

(44–46). Therefore anticoagulation with warfarin should be continued for a minimum of 4 weeks after reversion to sinus rhythm (28). New data from the AFFIRM trial, however, suggests that maintenance of sinus rhythm may not eliminate the need for anticoagulation therapy in high-risk patients. Warfarin may have to be continued indefinitely in these patients, as further discussed in Sec. VIII, below.

TEE has high degree of accuracy for detecting left atrial thrombi (47–49). Interest in using this modality to guide cardioversion arose in the early 1990s. The risk of thromboembolic events in the immediate postcardioversion period is thought to be due to preformed atrial thrombi. If a left atrial thrombus can be ruled out by TEE immediately prior to cardioversion, the risk of thromboembolism should be minimal. Based on this assumption, an alternative strategy of cardioversion was proposed in the mid-1990s. Intravenous heparin is started before cardioversion to achieve therapeutic anticoagulation. A TEE is performed, and if no atrial thrombus is detected, cardioversion is performed. Warfarin therapy should be continued for 4 weeks after cardioversion, as in conventional strategy. Several small-scale studies in the 1990s involving about 1300 patients consistently showed the safety of this strategy (31,50–52).

The largest prospective trial to compare the conventional strategy with this new strategy was published by Klein et al. in 2001 (53). In a multicenter, randomized, prospective clinical trial, 1222 patients with atrial fibrillation of more than 2 days' duration were enrolled and assigned to either treatment guided by the findings on TEE or conventional treatment. Thrombi were detected in 13.8% of patients assigned to the TEE arm of the study.

Rates of the composite endpoint of cerebrovascular accident, TIA, or peripheral embolism within 8 weeks of cardioversion were similar in the two groups. In the group undergoing TEE, the event rate was 0.8%, compared to an event rate of 0.5% in the patients managed in the conventional manner. The 8-week incidence of hemorrhagic events was significantly lower in the TEE-guided group (2.9 vs. 5.5%, $p = 0.03$). At 8 weeks, the two groups did not differ significantly in mortality (TEE-guided, 2.4%; conventional, 1.0%) or in maintenance of sinus rhythm (52.7 vs. 50.4%, respectively). More bleeding complications in the conventional strategy were thought to be related to the longer duration of anticoagulant therapy.

The cost-effectiveness of this strategy was studied by Seto et al. (54). Using a decision-analytic model, they ascertained the cost per quality-adjusted life-year of three strategies: (1) conventional therapy with transthoracic echocardiography (TTE) and warfarin therapy for 1 month before cardioversion; (2) initial TTE followed by TEE and early cardioversion if no thrombus is detected; and (3) initial TEE with early cardioversion if no thrombus is detected. They found that the TEE-guided early cardioversion (strategy 3) was the least costly, with similar effectiveness.

The findings of these studies support the use of TEE-guided early cardioversion as a safe and clinically effective alternative to the conventional strategy. This strategy is potentially cost-saving and may reduce the bleeding complications related to the longer anticoagulant therapy in the conventional strategy. It is important to emphasize that whatever strategy is used, warfarin should be continued for at least 4 weeks after cardioversion to prevent new clot formation (Fig. 1).

Spontaneous echo contrast is a dynamic, smoke-like signal that is detected by TEE. It is considered to be a marker for blood stasis and is a

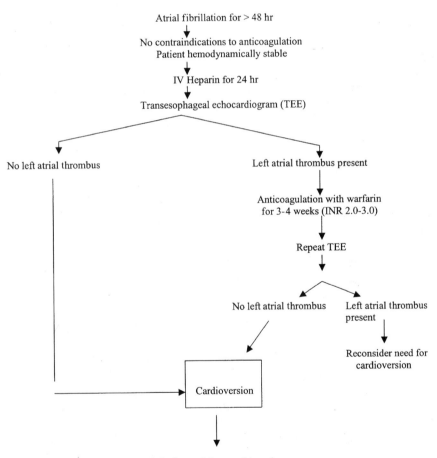

Figure 1 Proposed algorithm for the use of transesophageal echocardiography and cardioversion of AF.

common finding in patients with a left atrial thrombus. Patients with spontaneous echo contrast have a high likelihood of a previous thromboembolic event (55,56). There remains controversy concerning the wisdom of performing cardioversion in patients who have spontaneous echo contrast on TEE. Further studies are needed in this area.

More recently, there has been enthusiasm for the use of low-molecular-weight heparins for cardioversion. These heparins have several advantages over unfractionated heparin. They produce a more predictable response, are easier to administer, and allow outpatient therapy, which can potentially decrease the cost. The Anticoagulation in Cardioversion using Enoxaparin (ACE) study is being performed in Europe and has been reported at the European Society of Cardiology (57). ACUTE II is an ongoing multicenter trial being conducted in United States (58). This trial is comparing TEE-guided use of enoxaparin with TEE-guided use of unfractionated heparin in patients with AF of more than 2 days' duration undergoing early electrical and chemical cardioversion.

At present, the use of low-molecular-weight heparins for immediate or early cardioversion should be considered investigational, pending the results of large clinical trials.

VI. ANTICOAGULATION AND SURGERY

Surgery poses a special problem for patients with AF who are on long-term warfarin therapy. Temporary discontinuation of warfarin increases the risk of thromboembolism. This risk is related to underlying AF as well as a possible rebound hypercoagulable state caused by discontinuation of warfarin (59–61). Although surgery itself increases the risk of venous thromboembolism, there is no good evidence that it increases the risk of arterial embolism in patients with AF. On the other hand, continuation of warfarin during the perioperative period is associated with increased risk of bleeding. Immediate postoperative intravenous heparin therapy increases the risk of major bleeding (62–64). This risk is variable and depends on multiple factors, including the nature of surgery. Major bleeding rates of up to 7.5% have been reported in patients receiving postoperative intravenous heparin (64).

There are two different approaches in the management of these patients: (1) an aggressive approach in which warfarin is stopped few days before surgery and intravenous heparin, as a "bridge therapy," is started 2 days prior to surgery and continued for 2 days after surgery and (2) a conservative approach in which warfarin therapy is discontinued few days prior to surgery, no perioperative anticoagulation is given, and warfarin is resumed 2 to 3 days after surgery.

There are no randomized controlled trials to evaluate these two approaches. Most of the available studies are of small sample sizes, often without a control group, and have a variable follow-up (65). In the absence of controlled trials, most of the recommendations are based on the estimated risks of thromboembolism and major bleeding.

Patients with nonvalvular AF and no previous history of stroke or TIA have a low absolute risk of systemic thromboembolism and an increased risk of bleeding, which can offset any benefit of immediate postoperative intravenous heparin. Temporary discontinuation of anticoagulant therapy during the perioperative period may be all that is necessary in these patients. In patients with nonvalvular AF and previous history of stroke or TIA, especially within the first month of the event, the risk of systemic thromboembolism is relatively high and perioperative intravenous heparin as bridge therapy is a reasonable strategy. Patients with AF and valvular heart disease, especially mitral stenosis, and those with prosthetic heart valve are considered at high risk for thromboembolic events, and bridging with intravenous heparin during the perioperative period is commonly performed and recommended.

Low-molecular-weight heparins are being studied as a bridge therapy instead of intravenous unfractionated heparin in patients requiring temporary discontinuation of warfarin for surgery. There are two unique problems in their use in this setting, including the long duration of action of these agents and only partial reversal with protamine sulfate. Therefore their use may add to the difficulties of anticoagulation in this setting.

Two studies have evaluated the use of low-molecular-weight heparins instead of intravenous unfractionated heparin in patients with AF (66,67). The small number of these patients and the lack of a randomized, controlled design prevents any conclusions from being drawn. More data are needed before they can be considered for use in the clinical setting.

VII. ATRIAL FIBRILLATION AFTER CARDIAC SURGERY

AF is one of the most common complications of cardiac surgery and is associated with an increase in the risk of systemic thromboembolism (68). This risk varies according to the underlying cardiovascular disease, as discussed earlier; it should be weighed against the risk of bleeding in the early postoperative period. Anticoagulation strategy in this setting is not well studied. In general, AF lasting more than 48 hr should be treated as it is in nonsurgical patients. Long-term warfarin therapy should be individualized, as in nonsurgical patients.

VIII. WARFARIN IN CLINICAL PRACTICE

Based on the randomized clinical trials, it was anticipated that the use of warfarin would increase substantially in the 1990s. The National Ambulatory Medical Care surveys showed that the use of warfarin for patients with AF ranged from 3 to 20% between 1980 and 1985 (69) and increased to 35 to 40% between 1993 and 1996 (70). From 1996 to 2000, this survey estimated the use of warfarin in patients with atrial fibrillation to be only 40 to 50%. Although the use of warfarin did increase after publication of the clinical trials, its use was not as high as many experts had expected.

Before exploring reasons for the underutilization of warfarin, it is important to point out two problems with the randomized clinical trials of stroke prevention in AF. The first issue is that patients recruited for clinical trials tend to be healthier than those in clinical practice. For example, 1330 patients were enrolled in the SPAF I study. However, a total of 17,046 were screened but were not included in the study. Over 20% of patients refused entry into the study or were unable to have adequate follow-up. A number of other patients were excluded for cardiac reasons, such as a recent revascularization procedure. A number of patients were not included because of noncardiac exclusions mandated by the study, including the need for nonsteroidal anti-inflammatory drugs or an anticipated life expectancy of less than 2 years. The exclusion of so many patients may have affected the application of the results to patients with atrial fibrillation in clinical practice. Evans has commented on the fact that patients in clinical practice have more comorbid conditions than those in randomized trials (71).

Second, despite the inclusion of apparently more compliant patients, many of the clinical trials had a relatively high discontinuation rate during a relatively short follow-up period. The high discontinuation of warfarin in the AFASAK study has been cited previously (13). In the CAFA study, patients were followed for a mean of 5.2 months. However, early permanent discontinuation of warfarin, not due to a primary outcome event, occurred in 26.2% of patients (22). More recent studies have reported a lower dropout rate over an extended period of time. In the recently published Atrial Fibrillation and Follow-up of Rhythm Management (AFFIRM) study, more than 85% of patients were taking warfarin at each study visit (72).

IX. REASONS FOR LACK OF USE OF WARFARIN

The underutilization of warfarin for stroke prevention in patients with AF was noted in the early 1990s. From 1992 to 1994, only 32% of patients with AF admitted to six academic medical centers received warfarin (73). Surveys of Medicare patients discharged from hospitals in the mid-1990s reported warfarin use ranging from 32 to 49% (74,75). Patients in rural areas who were treated by generalists often were less likely to be using warfarin than those in metropolitan areas who were treated by cardiologists (75). The possibility that the message from the clinical trials was not being heard by many primary caregivers led to the implementation of medical education campaigns (76), which resulted in increased use of warfarin; but many workers in the field concluded that this highly effective therapy was used less often than expected. Elderly patients had a particularly low rate of warfarin use (77,78).

The main reason physicians give for failure to use warfarin is fear of bleeding (79). When warfarin is given for AF, the clinician must believe that the risks and consequences of stroke are greater than the risk of major bleeding, which arises when anticoagulants are prescribed. The Atrial Fibrillation Investigators reported that the risk of major bleeding with warfarin was 2.3% per year. Increasing age, the increased use of prescription medications (perhaps a marker for more advanced disease), and the intensity of anti-coagulation were all independent risk factors for bleeding (18). If physicians believe that the bleeding risk is substantially higher than this, they are less likely to prescribe anticoagulation. In the Anticoagulation and Risk Factors in Atrial Fibrillation (ATRIA) study, patients with a history of intracranial hemorrhage or gastrointestinal bleeding were less likely to receive warfarin. Other common reasons include dementia, hepatic or renal disease, and mechanical falls (77). These conditions are common among elderly patients. In these patients, the clinician may feel that the risk of bleeding outweighs the beneficial effect of anticoagulation.

A second major reason given for failure to use warfarin in patients with AF is the perception that the risk of stroke is too low to warrant anti-coagulation. Approximately 30% of patients with AF will have a low risk of stroke if they are given aspirin (80,81).

A third reason for failure to use warfarin may be misperceptions about the stroke risk of different varieties of AF. It should be recognized that the risk of stroke in intermittent AF is similar to the stroke risk with persistent AF and that clinical risk factors apply to patients with intermittent AF just as they apply to patients with chronic AF (82). A number of patients have asymp-tomatic AF and their risk of stroke may be higher than it is in symptomatic patients (83,84). Maintenance of sinus rhythm with antiarrhythmic drugs does not affect the need for continued antithrombotic therapy (72). In the AFFIRM study, patients at high risk for stroke were randomized either to a strategy involving rhythm control or to rate control. After 1, 3, and 5 years of follow-up, the prevalence of sinus rhythm in the rhythm-control group was 82.4, 73.3, and 62.6%, respectively. Ischemic strokes occurred in 80 patients in the rhythm-control group and in 77 patients in the rate-control group. Most strokes occurred in patients in whom warfarin had been stopped or was subtherapeutic. Consequently, warfarin should likely be continued in these high-risk patients even if sinus rhythm appears to be maintained. Studies involving Holter monitoring and transtelephonic recordings in selected groups of patients have demonstrated that a number of episodes of AF are asymptomatic (84–86). Clinicians may discontinue anticoagulation inappropriately based on the absence of symptomatic recurrences. Finally, it appears that patients with atrial flutter are also at risk for stroke, and anticoagulation is recommended for these patients (28).

To help manage patients receiving anticoagulation therapy, anticoagulation clinics have been established, and these clinics have been shown to reduce the number of thromboembolic rates and the risk of major bleeding. Publication of bleeding risks in anticoagulation clinics gives an idea about the risks of warfarin in a wide variety of clinical practices. For example, in an HMO model, the risk of major bleeding has been reported to be less than that reported in the clinical trials, as low as 0.65% per year (87). Other anticoagulation clinics, including those associated with academic institutions, have reported a risk of major bleeding of 0 to 8.1% per year (88,89). These trials have often compared the bleeding risk to that of patients receiving usual care, such as those receiving anticoagulation regulated by office practices. In one study, the yearly rate of significant bleeding was as high as 35% (89). If the yearly rate of major bleeding in community practices is anywhere near this figure, it is no wonder that physicians are reluctant to use warfarin.

Not only is warfarin underutilized, it is often used inappropriately. In the randomized trials, it was unusual for a patient to have a stroke if the INR was between 2 and 3. Hylek noted that the risk of stroke rose steeply as the INR became less than 2 (90). Despite this information, only one-third of patients in their anticoagulation clinic had an INR between 2 and 3, and nearly half had an INR value less than 2, making them more vulnerable to stroke. In the Stroke Prevention in Atrial Fibrillation III study (25), only 61% of INR values were between 2 and 3, despite the fact that a nurse followed monthly prothrombin times and adjusted warfarin doses with the use of a warfarin nomogram developed by the invetigators. In the AFFIRM study, 62.3% of INR values were between 2 and 3 (72).

X. NEW THERAPIES

The difficulties encountered with the use of warfarin have led to the quest for other pharmacological alternatives. Two agents being studied include a direct thrombin inhibitor and an antiplatelet agent.

Ximalagatran is an oral direct thrombin inhibitor that has been under investigation for stroke prevention in AF. It has predictable pharmacokinetics and has no known food or drug interactions. It does not require monitoring to prove efficacy.

In the Stroke Prevention by Oral Thrombin Inhibitor in Atrial Fibrillation (SPORTIF) II pilot study, patients at increased risk for stroke were randomized to receive 20, 40, or 60 mg twice daily of ximelagatran and compared with patients on adjusted-dose warfarin. In follow-up, 16 patients (8.6%) assigned to ximelagatran and 6 patients (9%) assigned to warfarin stopped study drug because of adverse events, usually bleeding. Major bleeding occurred in one patient receiving warfarin. No major bleeding occurred in patients receiving ximelagatran. Although this pilot study (91) was designed to test the safety of ximelagatran and not efficacy, it was noted that the incidence of stroke or transient ischemic attacks was low. Two patients assigned to ximelagatran had central nervous system (CNS) events (one stroke, one TIA) and two patients assigned to warfarin had CNS events (two TIAs).

As a result of this favorable pilot study, two large-scale clinical trials, SPORTIF III and SPORTIF V, involving over 7000 patients have completed enrollment and follow-up. In both trials patients with atrial fibrillation and at least one risk factor for stroke were randomized to receive either adjusted-dose warfarin with an INR goal of 2 to 3 or a fixed dose of 36 mg of ximelagatran twice a day. SPORTIF III enrolled 3407 patients from 23 nations. SPORTIF V enrolled 3913 patients from the United States and Canada. The protocols were identical except for the fact that therapy with ximelagatran and warfarin was blinded in SPORTIF V and nonblinded in SPORTIF III.

The primary endpoint was stroke (ischemic or hemorrhagic) and systemic embolic events. The study was designed to determine whether ximelagatran was "noninferior" to warfarin. All patients were followed for at least 12 months.

The event rate in the warfarin-treated patients was 2.3% per year, compared with an event rate in the ximelagatran patients of 1.6% per year, which satisfied the prespecified boundaries for "noninferiority." Major bleeding, including intracerebral hemorrhage, was similar in both groups. The combination of major and minor bleeding was less in the ximelagatran-treated patients. The rates of other endpoints—including heart failure, myocardial infarction, and total mortality—were low and not significantly different between the two groups. Importantly, ximelagatran-treated patients had an incidence of liver function abnormalities more than three times the upper limit of normal, of 6.5%, compared with 0.7% in warfarin-treated patients. The results of the SPORTIF V have been presented but not published and confirm that ximelagatran is not inferior to warfarin for stroke prevention in AF.

A second trial involving stroke prevention in atrial fibrillation is the Atrial Fibrillation Clopidogrel Trial with Irbesartan for Prevention of Vascular Events (ACTIVE). The premise of this trial is that although warfarin is highly effective in the prevention of stroke in AF, the effect of warfarin on other vascular events—including myocardial infarction and vascular events—is less impressive (92). Aspirin has been shown to have some effect in preventing stroke in AF, and aspirin and newer antiplatelet agents have a synergistic effect on platelet function. In addition, the angiotensin receptor blockers have been shown to have favorable effects on atrial structure and function as well as favorable blood pressure effects. Both of these effects may play a role in the prevention of vascular events. This study will enroll over 14,000 patients with AF, who are at high risk for vascular events, into two arms. One group that is eligible for anticoagulation will be randomized to 75 mg of clopidogrel plus 75 to 100 mg of aspirin and will be compared with a group on dose-adjusted oral anticoagulants (INR goal 2 to 3). Patients who are not eligible for anticoagulation will receive either aspirin and clopidogrel or aspirin. A number of patients will also be randomized to either irbesartan or placebo.

REFERENCES

1. Wolf PA, Dawber TR, Thomas HE, Kannel WB. Epidemiologic assessment of chronic atrial fibrillation and risk of stroke: the Framingham study. Neurology 1978; 28:973–977.
2. Graef I, Berger AR, Bunin JJ, de la Chapelle CE. Auricular thrombosis in rheumatic heart disease. Arch Pathol 1941; 24:344.
3. Garvin CF. Mural thrombi in the heart. Am Heart J 1941; 21:713.
4. Coulshed N, Epstein EJ, MacKendrick CS, Galloway RW, Walker E. Systemic embolism in mitral valve disease. Br Heart J 1970; 32:26.
5. Szekely P. Systemic embolism and anticoagulant prophylaxis in rheumatic heart disease. Br Med J 1964; 1:1209.
6. Griffith GC, Stragnell R, Levinson DC, Moore FJ, Ware AG. A study of the beneficial effects of anticoagulant therapy in congestive heart failure. Ann Intern Med 1952; 37:867.
7. Cosgriff SW. Chronic anticoagulation therapy in recurrent embolism of cardiac origin. Ann Intern Med 1953; 38:278.
8. Adams GF, Merrett JD, Hutchinson WM, Pollock AM. Cerebral embolism and mitral stenosis: survival with and without anticoagulants. J Neurol Neurosurg Psychiatry 1974; 37:378–383.

9. Wessler S, Gitel S. Seminars in Medicine of the Beth Israel Hospital, Boston: warfarin: from bedside to bench. N Engl J Med 1984; 311(10):645–652.

10. Roy D, Marchand E, Gagne P, Chabet M, Cartier R. Usefulness of anticoagulant therapy in the prevention of embolic complications of atrial fibrillation. Am Heart J 1986; 112:1039–1043.

11. Askey JM, Cherry CB. Thromboembolism associated with auricular fibrillation: Continuous anticoagulant therapy. JAMA 1950; 144(2):97–100.

12. Hart RG, Benavente O, McBride R, Pearce LA. Antithrombotic therapy to prevent stroke in patients with atrial fibrillation: a meta-analysis. Ann Intern Med 1999; 131:492–501.

13. Petersen P, Boysen G, Godtfredsen J, Andersen ED, Andersen B, for the Copenhagen AFASAK Study. Placebo-controlled, randomized trial of warfarin and aspirin for prevention of thromboembolic complications in chronic atrial fibrillation. Lancet 1989; 1:175–179.

14. Special Report. Preliminary report of the stroke prevention in atrial fibrillation study. N Engl J Med 1990; 322:863–868.

15. Stroke Prevention in Atrial Fibrillation Investigators. Stroke prevention in atrial fibrillation study: Final results. Circulation 1991; 84:527–539.

16. Miller VT, Rothrock JF, Pearce LA, Feinberg WM, Hart RG, Anderson DC, on behalf of the Stroke Prevention in Atrial Fibrillation investigators. Ischemic stroke in patients with atrial fibrillation: effect of aspirin according to stroke mechanism. Neurology 1993; 43:32–36.

17. Stroke Prevention in Atrial Fibrillation Investigators. Warfarin versus aspirin for prevention of thromboembolism in atrial fibrillation: stroke prevention in Atrial Fibrillation II Study. Lancet 1994; 343:687–691.

18. Stroke Prevention in Atrial Fibrillation Investigators. Bleeding during anti-thrombotic therapy in patients with atrial fibrillation. Arch Intern Med 1996; 156:409–416.

19. The Boston Area Anticoagulation Trial for Atrial Fibrillation Investigators. The effect of low-dose warfarin on the risk of stroke in patients with nonrheumatic atrial fibrillation. N Engl J Med 1990; 323:1505–1511.

20. Singer DE, Hughes RA, Gress DR, Sheehan MA, Oertel LB, Maraventano SW, Blewett DR, Rosner B, Kistler JP, for the BAATAF investigators. The effect of aspirin on the risk of stroke in patients with nonrheumatic atrial fibrillation: The BAATAF study. Am Heart J 1992; 124:1567–1573.

21. Ezekowitz MD, Bridgers SL, James KE, Carliner NH, Colling CL, Gornick CC, Krause-Steinrauf H, Kurtzke JF, Nazarian SM, Radford MJ, Rickles FR, Shabetai R, Deykin D, for the Beterans Affairs Stroke Prevention in Non-rheumatic Atrial Fibrillation Investigators. Warfarin in the prevention of stroke associated with nonrheumatic atrial fibrillation. N Engl J Med 1992; 327:1406–1412.

22. Connolly SJ, Laupacis A, Gent M, Roberts RS, Cairns JA, Joyner C, for the CAFA study coinvestigators. Canadian atrial fibrillation anticoagulation (CAFA) study. J Am Coll Cardiol 1991; 18:349–355.

23. EAFT (European Atrial Fibrillation Trial) Study Group. Secondary prevention

in non-rheumatic atrial fibrillation after transient ischemic attack or minor stroke. Lancet 1993; 342:1255–1262.

24. EAFT (European Atrial Fibrillation Trial) Study Group. Optimal oral anticoagulant therapy in patients with nonrheumatic atrial fibrillation and recent cerebral ischemia. N Engl J Med 1995; 333:5–10.

25. The Stroke Prevention in Atrial Fibrillation Investigators. Adjusted-dose warfarin verses low-intensity, fixed dose warfarin plus aspirin for high-risk patients with atrial fibrillation: Stroke Prevention in Atrial Fibrillation III. Lancet 1996; 348:633–638.

26. The SPAF III Writing Committee for the Stroke Prevention in Atrial Fibrillation Investigators. Patients with nonvalvular atrial fibrillation at low risk of stroke during treatment with aspirin: Stroke Prevention in Atrial Fibrillation III study. JAMA 1998; 279:1273–1277.

27. Atrial Fibrillation investigators. Risk factors for stroke and efficacy of antithrombotic therapy in atrial fibrillation. Arch Intern Med 1994; 154:1449–1457.

28. Albers GW, Dalen JE, Laupacis A, Manning WJ, Petersen P, Singer DE. Antithrombotic therapy in atrial fibrillation. Chest 2001; 119:194S–206S.

29. ACC/AHA/ESC guidelines for the management of patients with atrial fibrillation: executive summary. J Am Coll Cardiol 2001; 38:1231–1265.

30. The Stroke Prevention in Atrial Fibrillation investigators. Predictors of thromboembolism in atrial fibrillation:II-Echocardiographic features of patients at risk. Ann Intern Med 1992; 116:6–12.

31. Manning WJ, Silverman DI, Gordon SPK, Krumholz HM, Douglas PS. Cardioversion from atrial fibrillation without prolonged anticoagulation with use of transesophageal echocardiography to exclude the presence of atrial thrombi. N Engl J Med 1993; 328:750–755.

32. Daniel WG, Grote J, Freedberg RS, et al. Assessment of left atrial thrombi by transesophageal echo in non-valvular atrial fibrillation: a multicenter study [abstr]. Eur Heart J 1993; 14(suppl):355.

33. Black IW, Hopkins AP, Lee LCL, Walsh WF. Evaluation of transesophageal echocardiography before cardioversion of atrial fibrillation and flutter in nonanticoagulated patients. Am Heart J 1993; 126:375–381.

34. The Stroke Prevention in Atrial Fibrillation Investigators Committee on Echocardiography. Transesophageal echocardiographic correlates of thromboembolism in high-risk patients with nonvalvular Atrial Fibrillation. Ann Intern Med 1998; 128:639–647.

35. Collins LJ, Silverman DI, Douglas PS, Manning WJ. Cardioversion of nonrheumatic atrial fibrillation: reduced thromboembolic complications with 4 weeks of precardioversion anticoagulation are related to atrial thrombus resolution. Circulation 1995; 92:156–159.

36. Kopecky SL, Gersh BJ, McGoon MD, et al. The natural history of lone atrial fibrillation: a population-based study over three decades. N Engl J Med 1987; 317:669–674.

37. Brand FN, Abbott RD, Kannell WB, et al. Characteristics and prognosis of lone

atrial fibrillation: 30 year follow-up in the Framingham study. JAMA 1985; 254:3449–3453.

38. Bjerkelund CJ, Ornig OM. The efficacy of anticoagulant therapy in preventing embolism related to DC electrical conversion of atrial fibrillation. Am J Cardiol 1969; 23:208–216.

39. Weinberg DM, Mancini GBJ. Anticoagulation for cardioversion of atrial fibrillation. Am J Cardiol 1989; 63:745–746.

40. Arnold AZ, Mick MJ, Mazurek RP, Loop FD, Trohman RG. Role of prophylactic anticoagulation for direct current cardioversion in patients with atrial fibrillation or atrial flutter. J Am Coll Cardiol 1992; 19:851–855.

41. Falk RH, Podrid PJ. Electrical conversion of atrial fibrillation. In: Falk RH, Podrid PJ, eds. Atrial Fibrillation: Mechanisms and Management. New York: Raven Press, 1992:188.

42. Kinch JW, Davidoff R. Prevention of embolic events after cardioversion of atrial fibrillation. Arch Intern Med 1995; 155:1353–1360.

43. Weigner MJ, Caulfield TA, Danias PG, Silverman DI, Manning WJ. Risk for clinical thromboembolism associated with coversion to sinus rhythm in patients with atrial fibrillation lasting less than 48 hours. Ann Intern Med 1997; 126:615–620.

44. Manning WJ, Leeman DE, Gotch PJ, Come PC. Pulsed Doppler evaluation of atrial mechanical function after electrical cardioversion of atrial fibrillation. J Am Coll Cardiol 1989; 13:617–623.

45. Grimm RA, Stewart WJ, Maloney JD, et al. Impact of electrical cardioversion for atrial fibrillation on left atrial appendage function and spontaneous echo contrast: characterization by simultaneous transesophageal echocardiography. J Am Coll Cardiol 1993; 22:1359–1366.

46. Fatkin D, Kuchar DL, Thorburn CW, et al. Transesophageal echocardiography before and during direct current cardioversion of atrial fibrillation: evidence for "atrial stunning" as a mechanism of thromboembolic complications. J Am Coll Cardiol 1994; 23:307–316.

47. Aschenberg W, Schluter M, Kremer P, Schroder E, Siglow V, Bleifeld W. Transesophageal two-dimensional echocardiography for the detection of left atrial appendage thrombus. J Am Coll Cardiol 1986; 7:163–166.

48. Manning WJ, Weintraub RM, Waksmonski CA, et al. Accuracy of trans-esophageal echocardiography for identifying left atrial thrombi: a prospective, intraoperative study. Ann Intern Med 1995; 123:817–822.

49. Fatkin D, Scalia G, Jacobs N, et al. Accuracy of biplane transesophageal echo-cardiography in detecting left atrial thrombus. Am J Cardiol 1996; 77:321–323.

50. Manning WJ, Silverman DI, Keighley CS, Oettgen P, Douglas PS. Trans-esophageal echocardiography facilitated early cardioversion from atrial fibrilla-tion using short-term anticoagulation: final results of a prospective 4.5-year study. J Am Coll Cardiol 1995; 25:1354–1361.

51. Stoddard MF, Dawkins PR, Prince CR, Longaker RA. Transesophageal echocardiographic guidance of cardioversion in patients with atrial fibrillation. Am Heart J 1995; 129:1204–1215.

52. Klein AL, Grimm RA, Black IW, et al. Cardioversion guided by transesophageal echocardiography: the ACUTE Pilot Study: a randomized, controlled trial: Assessment of Cardioversion Using Transesophageal Echocardiography. Ann Intern Med 1997; 126:200–209.

53. Klein AL, Grimm RA, Murray RD, et al., for the Assessment of Cardioversion Using Transesophageal Echocardiography Investigators. Use of transesophageal echocardiography to guide cardioversion in patients with atrial fibrillation. N Engl J Med 2001; 344:1411–1420.

54. Seto TB, Taira DA, Tsevat J, et al. Cost effectiveness of transesophageal echocardiographic-guided early cardioversion for patients admitted to the hospital with atrial fibrillation. J Am Coll Cardiol 1997; 29(1):122–130.

55. De Belder MA, Lovat LB, Tourikis L, et al. Left atrial spontaneous contrast echoes—markers of thromboembolic risk in patients with atrial fibrillation. Eur Heart J 1993; 14(3):326–335.

56. Chimowitz MI, DeGeorgia MA, Poole RM, et al. Left atrial spontaneous echo contrast is highly associated with previous stroke in patients with atrial fibrillation or mitral stenosis. Stroke 1993; 24(7):1015–1019.

57. Stellbrink C, Hanrath P, Nixdorff U, et al. Low molecular weight heparin for prevention of thromboembolic complications in cardioversion—rationale and design of the ACE study (Anticoagulation in Cardioversion using Enoxaparin). Z Kardiol 2002; 91(3):249–254.

58. Murray RD, Shah A, Jasper SE, et al. The ACUTE II pilot study. Transesophageal echocardiography–guided enoxaparin antithrombotic strategy for cardioversion of atrial fibrillation. Am Heart J 2000; 139:e5.

59. Palareti G, Legnani C, Guazzaloca G, et al. Activation of blood coagulation after abrupt or stepwise withdrawal of oral anticoagulants—a prospective study. Thromb Haemost 1994; 72:222–226.

60. Genewein U, Haeberli A, Straub PW, Beer JH. Rebound after cessation of oral anticoagulant therapy: the biochemical evidence. Br J Haematol 1996; 92:479–485.

61. Grip L, Blomback M, Schulman S. Hypercoagulable state and thromboembolism following warfare withdrawal in post–myocardial-infarction patients. Eur Heart J 1991; 12:1225–1233.

62. Levine MN, Hirsh J, Gent M. Prevention of deep vein thrombosis after elective hip surgery: a randomized trial comparing low molecular weight heparin with standard unfractionated heparin. Ann Intern Med 1991; 114:545–551.

63. Treiman RL, Cossman DV, Foran RF, Levin PM, Cohen JL, Wagner WH. The influence of neutralizing heparin after carotid endarterectomy on postoperative stroke and wound hematoma. J Vasc Surg 1990; 12:440–446.

64. Wilson JR, Lampman J. Heparin therapy: a randomized prospective study. Am Heart J 1979; 97:155–158.

65. Dunn AS, Turpie AGG. Perioperative management of patients receiving oral anticoagulants. Arch Intern Med 2003; 163:901–908.

66. Johnson J, Turpie AGG. Temporary discontinuation of oral anticoagulants: role of low molecular weight heparin (dalteparin) [abstr]. Thromb Haemost 1999; 82(suppl):62–63.

67. Spandorfer JM, Lynch S, Weitz HH, Fertel S, Merli GT. Use of enoxaparin for the chronically anticoagulated patient before and after procedures. Am J Cardiol 1999; 84(4):478–480.

68. Creswell LL, Schuessler RB, Rosenbloom MH, Cox JL. Hazards of postoperative atrial arrhythmias. Ann Thorac Surg 1993; 56(3):539–549.

69. Stafford RS, Singer DE. National patterns of warfarin use in atrial fibrillation. Arch Intern Med 1996; 156:2537–2541.

70. Stafford RS, Singer DE. Recent national patterns of warfarin use in atrial fibrillation. Circulation 1998; 97:1231–1233.

71. Evans A, Kalra L. Are the results of randomized controlled trials on anticoagulation in patients with atrial fibrillation generalizable to clinical practice? Arch Intern Med 2001; 161:1447.

72. AFFIRM Investigators. A comparison of rate control and rhythm control in patients with atrial fibrillation. N Engl J Med 2002; 347:1825–1833.

73. Albers GW, Yim JM, Belew KM, Bittar N, Hattemer CR, Phillips BG, Kemp S, Hall EA, Morton DJ, Vlasses PH. Status of antithrombotic therapy for patients with atrial fibrillation in university hospitals. Arch Intern Med 1996; 156:2311–2316.

74. Malach M. Use of anticoagulant and antiplatelet agents in trial fibrillation in New York State: the IPRO study. Cardiovascular Reviews and Reports, January 1997:12–15.

75. Flaker GC, McGowan DJ, Boechler M, Fortune G, Gage B. Underutilization of antithrombotic therapy in elderly rural patients with atrial fibrillation. Am Heart J 1999; 137:307–312.

76. Gage BF, Boechler M, Doggette AL, Fortune G, Flaker GC, Rich MW, Radford MJ. Adverse outcomes and predictors of underuse of antithrombotic therapy in Medicare beneficiaries with chronic nonvalvular atrial fibrillation. Stroke 2000; 31:822–827.

77. Go AS, Hylek EM, Borowsky LH, Phillips KA, Selby JV, Singer DE. Warfarin use among ambulatory patients with nonvalvular atrial fibrillation: the anticoagulation and Risk Factors in Atrial Fibrillation (ATRIA) study. Ann Intern Med 1999; 131:927–934.

78. Smith NL, Psaty BM, Furberg CD, White R, Lima JC, Newman AB, Manolio TA. Temporal trends in the use of anticoagulants among older adults with atrial fibrillation. Arch Intern Med 1999; 159:1574–1578.

79. McCrory DC, Matchar DB, Samsa G, Sanders LL, Pritchett ELC. Physician attitudes about anticoagulation for nonvalvular atrial fibrillation in the elderly. Arch Intern Med 1995; 155:277–281.

80. Go AS, Hylek EM, Phillips KA, Borowsky LH, Henault LE, Chang Y, et al. Implications of stroke risk criteria on the anticoagulation decision in nonvalvular atrial fibrillation: the Anticoagulation and Risk Factors in Atrial Fibrillation (ATRIA) study. Circulation 2000; 102:11–13.

81. Hart RG, Halperin JL, Pearce LA, Anderson DC, Kronmal RA, McBride R, Nasco E, Sherman DG, Talbert RL, Marler JR, for the Stroke Prevention in Atrial Fibrillation Investigators. Lessons from the stroke prevention in atrial fibrillation trials. Ann Intern Med 2003; 138:831–838.

82. Hart RG, Pearce LA, Rothbart RB, McAnulty JH, Asinger RW, Halperin JL, for the Stroke Prevention in Atrial Fibrillation Investigators. Stroke with intermittent atrial fibrillation: incidence and predictors during aspirin therapy. J Am Coll Cardiol 2000; 35:183–187.

83. Flaker GC, Belew K, Beckman K, Vidaillet H, Kron J, Safford R, Mickel M, Barrell P, for the AFFIRM Investigators. Asymptomatic atrial fibrillation: demographic features and prognostic information from the Atrial Fibrillation Follow-up Investigation of Rhythm Management (AFFIRM) study. PACE 2003; 26:966.

84. Glotzer TV, Hellkamp AS, Zimmerman J, et al. Symptoms are an unreliable predictor of clinically important supraventricular tachycardias: report of the atrial diagnostics ancillary study of MOST. Circulation 2003; 107:1614–1619.

85. Page RL, Wilkinson WE, Clair WK, McCarthy EA, Pritchett ELC. Asymptomatic arrhythmias in patients with symptomatic paroxysmal atrial fibrillation and paroxysmal supraventricular tachycardia. Circulation 1994; 89:224–227.

86. Neumann T, Kurzidim K, Berkowitsch A, Sperzel J, Pitschner HF. Occurrence of silent atrial fibrillation after catheter ablation of the pulmonary veins. Circulation 2002; 106(19)(suppl II):542.

87. Gottlieb LK, Salen-Schatz S. Anticoagulation in atrial fibrillation. Arch Intern Med 1994; 154:1945–1953.

88. Chiquette E, Amato MG, Bussey HI. Comparison of an anticoagulation clinic with usual medical care. Arch Intern Med 1998; 158:1641–1647.

89. Wilt VM, Gums JG, Ahmed OI, Moore LM. Outcome analysis of a pharmacist-managed anticoagulation service. Pharmacotherapy 1995; 15(6):732–739.

90. Hylek EM, Skates SJ, Sheehan MA, Singer DE. An analysis of the lowest effective intensity of prophylactic anticoagulation for patients with nonrheumatic atrial fibrillation. N Engl J Med 1996; 335:540–546.

91. Petersen P, Grind M, Adler J, for the SPORTIF Investigators. Ximelagatran versus warfarin for stroke prevention in patients with nonvalvular atrial fibrillation. J Am Coll Cardiol 203; 41:1445–1451.

92. Taylor FC, Cohen H, Ebrahim S. Systemic review of long term anticoagulation or antiplatelet treatment in patients with non-rheumatic atrial fibrillation. BMJ 2001; 322:321–326.

8
Cardioversion

Carl Timmermans, Luz-Maria Rodriguez, and Harry J. G. M. Crijns
University Hospital Maastricht, Maastricht, The Netherlands

For more than 40 years, electrical cardioversion, or the discharge of electrical energy synchronized on the R wave of atrial fibrillation (AF), has been the most effective and safest method of restoring sinus rhythm. Only recently, new technical developments, a reappraisal of the initial energy settings, pretreatment with antiarrhythmic drugs, and a better identification of the different types of postshock recurrences have further refined the technique and improved the outcome of cardioversion. Also, our understanding of stroke risk in relation to cardioversion and the development of new antithrombotic strategies, including cardioversion guided by transesophageal echocardiography, have improved the speed and safety of cardioversion.

I. TECHNIQUES

Although electrical cardioversion of AF is routinely performed by many clinicians, an optimal awareness of the subtleties of the technique may prevent unnecessary failures and eventual complications.

Before elective cardioversion, the patient should be informed about the procedure and physically examined. Patients should be cardioverted in a fasting state with a reliable intravenous access and without dentures. The serum potassium level should be normal in order to avoid the induction of arrhythmias. In case of digitalis toxicity, the procedure must be postponed. The normal use of digitalis is, however, not a contraindication. The cardioversion should be carried out in an area with facilities for cardiopulmonary resuscitation, should this be needed. Light general anesthesia using a short-acting anesthetic or sedative drug, administrated by a qualified physician, is preferred, because most such procedures can be performed on an outpatient basis. During cardioversion and at least for the first minutes thereafter, the heart rhythm should be carefully monitored and recorded to detect possible postshock arrhythmias, conduction disturbances, or immediate reinitiation of AF. The resumption of AF after some sinus beats may lead to a failed cardioversion or unnecessary additional shocks if this phenomenon recurs during the same procedure. As discussed below, a detailed classification of several time-dependent cardioversion outcomes may serve to improve management strategy.

II. SYNCHRONIZATION

Synchronization of shock delivery with the R wave of the QRS complex is essential during cardioversion. Although properly synchronized shocks rarely, if ever, induce ventricular fibrillation, unsynchronized shocks may be delivered in the ventricular vulnerable period of the preceding beat (near the apex of the T wave) and result in ventricular fibrillation. The lead with the highest R-wave amplitude should be selected for synchronization. The appropriateness of synchronization of each shock delivery should always be verified, since a large or tall T or P wave, artifacts, or noise can be misidentified as the R wave. Improper synchronization may also occur when the QRS complex shows a right bundle branch block configuration with a tall secondary R wave. Electrocardiographic tracings derived from paddle electrodes may produce motion artifacts and errors in R-wave sensing.

The paddle electrodes can be placed at the anterolateral or anteroposterior position. In the anterolateral position, the anterior electrode is placed parasternally over the right second and third intercostal spaces and the lateral electrode just below the fourth intercostal space in the midaxillary line. In the anteroposterior position, the anterior electrode is placed as previously mentioned and the posterior electrode is positioned just below the left scapula. Recently, some authors have provided convincing data that favor the anteroposterior electrode position for cardioversion of persistent AF. The anteroposterior configuration includes both atria directly within its shock field and therefore a more homogeneous shock field, especially within the posteriorly positioned left atrium, is created (1,2).

Successful cardioversion requires sufficient flow of electrical current through the appropriate chambers of the heart. Current flow is determined by the shock strength and the transthoracic impedance. If the impedance is high, low-energy shocks will fail to terminate the arrhythmia. Several authors have reported on the different factors that influence transthoracic impedance, including the electrode size, the contact medium used, adequate contact between electrode and skin, the phase of respiration, a recent sternotomy, and previous shocks (3–5). Optimal electrode size seems to be 8 to 12 cm in diameter for adults. This size should also be used for children weighing more than 10 kg. The slightly higher impedance of self-adhesive disposable electrode pads makes their use not optimal in patients predisposed to a high transthoracic impedance. Firm electrode pressure with the patient in full expiration reduces transthoracic impedance and enhances the likelihood of success (6). Even shaving the chest in patients undergoing elective cardioversion may improve outcome. A sternotomy reduces transthoracic impedance for at least 1 month after the procedure. Finally, impedance also becomes lower with repeated shock delivery.

III. MONOPHASIC VS. BIPHASIC SHOCK WAVEFORM

Until recently, clinical transthoracic defibrillation and cardioversion for AF was performed exclusively with a monophasic waveform. The one most frequently used is the monophasic damped sinusoidal waveform. This is obtained by a single capacitor discharge, generating a high-voltage peaked wave with an exponential decay, in combination with rounding of the initial peak using an inductor. Further development of alternative waveforms was driven by the advent of implantable cardioverter/defibrillators. Previous experimental studies showed that biphasic waveforms, delivering current first flowing in a positive direction and thereafter in a negative direction for a specific duration, achieved the same success rates as monophasic waveforms but at significantly lower energy levels. These lower-energy waveforms offered several technical advantages over a monophasic waveform: they allowed the development not only of small implantable cardioverter/defibrillators but also of small, lightweight, low-maintenance automatic external defibrillators. Until now, only a few impedance-compensating biphasic waveforms have been evaluated for the treatment of AF (see Sec. V). Biphasic defibrillators with this feature automatically ensure a constant current and/or adjust the duration of the waveform during shock delivery based on real-time measurement of the patient's transthoracic impedance.

IV. ENERGY SETTING

A. Monophasic Waveform

Since evidence of myocardial injury during the cardioversion of AF with standard energies is lacking and initial shocks of 100 J often fail, the current

American College of Cardiology/American Heart Association/European Society of Cardiology guidelines recommend a first shock of at least 200 J (7). If atrial fibrillation persists, a 360-J shock should be delivered and, if necessary, repeated. Shocks lower than 200 J are likely to be effective only when the duration of atrial fibrillation is shorter than 24 hr, when the patient does not have structural heart disease, or when he or she is not receiving antiarrhythmic drugs (8). In overweight patients or those with AF for more than 6 months, an initial setting of ≥ 300 J is appropriate (9).

B. Biphasic Waveform

Although experience with biphasic shocks for the cardioversion of AF is limited, a shock of 150 J may be the appropriate first choice. Failure with this first shock would warrant advancing to 200 J. For AF of less than 48 hr, a first shock of 100 J seems justified, as it results in the efficient achievement of conversion (10). Differences between devices with maximum output varying between 180 and 360 J preclude giving definitive recommendations for the appropriate energy levels in this new area.

V. ACUTE OUTCOME OF ELECTRICAL CARDIOVERSION

The immediate success rate of external cardioversion using a monophasic waveform varies between 70% and 94% (11,12). This variation in outcome may be due to heterogeneous clinical characteristics of the patients, the concomitant use of different antiarrhythmic drugs, and the absence of a generally accepted definition for a successful cardioversion. The probability of a successful cardioversion depends mainly on the duration of the atrial fibrillation episode (11,12). Other factors—such as the transthoracic impedance (13), left atrial size, and the patient's age (14)—are also important for acute success.

As previously mentioned, the literature does not provide a uniform definition of a successful or failed cardioversion. Recent internal atrial cardioversion and day-to-day postconversion studies have identified several distinct types of time-dependent cardioversion outcomes of persistent AF, which require different management strategies (Fig. 1). The electrocardiogram recorded immediately after the application of a cardioversion shock may or may not reveal sinus rhythm. The inability to interrupt atrial fibrillatory activity, even not for a single sinus beat, represents shock failure. If sinus rhythm is obtained, immediate (within some minutes after a successful cardioversion) reinitiation of atrial fibrillation (IRAF) may occur. The prevalence of IRAF after external cardioversion has been reported to range

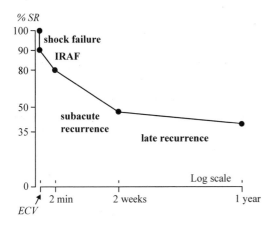

Figure 1 Hypothetical curve illustrating the time course of the electrical cardioversion outcomes of persistent AF. ECV, external cardioversion; IRAF, immediate reinitiation of atrial fibrillation after a successful cardioversion; SR, sinus rhythm. (Adapted from Ref. 73.)

from 5% to 26% (15,16). IRAF may occur in patients with persistent AF as well as in those with paroxysmal AF. Recently, it was shown that the probability of IRAF, in contrast to the other time-dependent types of recurrence, was inversely related to the duration of the AF episode (17). If the shock restores sinus rhythm and no IRAF occurs, most patients will remain free from AF for 24 hr. However, from the next day until 1 to 2 weeks after the cardioversion, subacute recurrences may follow (18). These occur more frequently than IRAF and dramatically further reduce the outcome of the cardioversion. Finally, the third time-dependent type of recurrence, the late recurrence, gradually follows over the next months. These different time-dependent types of recurrence suggest different pathophysiological mechanisms. IRAF may be due to a transient ultrashort atrial effective refractory period and a decreased conduction velocity in combination with short-coupled atrial premature beats (19,20). The subacute recurrences most likely occur due to heterogeneous ongoing reversed electrical and mechanical atrial remodeling, resulting in a pronounced dispersion of refractoriness, in combination with stretch-induced triggers. It is possible that late recurrences coincidentally occur (e.g., in patients with only sporadic triggers) or are related to intercurrent events like ischemia or heart failure. The implication of this classification of recurrences for the management strategy is discussed in Sec. VI, below.

In case of shock failure, three alternative electrical approaches are possible: a high-energy (720 J) monophasic shock, a biphasic shock, or internal cardioversion. A high-energy (720 J) monophasic shock, using two external defibrillators, has been shown to effectively restore sinus rhythm in patients with AF refractory to standard cardioversion energies. Nevertheless, the authors recommended the use of a 720-J shock only in patients with a large body habitus because of the potential risk of myocardial injury (21). Despite methodological differences, the presently performed studies comparing monophasic and biphasic shock waveforms for external cardioversion of atrial fibrillation demonstrate the superiority of biphasic shocks. Two prospective, randomized, multicenter studies showed that the efficacy of the first shock with a biphasic waveform was significantly greater than that with a monophasic waveform. Mittal et al. reported a rate of initial shock success with a 70-J biphasic waveform of 68% compared to 21% with a 100-J monophasic waveform (22). Page et al. showed that the efficacy for a first 100-J biphasic shock was 60% and for a first 100-J monophasic shock 22% (10). Biphasic shock waveforms also required significantly lower delivered current to convert AF and produced less dermal injury. The small difference in cumulative efficacy with the biphasic waveform between both studies (91% and 94%) may be due to a longer duration of AF. The technique, efficacy, and indications for internal cardioversion are discussed below.

VI. ADMINISTRATION OF ANTIARRHYTHMIC DRUGS BEFORE CARDIOVERSION

Although not without risk (see Chap. 10), the administration of antiarrhythmic drugs before cardioversion may have a beneficial effect on the different time-dependent types of cardioversion outcomes.

Shock failure can be prevented by ibutilide. In 100 patients with persistent atrial fibrillation, placebo and intravenous ibutilide, administered 10 min before external cardioversion, were compared. Electrical cardioversion had a 100% success rate in the ibutilide-pretreated patients compared to 72% in the placebo group. It is noteworthy that in all the patients in the placebo group in whom cardioversion initially could not restore sinus rhythm, resumption of sinus rhythm was obtained when ibutilide was given before a second cardioversion attempt. Nevertheless, due to the risk of prolongation of the QT interval and torsades de pointes, the authors recommended the avoidance of ibutilide in patients with a very low ejection fraction (23). Other antiarrhythmic drugs may also affect the energy required for atrial cardioversion, but due to the small-scaled, uncontrolled nature of some of these studies and their sometimes conflicting results, no firm conclusions can be drawn (24–28).

Most studies of electrical cardioversion of AF do not distinguish shock failure from IRAF. Shock failure may require an alternative electrical approach or the administration of ibutilide, but IRAF is, most of the time, not prevented by a repeated shock and seems not to be affected by ibutilide (29,30). Because the long-term recurrence of the arrhythmia in patients in whom IRAF could be suppressed or prevented was the same as that in patients without IRAF, pretreatment with other antiarrhythmic drugs may be considered (20,31). In 1967, the beneficial effect of a class IA antiarrhythmic drug on preventing the prompt relapse of AF after electrical cardioversion was reported. Fifty consecutive patients with chronic AF were randomly assigned to a control or quinidine (1.2 g for 1 day) group prior to cardioversion. IRAF occurred in 7 of 23 (30%) successfully cardioverted patients of the control group and in only 1 of 24 (4%) successfully cardioverted patients of the quinidine group (27). Pretreatment with class IC antiarrhythmic drugs may also prevent IRAF. In a randomized, placebo-controlled study of 100 patients with chronic atrial fibrillation scheduled for external cardioversion, no patient given oral propafenone (750 mg/day for 2 days) had IRAF. In the placebo group of this study, IRAF occurred in 17% of the patients, and the majority were also successfully treated with propafenone (intravenous bolus of 1.5 mg/kg) followed by a repeated shock (32). More recent studies have shown a favorable effect of class III and IV antiarrhythmic drugs on the suppression of IRAF. In a retrospective study, IRAF occurred in 20 (31%) of 64 patients after internal cardioversion of chronic AF. Repeated cardioversion was effective at preventing IRAF in only two patients, and intravenous sotalol (1.5 mg/kg) given before a repeated internal shock suppressed IRAF in 15 of the remaining 18 patients (83%) (29). Another unrandomized study demonstrated that 5 of 11 patients (46%) with IRAF after external cardioversion converted to sinus rhythm during loading with amiodarone (600 mg/day for 4 weeks), compared to only 1 of 16 patients (6%) with shock failure. Of interest is that 1 month after either pharmacological or a second electrical cardioversion, 91% of the patients with IRAF after the initial electrical cardioversion vs. 31% of the patients with shock failure were in sinus rhythm. This study suggests that IRAF identifies patients in whom amiodarone loading with or without repeated electrical cardioversion successfully restores and maintains sinus rhythm (31). In another study, intravenous verapamil (10 mg over 5 to 10 min) followed by a fourth cardioversion could suppress IRAF in approximately half of the 19 patients with reproducible IRAF after each of three consecutive external cardioversions. This favorable effect of a calcium channel blocker probably occurred due to the fact that all patients were on a class I antiarrhythmic drug or sotalol during the procedure (15). The role of antiarrhythmic drugs to prevent or suppress subacute and late recurrences after electrical cardioversion is discussed in

Chap. 9. The selection of the appropriate antiarrhythmic drug to be administered before the electrical cardioversion depends not only on the type of the time-dependent recurrence but also on the presence of structural heart disease (7).

VII. INTERNAL CARDIOVERSION

A transvenous electrode system, by delivering energy closer to the atrial myocardium, improves the efficacy and considerably reduces the amount of energy required for cardioversion of atrial fibrillation. The same preprocedural recommendations should be used for internal cardioversion as previously discussed for external cardioversion except that the anticoagulation therapy must be temporarily interrupted before the procedure if a safe venous puncture is to be performed. General anesthesia is not needed but, whenever required, conscious sedation should be provided while monitoring the blood pressure and transcutaneous oxygen saturation. Although several techniques are used for internal cardioversion, the following is the most frequently used. Three temporary catheters are inserted in the venous system and positioned under fluoroscopic guidance. Two large-surface-area catheters are used for shock delivery as well as a third bipolar catheter for R-wave synchronization and temporary ventricular postshock pacing. Previous animal studies have shown that biatrial shocks are safe if they are synchronized to the R wave, not preceded by a long–short sequence, and delivered after an R-R interval of at least 300 ms (33,34). During clinical application, intracardiac shocks are delivered only after R-R intervals above 500 ms, so as to allow a safety margin. The first cardioversion catheter is advanced in the distal coronary sinus and the second is preferably positioned in the right atrial appendix or in the lateral wall of the right atrium. The cardioversion catheters are connected to an external defibrillator delivering biphasic shocks. The bipolar catheter is placed in the apex of the right ventricle and also connected to an external pacemaker. An alternative position for a cardioversion catheter placed in the distal coronary sinus is the left pulmonary artery or the left atrium through a patent foramen ovale. During the procedure, intravenous heparin should always be administrated.

Although the invasive nature of this procedure, requiring a brief hospitalization, remains the main limitation for its widespread use, internal cardioversion of AF has several clinical applications. The treatment of patients in whom external cardioversion has failed to restore sinus rhythm (35) is the most accepted indication for catheter-based restoration of sinus rhythm. After internal cardioversion, the long-term outcome of the arrhythmia in patients refractory to external cardioversion is good, especially if total arrhythmia duration has been brief (Fig. 2) (36). Patients in whom general anesthesia is contraindicated or hazardous—as, for example, patients with severe obstructive lung disease—may also be considered for a low-energy intracardiac shock. Atrial fibrillation may complicate a diagnostic electro-physiologic study or ablation procedure. Provided that the appropriate catheters are already in place, internal cardioversion is the method of choice to restore sinus rhythm and allows completion of the study or treatment with no need for general anesthesia or the intravenous administration of antiar-rhythmic drugs, which may prolong or complicate these procedures. On the other hand, the repetitive occurrence of IRAF after low-energy intracardiac shocks may help to identify and ablate the trigger(s) in patients with focal atrial fibrillation (37). Another possible indication for transvenous cardio-version is present in patients with suspected atrioventricular conduction disturbances in whom cardioversion can be performed only after insertion of a temporary pacing lead.

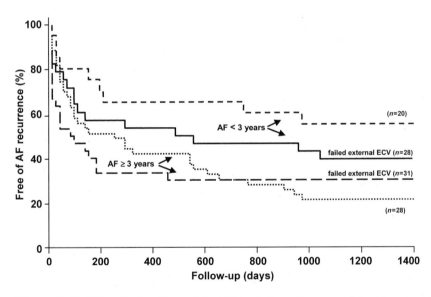

Figure 2 In 122 patients with persistent AF, of whom 59 were resistant to external cardioversion, the time to the first recurrence after a single internal cardioversion was recorded. The two patient populations were subdivided into two groups according to the duration of AF (< or ≥ 3 years). Kaplan Meier curves were constructed for the first 3 months of follow-up. This study suggests that internal cardioversion can be attempted in patients with persistent atrial fibrillation refractory to external cardioversion, especially if the arrhythmia exists for a short time. AF, atrial fibrillation; ECV, electrical cardioversion; n, number of patients.

A comparison of the reported success rates and energy requirements for internal cardioversion is not only difficult because of the variable use of a preestablished energy limit for termination of the procedure but also because of the heterogeneous populations treated, the evaluation of several technological improvements of the cardioversion system, and the differences in lead configurations. In general, energies of 6 to 10 J convert most episodes of AF. The efficacy for terminating episodes of paroxysmal AF varies between 92% and 100% and for persistent AF between 70% and 100% (38). Although internal cardioversion has a higher acute efficacy in restoring sinus rhythm with remarkably low amounts of energy compared with external cardioversion, the long-term outcome seems to be independent of the method of cardioversion.

Complications of internal cardioversion are rare and, if they occur, are related to the insertion and manipulation of catheters and improper synchronization and anticoagulation.

VIII. COMPLICATIONS

Complications after external cardioversion are reported to vary from 5% to 27% (12,39–41). The most commonly observed complications are discussed below.

No myocardial injury occurs following cardioversion with the energies used in a regular clinical situation, as detected by the cardiac regulatory protein troponin I (42). Immediately after cardioversion, ST-segment elevation and negative T waves may be observed. The time frame for normalization of these electrocardiographic changes may vary from minutes (ST-segment elevation) to days (negative T waves). The exact mechanism of these electrocardiographic changes remain unknown. However, they have been associated with the amount of energy delivered (43,44). Furthermore, it has been postulated that postshock transient enhanced permeability of the cellular membrane occurs, allowing ionic exchange that leads to membrane depolarization (electroporation) (45). This phenomenon is macroscopically manifest as ST-segment changes.

Ventricular arrhythmias are the most common complications after electrical cardioversion. They are related to the presence of hypokalemia, digitalis toxicity, severity of heart disease, improper synchronization, and the repeated use of high levels of energy. If atrioventricular conduction disturbances are suspected—for example, a slow ventricular response to atrial fibrillation without antiarrhythmic drug treatment—cardioversion should be avoided, as asystole may result or should be performed after the insertion of a temporary transvenous pacing lead. Atropine should always be available before cardioversion.

Thromboembolic events have been reported in about 3% to 5% of patients who did not receive anticoagulation before cardioversion, whereas it is only 0% to 1% in anticoagulated subjects (46,47). Thromboembolism is discussed below.

Minor complications, such as first-degree skin burns and chest muscle or skeleton pain, may occur and are related to the amount of energy used.

IX. SPECIAL SITUATIONS

In patients with hyperthyroidism, cardioversion should be deferred until approximately the fourth month of maintaining a euthyroid state, because more than half of AF spontaneously reverts to sinus rhythm when the thyroid hormone levels start to decline. After cardioversion, almost all of these patients maintain sinus rhythm (48).

Heart failure should as much as possible be controlled before cardioversion (49).

Damage to the electrical circuitry of an implanted device (pacemaker/ implantable cardioverter defibrillator) or to the electrode–myocardial interface may occur following cardioversion (50). The cardioversion electrodes should be placed as far from the implanted device as possible, preferably in the anteroposterior position. This also helps to avoid a maximum electrical field parallel to the direction of the lead system. After the cardioversion, the pacemaker system should be checked. Because pacing thresholds may increase gradually over weeks, with subsequent loss of capture by the device, serial pacing threshold measurements for 2 months are recommended.

Atrial fibrillation during pregnancy is rarely observed. However, if this occurs in the presence of organic heart disease (e.g., mitral stenosis), it may be associated with severe hemodynamic deterioration. Electrical cardioversion is necessary in all patients who are hemodynamically unstable and does not appear to adversely affect the fetus (51,52).

X. INDICATIONS FOR ELECTRICAL CARDIOVERSION

The primary goal of electrical cardioversion is amelioration of arrhythmia-related complaints (7). This is most evident in *acute-onset* AF but also relatively asymptomatic patients with *persistent* AF may benefit. Acute cardioversion for hypotension, angina pectoris, or heart failure induced by AF is rarely needed. Under those circumstances, the procedure is not without significant risk, and recurrence is frequent due to clinical instability. In most cases, aggressive rate control suffices.

There is no proof that, in the long run, cardioversions help to reduce heart failure or thromboembolism. By contrast, the evidence is in favor of a lack of benefit (53–56). Nevertheless, electrical cardioversion is indicated in (1) relatively stable patients with symptomatic attacks of AF and in (2) patients with first-ever AF whether or not they are reporting symptoms. In all these patients, rhythm-control drugs may be tried first to see whether (concealed) symptoms can be alleviated by restoration of sinus rhythm. The third group is (3) patients with symptomatic persistent AF in whom arrhythmia recurrence is unlikely. Electrical rather than pharmacological cardioversion is preferred, since rhythm-control drugs are usually ineffective in persistent AF. Finally, electrical cardioversion may be indicated in (4) patients with persistent AF and a relatively high recurrence risk who can safely sustain prophylactic rhythm-control drugs.

XI. ANTICOAGULATION

Cardioversion without anticoagulation carries a substantial risk of thromboembolism (46,47), particularly when the arrhythmia has lasted longer than 48 hr. The embolic events usually occur from hours after conversion up until 10 days, with a maximum of 18 days (57). Routine anticoagulation includes the effective use of warfarin or another vitamin K antagonist for 3 to 4 weeks before and until 4 weeks after the procedure (7,58). The decision to stop anticoagulation depends on whether or not the patient has stroke risk factors (7).

The guidelines (7,58) also indicate that, for AF lasting less than 48 hr, anticoagulation is not needed during cardioversion. Thrombi may form within that time period. However, the risk of clinical thromboembolism with either spontaneous, pharmacological, or electrical conversion of AF with a known duration shorter than 48 hr is low, justifying an unanticoagulated approach (59). Firm data are still lacking. Therefore, we suggest considering stroke risk factors before cardioversion and, in case these are present, acute follow-up anticoagulation with (low-molecular-weight) heparin. The reason to pretreat with anticoagulation is to allow for either thrombus organization and adherence to the atrial wall or resolution of thrombus. These processes take approximately 4 weeks of anticoagulation (60). Anticoagulation after conversion is needed, since thrombi may form, and these may dislodge with the return of atrial contraction. The return of normal mechanical atrial contraction may take several weeks because of time-dependent reverse remodeling of the atria (61–64). The structural and mechanical remodeling associated with long-lasting forms of AF has been called "stunning" (65) and is characterized by absent or diminished atrial contraction while blood flow is sufficient and the rate is normal. Restoration of the mechanical function of the atria is related to the duration of atrial fibrillation (61–64). The prolonged recovery from stunning explains the time lag between conversion and occurrence of stroke.

There is no solid clinical evidence that cardioversion followed by chronic sinus rhythm effectively reduces thromboembolism in patients with AF. A post hoc analysis of the four rhythm- vs. rate-control studies (66) has shown that the current rhythm-control strategies increase rather than decrease the stroke rate. Until more effective and less toxic rhythm-control strategies become available, rhythm control cannot be advised for the patient with the arguments that stroke rate can be reduced and that this approach obviates the need for anticoagulation. Concerning the latter, there is an extremely fixed misconception among physicians that patients with chronic sinus rhythm after cardioversion may terminate anticoagulation. However, the stroke risk is not determined by the rhythm but by stroke risk factors such as previous stroke, hypertension, heart failure, increasing age, coronary artery disease, and diabetes mellitus (7). The actual rhythm—sinus rhythm or atrial fibrillation—is not in this list.

XII. RESCUE ELECTRICAL CARDIOVERSION

After failed pharmacological conversion for an episode of AF, a rescue electrical cardioversion may be carried out to prevent patients from crossing the 48-hr anticoagulation boundary. This strategy is essential mainly in patients with paroxysmal AF with prolonged attacks, lasting longer than 48 hr to usually less than 1 week, in whom full anticoagulation may thus be avoided. However, if these patients have crossed the 48-hr boundary, transesophageal echocardiography may be helpful to exclude a low-flow state or thrombi and allow for immediate electrical cardioversion with heparin.

XIII. THE ROLE OF TRANSESOPHAGEAL ECHOCARDIOGRAPHY

Transesophageal echocardiography–guided cardioversion is being used to avoid prolonged anticoagulation before cardioversion. The potential advantages are immediate amelioration of complaints and shortening of the time spent in AF, thereby reducing atrial remodeling as well as bleeding risk. The clinical role of transesophageal echocardiography is, however, rather limited. The Assessment of Cardioversion Using Transesophageal Echocardiography (ACUTE) trial was designed to compare prospectively conventional anticoagulation with transesophageal echocardiography–guided short-term anticoagulation in patients with AF of more than 2 days' duration undergoing electrical cardioversion (67). The transesophageal echocardiography–guided group (n = 619) received heparin before cardioversion and warfarin for 4 weeks following cardioversion. Cardioversion was postponed when a thrombus was identified, and warfarin was administered for 3 weeks before transesophageal echocardiography was repeated. The conventional group (n = 603) received oral anticoagulation for 3 weeks before and 4 weeks after cardioversion. The 8-week stroke rate was low: 0.81% with the transesophageal echocardiography approach and 0.50% with the conventional approach. There was slightly less bleeding with the transesophageal echocardiography–guided approach but no difference in the proportion of cardioverted subjects. Combined major and minor bleeding was lower in the invasive arm (2.9 vs. 5.5%) (68). Thus, transesophageal echocardiography–guided cardioversion may be used to foreshorten conversion to sinus rhythm in patients who lack intra-atrial thrombi or spontaneous echo contrast. At the same time, bleeding may be avoided. These patients may undergo cardioversion immediately after the start of heparin, including low-molecular-weight heparin (69).

Despite these potential advantages, compared to routine cardioversion, there is no advantage in terms of limiting atrial remodeling and improving the prognosis of the long-term arrhythmia. In addition, the advantage of shorter term of oral anticoagulation with less bleeding compared to the conventional approach holds only for the very limited number of patients who do not need chronic anticoagulation. Of note, most candidates for electrical cardioversion have concurrent stroke risk factors; hence, an acute strategy does not provide an advantage in this respect. In view of the above, the main indication for transesophageal echocardiography–guided cardioversion is foreshortening restoration of sinus rhythm in patients with paroxysmal AF with significant arrhythmic complaints during the attack but who have crossed the 48-hr anticoagulation boundary or who have a high perceived stroke risk. In these patients pharmacological or electrical cardioversion may be carried out with heparin treatment immediately after transesophageal echocardiography has excluded abnormalities in the atria. Needless to say, whatever conversion strategy is followed in this subgroup of patients, 1 month of full anticoagulation (and lifelong anticoagulation if stroke risk factors are present) after conversion remains indicated.

XIV. LOW-MOLECULAR-WEIGHT HEPARIN

In patients undergoing transesophageal echocardiography-guided cardioversion, low-molecular-weight heparin is an attractive alternative to unfractionated heparin. Some of these advantages include more predictable anticoagulation and no requirement for monitoring (70) as well as potential cost savings due to an earlier hospital discharge or cardioversion in the outpatient setting (71). The recently reported Anticoagulation for Cardioversion using Enoxaparin (ACE) trial (69) compared subcutaneous enoxaparin (212 patients) with conventional intravenous unfractionated heparin followed by coumarin (216 patients) in association with cardioversion. Transesophageal echocardiography-guided cardioversion was performed in 87% of the patients. The 4-week combined primary endpoint (cerebral ischemic neurological events, systemic thromboembolism, death from any cause, and major bleeding) was observed in 7 enoxaparin patients (3.3%) and in 12 patients of the unfractionated heparin/coumarin group (5.6%) ($p < 0.02$). The ACE trial shows that low-molecular-weight enoxoparin is at least as effective as conventional anticoagulation, if not more so, in the cardioversion of AF. The ongoing ACUTE II pilot study may support the findings of the ACE trial (72).

XV. HOW TO APPLY ANTICOAGULATION WITH CARDIOVERSION

Based on the ACC/AHA/ESC guidelines for the management of patients with atrial fibrillation (7) as well as the ACCP guideline (see also Chap. 7, Tables 1 and 2) (58), all patients with AF lasting more than 48 hr or of unknown duration should receive anticoagulation with an INR between 2 and 3 for at least 3 to 4 weeks before and after cardioversion. For patients with acute AF needing prompt cardioversion, the procedure may be carried out without pretreatment. If not contraindicated, heparin should be given, first a bolus and then a continuous infusion in a dose adjusted to prolong the activated partial thromboplastin time 1.5 to 2.0 times the reference control value. Oral anticoagulation should then be given for at least 3 to 4 weeks and lifelong if stroke risk factors are present. Instead of heparin, low-molecular-weight heparin may be given subcutaneously. Fast-track cardioversion under (low-molecular-weight) heparin followed by oral anticoagulation may be performed in patients without thrombi or spontaneous echocontrast as detected by transesophageal echocardiography. If transesophageal echocardiography reveals a thrombus, pretreatment with oral anticoagulants, usually followed by a repeat transesophageal echocardiography before cardioversion, is needed.

Four weeks after cardioversion, anticoagulation may be stopped only in patients who do not have stroke risk factors. Note that if the actual rhythm is AF, it is not an established stroke risk factor. Patients with AF shorter than 48 hr in duration may undergo conversion without anticoagulation. However, if these patients show evidence of stroke risk factors, lifelong anticoagulation is recommended.

REFERENCES

1. Botto GL, Politi A, Bonini W, Broffoni T, Bonatti R. External cardioversion of atrial fibrillation: role of paddle position on technical efficacy and energy requirements. Heart 1999; 82:726–730.
2. Kirchhof P, Eckardt L, Loh P, Weber K, Fischer RJ, Seidl KH, Böcker D, Breithardt G, Haverkamp W, Borggrefe M. Anterior–posterior versus anterior–lateral electrode positions for external cardioversion of atrial fibrillation: a randomised trial. Lancet 2002; 360:1275–1279.
3. Ewy GA. Optimal technique for electrical cardioversion of atrial fibrillation. Circulation 1992; 86(5):1645–1647.
4. Kerber RE, Grayzel J, Hoyt R, Marcus M, Kennedy J. Transthoracic resistance in human defibrillation. Influence of body weight, chest size, serial shocks, paddle size and paddle contact pressure. Circulation 1981; 63(3):676–682.
5. Cohen TJ, Ibrahim B, Denier D, Haji A, Quan W. Active compression cardioversion for refractory atrial fibrillation. Am J Cardiol 1997; 80(3):354–355.
6. Bissing JW, Kerber RE. Effect of shaving the chest of hirsute subjects on transthoracic impedance. Am J Cardiol 2000; 86:587–589.
7. Committee to develop guidelines for the management of patients with atrial fibrillation: executive summary. A report of the American College of Cardiology/American Heart Association task force on practice guidelines and the European Society of Cardiology committee for practice guidelines and policy conferences. Circulation 2001; 104:2118–2150.
8. Ricard P, Lévy S, Trigano J, Paganelli F, Daoud E, Man KC, Strickberger SA, Morady F. Prospective assessment of the minimum energy needed for external electrical cardioversion of atrial fibrillation. Am J Cardiol 1997; 79(6): 815–816.
9. Gallagher MM, Guo XH, Poloniecki JD, Yap YG, Ward D, Camm J. Initial energy setting, outcome and efficiency in direct current cardioversion of atrial fibrillation and flutter. J Am Coll Cardiol 2001; 38(5):1498–1504.
10. Page RL, Kerber RE, Russell JK, Trouton T, Waktare J, Gallik D, Olgin JE, Ricard P, Dalzell GW, Reddy R, Lazzara R, Lee K, Carlson M, Halperin B,

Bardy GH. Biphasic versus monophasic shock waveform for conversion of atrial fibrillation. J Am Coll Cardiol 2002; 39:1956–1963.

11. Lown B. Electrical reversion of cardiac arrhythmias. Br Heart J 1967; 29:469–489.

12. van Gelder IC, Crijns HJ, van Gilst WH, Verwer R, Lie KI. Prediction of uneventful cardioversion and maintenance of sinus rhythm from direct-current electrical cardioversion of chronic atrial fibrillation and flutter. Am J Cardiol 1991; 68:41–46.

13. Kerber RE, Martins JB, Kienzle MG, Constantin L, Olshansky B, Hopson R, Charbonnier F. Energy, current, and success in defibrillation and cardioversion: clinical studies using an automated impedance-based method of energy adjustment. Circulation 1988; 77(5):1038–1046.

14. van Gelder IC, Crijns HJGM, Tieleman RG, Brügemann J, de Kam PJ, Gosselink ATM, Verheugt FWA, Lie KI. Chronic atrial fibrillation. Success of serial cardioversion therapy and safety of oral anticoagulation. Arch Intern Med 1996; 156:2585–2592.

15. Daoud EG, Hummel JD, Augostini R, Williams S, Kalbfleisch SJ. Effect of verapamil on immediate recurrence of atrial fibrillation. J Cardiovasc Electrophysiol 2000; 11:1231–1237.

16. Yu WC, Lin YK, Tai CT, Tsai CF, Hsieh MH, Chen CC, Hsu TL, Ding YA, Chang MS, Chen SA. Early recurrence of atrial fibrillation after external cardioversion. PACE 1999; 22:1614–1619.

17. Oral H, Ozaydin M, Sticherling C, Tada H, Scharf C, Chugh A, Lai SWK, Pelosi F, Knight BP, Strickberger SA, Morady F. Effect of atrial fibrillation duration on probability of immediate recurrence after transthoracic cardioversion. J Cardiovasc Electrophysiol 2003; 14:182–185.

18. Tieleman RG, van Gelder IC, Crijns HJGM, de Kam PJ, van den Berg MP, Haaksma J, van der Woude HJ, Allessie MA. Early recurrences of atrial fibrillation after electrical cardioversion: a result of fibrillation-induced electrical remodeling of the atria? J Am Coll Cardiol 1998; 37:167–173.

19. Duytschaever M, Danse P, Allessie M. Supervulnerable phase immediately after termination of atrial fibrillation. J Cardiovasc Electrophysiol 2002; 13:267–275.

20. Timmermans C, Rodriguez LM, Smeets JLRM, Wellens HJJ. Immediate reinitiation of atrial fibrillation following internal atrial defibrillation. J Cardiovasc Electrophysiol 1998; 9:122–128.

21. Saliba W, Juratli N, Chung MK, Niebauer MJ, Erdogan O, Trohman R, Wilkoff BL, Augostini R, Mowrey KA, Nadzam GR, Tchou PJ. Higher energy synchronized external direct current cardioversion for refractory atrial fibrillation. J Am Coll Cardiol 1999; 34:2031–2034.

22. Mittal S, Ayati S, Stein KM, Schwartzman D, Cavlovich D, Tchou PJ, Markowitz SM, Slotwiner DJ, Scheiner MA, Lerman BB. Transthoracic cardioversion of atrial fibrillation. Comparison of rectilinear biphasic versus damped sine wave monophasic shocks. Circulation 2000; 101:1282–1287.

23. Oral H, Souza JJ, Michaud GF, Knight BP, Goyal R, Strickberger SA, Morady

F. Facilitating transthoracic cardioversion of atrial fibrillation with ibutilide pretreatment. N Engl J Med 1999; 340(No 24):1849–1854.

24. Lau CP, Lok NS. A comparison of transvenous atrial defibrillation of acute and chronic atrial fibrillation and the effect of intravenous sotalol on human atrial defibrillation threshold. PACE 1997; 20:2442–2452.

25. van Gelder IC, Crijns HJGM, van Gilst WH, de Langen CDJ, van Wijk LM, Lie KI. Effects of flecainide on the atrial defibrillation threshold. Am J Cardiol 1989; 63:112–114.

26. Boriani G, Biffi M, Capucci A, Bronzetti G, Ayers GM, Zannoli R, Branzi AA, Magnani B. Favorable effects of flecainide in transvenous internal cardioversion of atrial fibrillation. J Am Coll Cardiol 1999; 33:333–341.

27. Rossi M, Lown B. The use of Quinidine in cardioversion. Am J Cardiol 1967; 19:234–238.

28. Hillestad L, Dale J, Storstein O. Quinidine before direct current countershock. A controlled study. Br Heart J 1972; 34:139–142.

29. Tse HF, Lau CP, Ayers GM. Incidence and modes of onset of early reinitiation of atrial fibrillation after successful interal cardioversion, and its prevention by intravenous sotalol. Heart 1999; 82:319–324.

30. van Noord T, van Gelder IC, Crijns HJGM. How to enhance acute outcome of electrical cardioversion by drug therapy: importance of immediate reinitiation of atrial fibrillation. J Cardiovasc Electrophysiol 2002; 13:822–825.

31. van Noord T, van Gelder IC, Schoonderwoerd BA, Crijns HJGM. Immediate reinitiation of atrial fibrillation after electrical cardioversion predicts subsequent pharmacologic and electrical conversion to sinus rhythm on amiodarone. Am J Cardiol 2000; 86:1384–1385.

32. Bianconi L, Mennuni M, Lukic V, Castro A, Chieffi M, Santini M. Effects of oral propafenone administration before electrical cardioversion of chronic atrial fibrillation: a placebo-controlled study. J Am Coll Cardiol 1996; 28:700–706.

33. Ayers GM, Alferness CA, Ilina M, Wagner DO, Sirokman WA, Adams JM, Griffin JC. Ventricular proarrhythmic effects of ventricular cycle length and shock strength in a sheep model of transvenous atrial defibrillation. Circulation 1994; 89:413–422.

34. Keelan ET, Krum D, Hare J, Mughal K, Li H, Akhtar M, Jazayeri MR. Safety of atrial defibrillation shocks synchronized to narrow and wide QRS complexes during atrial pacing protocols simulating atrial fibrillation in dogs. Circulation 1997; 96:2022–2030.

35. Schmitt C, Alt E, Plewan A, Ammer R, Leibig M, Karch M, Schömig A. Low energy intracardiac cardioversion after failed conventional external cardioversion of atrial fibrillation. J Am Coll Cardiol 1996; 28:994–999.

36. Timmermans C, Rodriguez LM, Efremidis M, Hahnraths E, Philippens S, Nabar A, Wellens HJJ. Long-term outcome in patients with permanent atrial fibrillation after internal cardioversion [abstr]. Circulation 2000; 102:II-482.

37. Lau CP, Tse HF, Ayers GM. Defibrillation-guided radiofrequency ablation of atrial fibrillation secondary to an atrial focus. J Am Coll Cardiol 1999; 33:1217–1226.

38. Boriani G, Biffi M, Gamainin C, Luceri RM, Branzi A. Transvenous low energy internal cardioversion for atrial fibrillation: a review of clinical application and future developments. PACE 2001; 24:99–107.

39. Rabinno MD, Lokoff W, Dreiffus LS. Complications and limitations of direct current countershock. JAMA 1964; 190:417–420.

40. Åberg H, Culihed I. Direct current countershock complications. Acta Med Scand 1968; 183:415–421.

41. Resnekov L, McDonald L. Complications in 220 patients with cardiac dysrhythmias treated by phased direct current shock and indications for electrocardioversion. Br Heart J 1967; 29:926.

42. Bonnefoy E, Chevalier P, Kirkorian G, Guidolet J, Marchand A, Touboul P. Cardiac troponin I does not increase after cardioversion. Chest 1997; 111:15–18.

43. van Gelder IC, Crijns HJ, van der Laarse A, van Gilst WH, Lie KI. Incidence and clinical significance of ST segment elevation after electrical cardioversion of atrial fibrillation and atrial flutter. Am Heart J 1991; 121:51–56.

44. Chun PKC, Davia JE, Donohue DJ. ST segment elevation with elective DC cardioversion. Circulation 1981; 63:220–224.

45. Jones JL, Jones RE, Balasky G. Microlesion formation in myocardial cells by high-intensity electric field stimulation. Am J Physiol 1987; 253:H480–H486.

46. Bjerkeland CI, Orning OM. The efficacy of anticoagulant therapy in preventing embolism related to DC electrical conversion of atrial fibrillation. Am J Cardiol 1969; 23:208–216.

47. Arnold AZ, Mick MJ, Mazurck RP, Loop FD, Trohman RG. Role of prophylactic anticoagulation for direct current cardioversion in patients with atrial fibrillation or atrial flutter. J Am Coll Cardiol 1992; 19:851–855.

48. Shimizu T, Koide S, Noh JY, Sugino K, Ito K, Nakazawa H. Hyperthyroidism and the management of atrial fibrillation. Thyroid 2002; 12:489–493.

49. van den Berg MP, Tuinenburg AE, van Veldhuisen DJ, de Kam PJ, Crijns HJGM. Cardioversion of atrial fibrillation in the setting of mild to moderate heart failure. Int J Cardiol 1998; 63:63–70.

50. Altamura G, Bianconi L, Bianco FL, Toscano S, Ammirati F, Pandozi C, Castro A, Cardinale M, Mennuni M, Santini M. Transthoracic DC shock may represent a serious hazard in pacemaker dependent patients. Pacing Clin Electrophysiol 1995; 18:194–198.

51. Gowda RM, Khan IA, Mehta NJ, Vasavada BC, Sacchi TJ. Cardiac arrhythmias in pregnancy: clinical and therapeutic considerations. Int J Cardiol 2003; 88:129–133.

52. Schroeder JS, Harrison DC. Repeated cardioversion during pregnancy. Am J Cardiol 1971; 27:445–446.

53. Hohnloser SH, Kuck KH, Lilienthal J. Rhythm or rate control in atrial fibrillation—pharmacological intervention in atrial fibrillation (PIAF): a randomized trial. Lancet 2000; 356:1789–1794.

54. Carlsson J, Miketic S, Windeler J, Cuneo A, Haun S, Micus S, et al., for the

STAF investigators. Randomized trial of rate-control versus rhythm-control in persistent atrial fibrillation. J Am Coll Cardiol 2003; 41:1690–1696.

55. Van Gelder IC, Hagens VE, Bosker HA, Kingma JH, Kamp O, Kingma T, et al. A comparison of rate control and rhythm control in patients with recurrent persistent atrial fibrillation. N Engl J Med 2002; 347:1834–1840.

56. The atrial fibrillation follow-up investigation of rhythm management (AF-FIRM) investigators. A comparison of rate control and rhythm control in patients with atrial fibrillation. N Engl J Med 2002; 347:1825–1833.

57. Berger M, Schweitzer P. Timing of thromboembolic events after electrical cardioversion of atrial fibrillation or flutter: a retrospective analysis. Am J Cardiol 1998; 82:1545–1547.

58. Albers GW, Dalen JE, Laupacis A, Manning WJ, Petersen P, Singer DE. Antithrombotic therapy in atrial fibrillation. Chest 2001; 119:S194–206.

59. Weigner MJ, Caulfield TA, Danias PG, Silverman DI, Manning WJ. Risk for clinical thromboembolism associated with conversion to sinus rhythm in patients with atrial fibrillation lasting less than 48 hours. Ann Intern Med 1997; 126:615–620.

60. Corrado G, Tadeo G, Beretta S, et al. Atrial thrombi resolution after prolonged anticoagulation in patients with atrial fibrillation: a transesophageal echocardiographic study. Chest 1999; 115:140–143.

61. Manning WJ, Silverman DI, Katz SE, et al. Impaired left atrial mechanical function after cardioversion: relation to the duration of atrial fibrillation. J Am Coll Cardiol 1994; 23:1535–1540.

62. Manning WJ, Silverman DI, Katz SE, et al. Temporal dependence of the return of atrial mechanical function on the mode of cardioversion of atrial fibrillation to sinus rhythm. Am J Cardiol 1995; 75:624–626.

63. Grimm RA, Leung DY, Black IW, Stewart WJ, Thomas JD, Klein AL. Left atrial appendage "stunning" after spontaneous conversion of atrial fibrillation demonstrated by transesophageal Doppler echocardiography. Am Heart J 1995; 130:174–176.

64. Mitusch R, Garbe M, Schmucker G, Schwabe K, Stierle U, Sheikhzadeh A. Relation of left atrial appendage function to the duration and reversibility of nonvalvular atrial fibrillation. Am J Cardiol 1995; 75:944–947.

65. Manning WJ, Leeman DE, Gotch PJ, Come PC. Pulsed Doppler evaluation of atrial mechanical function after electrical cardioversion of atrial fibrillation. J Am Coll Cardiol 1989; 13:617–623.

66. Verheugt FWA, van Gelder IC, Wyse DG, Hohnloser SH, Carlsson J, Crijns HJGM. Stroke prevention by rhythm versus rate control in atrial fibrillation: insight from the randomized studies [abstr]. Circulation 2002; 106(suppl II):546.

67. Klein AL, Grimm RA, Murray RD, et al., for the Assessment of Cardioversion Using Transesophageal Echocardiography Investigators. Use of transesophageal echocardiography to guide cardioversion in patients with atrial fibrillation. N Engl J Med 2001; 344:1411–1420.

68. Klein AL, Murray RD, Grimm RA, Li J, Apperson-Hansen C, Jasper SE, Goodman-Bizon AS, Lieber EA, Black IW, for the ACUTE Investigators.

Bleeding complications in patients with atrial fibrillation undergoing cardioversion randomized to transesophageal echocardiographically guided and conventional anticoagulation therapies. Am J Cardiol 2003; 92:161–165.

69. Stellbrink C. Anticoagulation for cardioversion using enoxaparin. Oral Presentation at the European Society of Cardiology Congress, Berlin, Germany, Aug 31–Sept 4, 2002. Available from www.escardio.org.

70. Hirsch J, Warkentin TE, Shaughnessy SG, et al. Heparin and low-molecular-weight heparin: mechanisms of action, pharmacokinetics, dosing, monitoring, efficacy, and safety. Chest 2001; 119:S64–S94.

71. Murray RD, Deitcher SR, Shah A, et al. Potential clinical efficacy and cost benefit of a transesophageal echo-cardiography-guided low-molecular-weight heparin (enoxaparin) approach to antithrombotic therapy in patients undergoing immediate cardioversion from atrial fibrillation. J Am Soc Echocardiogr 2001; 14:200–208.

72. Murray RD, Shah A, Jasper SE, et al. Transesophageal echocardiography guided enoxaparin antithrombotic strategy for cardioversion of atrial fibrillation: the ACUTE II pilot study [online exclusive article]. Am Heart J 2002; 139.e5. Available at www.mosby.com\ahj.

73. van Gelder IC, Tuinenburg AE, Schoonderwoerd BS, Tieleman RG, Crijns HJGM. Pharmacologic versus direct-current electrical cardioversion of atrial flutter and fibrillation. Am J Cardiol 1999; 84:147R–151R.

9
Pharmacological Cardioversion of Atrial Fibrillation

Joachim R. Ehrlich and Stefan H. Hohnloser
Johann Wolfgang Goethe-University, Frankfurt, Germany

I. INTRODUCTION

Atrial fibrillation (AF) is the most commonly encountered clinical arrhythmia, with an age-dependent prevalence of 0.5 to 8% (1). Although the arrhythmia is initially often present in a paroxysmal form, it progresses to persistent or permanent AF in most patients (2). According to this definition, persistent AF is continually present but may still be converted by medical treatment, whereas permanent AF cannot be terminated, and only rate-control with anticoagulation remains as a therapeutic option.

In patients in whom AF does not spontaneously revert to sinus rhythm, termination of AF must be achieved by pharmacological or electrical cardioversion. This chapter focuses on pharmacological interventions and reviews mechanisms of antiarrhythmic drug action for stopping AF.

II. PATHOPHYSIOLOGY AND ROLE OF AF-INDUCED REMODELING

In order to understand the effects of class I and III antiarrhythmic drugs on AF termination, one must consider the changes in atrial electrophysiology due to tachycardia-induced remodeling and theoretical concepts that help explain the effects of antiarrhythmics. For further detailed information, please refer to Chapter.

In persistent AF, multiple-wavelet reentry is a final common pathway of various AF pathomechanisms (3). Maintenance of reentry is critically dependent on short wavelengths (WL) of the reentrant circuits. WL is defined as the distance traveled by an impulse during the effective refractory period (ERP) and is given by the product of conduction velocity times ERP (4). The larger the WL, the fewer circuits can coexist and the more likely it is that the circulating impulse will encounter refractory tissue and die out.

AF creates an atrial substrate that facilitates its own persistence and induces a number of electrophysiological, structural, and mechanical changes. The electrophysiological changes occur early in AF and are centered around a self-protective reduction of L-type calcium currents ($I_{Ca,L}$) (5,6). They lead to shortened ERP and reduced WL, ultimately promoting reentry (3). Figure 1 summarizes some key features of AF-induced remodeling and puts changes in ERP in perspective with the likelihood of spontaneous or pharmacological cardioversion and the risk of AF relapse.

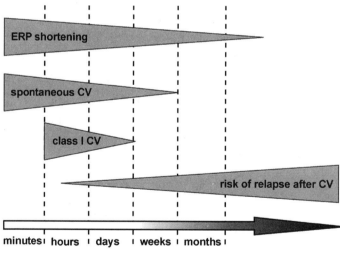

Figure 1 This Figure schematically demonstrates the interlude between shortening of the effective refractory period (ERP) as a key feature of AF-induced remodeling and the probability that an AF episode may end spontaneously. Pharmacological cardioversion (CV) with class I agents is readily possible within a time frame of hours to a few days, with decreasing efficacy after prolonged periods of AF. The risk of an AF relapse increases conversely.

III. MECHANISMS OF AF TERMINATION BY CLASS III ANTIARRHYTHMIC DRUGS

Action potential duration (APD) is the single most important cellular determinant of ERP. APD prolongation is the defining prerequisite for the classification of drugs as having class III efficacy (7). Antiarrhythmic drugs that prolong APD and hence ERP are effective agents for pharmacological cardioversion of AF. According to the multiple-wavelet theory, a shorter WL tends to promote AF. As a consequence of WL prolongation, multiple wavelets are unable to coexist simultaneously in the atria.

This is most impressively exemplified by the experimental congestive heart failure models of AF. Since congestive heart failure leads to significant downregulation of the slow delayed rectifier potassium current (I_{Ks}), I_{Kr} contributes more importantly to repolarization (8). Accordingly, application of dofetilide, a pure class III agent that blocks I_{Kr}, leads to significant prolongation of ERP in this setting leaving conduction velocity essentially unaffected (9). The subsequent increase in WL efficiently terminates AF episodes in this experimental model.

The efficacy of these agents in rapidly activated tissues is limited by the "reverse use dependence" shared by many class III drugs (10). This property leads to a relatively lower increase in ERP at higher stimulation frequencies or heart rates, making effective arrhythmia termination less likely.

IV. MECHANISMS OF AF TERMINATION BY CLASS I ANTIARRHYTHMIC DRUGS

From a theoretical point of view, the effect of sodium channel–blocking drugs is incompatible with the classical multiple-wavelet theory. These agents are effective in terminating AF, but they should rather promote AF by decreasing CV due to reduced availability of Na^+ channels and consecutively decreased WL. Contrary to these predictions, flecainide and propafenone are effective in converting high percentages of recent-onset AF (11,12).

Excitation of the atria in AF can be viewed as spiral waves with rotors that meander through the atria with a gradient of excitability that makes activation in the center of a rotor slower than in the periphery (13). Once excitability is reduced by Na^+-channel blockade, the rotor can no longer turn in a small radius. With increasing radius, it loses the ability to maintain itself, finally resulting in conversion of AF (14). This is evidenced by a decrease in WL during application of class I drugs in experimental animals, with an increase in the temporal excitable gap (difference between AF cycle length and atrial refractoriness during AF) (15). Along with the increase in the excitable gap, the core perimeter of the mother rotor increases and may lead to conversion, as shown in experiments using the Na^+-channel blocker pilsicainide (16). These experimental findings are in line with theoretical predictions made on the basis of mathematical models (14).

It remains to be determined why class I antiarrhythmics are effective in recent-onset AF whereas long-lasting AF remains quite resistant to drug therapy. A simple possibility may be that, with longer AF duration, remodeling becomes more prominent and ERPs are shortened to an extent where reduced excitability induced by Na^+-channel blockade does not suffice to stop AF.

V. CLINICAL PRINCIPLES OF PHARMACOLOGICAL CARDIOVERSION

Pharmacological cardioversion is primarily used to revert paroxysmal AF of recent onset, particularly if the arrhythmia is of less than 48-hr duration. Many controlled trials have shown the usefulness of class I and III antiarrhythmic drugs for this purpose. These drugs shorten the time to conversion when compared to placebo and increase the number of patients who revert acutely (within 30 to 60 min) or subacutely (within a few hours to days). On the other hand, digoxin, beta blockers, or calcium channel blockers are usually ineffective in reverting AF. The most important antiarrhythmic drugs for pharmacological cardioversion include procainamide, flecainide, and propafenone and the class III substances ibutilide, dofetilide, and amiodarone. Sotalol has been shown to have only very limited cardioversion efficacy, but it has the advantage of rapid rate control due to its beta blocking effects.

In evaluating the potential of a drug to cardiovert AF to normal sinus rhythm, the conversion rate and time from start of drug administration must be considered. Furthermore, the route of drug administration (i.e., single bolus intravenous administration vs. prolonged oral treatment) must be taken into account. Paroxysmal AF will convert earlier after initiation of therapy than persistent AF. Usually, paroxysmal AF converts within an hour, although some studies have reported conversion only after several hours to 1 to 2 days.

The most important question to answer before choosing a specific antiarrhythmic drug to convert AF acutely is whether or not the patient is affected by underlying structural heart disease. In patients with structural heart disease—particularly in the presence of coronary artery disease, arterial hypertension with left ventricular (LV) hypertrophy, or congestive heart failure—administration of class I antiarrhythmic drugs should be avoided due to the increased risk of ventricular proarrhythmia associated with these

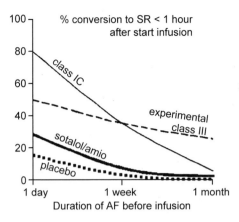

Figure 2 This Figure emphasizes the efficacy of class I and III drugs in terminating AF of various durations. With increasing duration of an AF episode, the likelihood of cardioversion by class I drugs decreases and the efficacy of class III drugs increases to a similar extent. (Modified from Ref. 48.)

drugs under these circumstances (17,18). In the absence of structural heart disease, sodium-channel blocking drugs are the preferred substances in many institutions.

Another important determinant of successful pharmacological cardioversion is the duration of the arrhythmic episode (19,20). Class IC drugs are particularly effective in the conversion of short-lasting AF. If the arrhythmia persists for less than 24 hr, the conversion rate may be as high as 90% at 1 hr after intravenous administration of flecainide or propafenone. The same drugs, however, are significantly less effective in converting AF that persisted for days or weeks. Class III antiarrhythmic drugs appear to be somewhat less effective than class IC drugs in converting short-lasting AF but may be superior in patients in whom AF had persisted for a few weeks or months (21) (Fig. 2).

VI. POTENTIAL LIMITATIONS OF PHARMACOLOGICAL CARDIOVERSION

All antiarrhythmic drugs may cause new arrhythmias or aggravate preexisting ones, an effect called proarrhythmia. On the ventricular side, class IC drugs may cause broad-complex incessant ventricular tachycardia (VT), whereas class III agents may cause polymorphic VT of the torsades de pointes type. On the atrial level, antiarrhythmic drugs may convert AF to atrial flutter. Atrial flutter with a reduced rate of atrial activation may subsequently be conducted to the ventricles in a 1:1 fashion, causing hemodynamic deterioration and syncope (22,23). This complication may occur in up to 5% of patients treated with class I drugs, and it is recommended to pretreat patients with beta blockers before application of class I drugs to slow atrioventricular (AV) conduction. Similarly, antiarrhythmic drugs are often associated with sinus bradycardia immediately after successful termination of AF. This effect is particularly often observed in patients with preexisting sinus node disease.

Another important consideration relates to the potential negative hemodynamic effects of antiarrhythmic drugs. Particularly class IC drugs have significant negative inotropic side effects, which limits their use in patients with impaired LV function. The one exception in this regard is represented by amiodarone, since this compound is essentially free of negative inotropic or other adverse hemodynamic effects.

Finally, the obvious disadvantage of pharmacological cardioversion is that it is often not applicable to patients with severe complaints directly related to AF. This form of cardioversion is time-consuming and may necessitate rather extensive surveillance of the patient, including continuous electrocardiographic (ECG) monitoring for several hours. In such instances, therefore, rapid electrical cardioversion may be the preferred treatment modality.

VII. FLECAINIDE AND PROPAFENONE FOR PHARMACOLOGICAL CARDIOVERSION

Flecainide and propafenone are two class IC antiarrhythmic drugs that have been extensively studied for the pharmacological conversion of AF. Particularly in patients with short-lasting, recent onset AF, these drugs restore sinus rhythm in up to 90% of treatment attempts. In most studies, flecainide has been administered as a short bolus infusion at dosages of 1 to 2 mg/kg. Unfortunately, the intravenous preparation is not available in the United States. There are only limited data in the literature concerning the effectiveness of single large oral doses of flecainide for pharmacological cardioversion. For instance, one study randomized 79 patients to intravenous or large oral dose of flecainide and found comparable conversion rates at 2 and 8 hr after the start of therapy (24). However, a shorter time to reversion was associated with the intravenous infusion.

Unlike flecainide, propafenone has been studied in several investigations in its oral form (12,25–28). For instance, one of the largest studies randomized 240 patients with AF of < 8 days' duration either to a single oral dose of propafenone (600 mg) or to matching placebo (27). The conversion rate with propafenone was approximately 45 and 76% at 3 and 8 hr, respectively, compared to 18 and 37% of control patients ($p < 0.02$). The conversion time was 181 ± 112 min in the propafenone group. Importantly, the efficacy of propafenone was similar in patients with or without structural heart disease; however, patients with documented conduction disturbances, recent myocardial infarction, or congestive heart failure were excluded from this trial. A recent comprehensive review by Khan (29) on the efficacy of a single oral loading dose of propafenone for conversion of recent-onset AF revealed conversion rates between 56 and 83%, thus confirming the usefulness of this therapeutic approach, which has been termed "the pill-in-the-pocket approach" to the treatment of AF. The same review also demonstrated that propafenone was well tolerated by the patients and that serious side effects, including potential proarrhythmic reactions, were noted no more frequently than in the control groups. Importantly, according to the present evidence derived from controlled trials, the administration of propafenone seems to be contraindicated in patients with congestive heart failure, disorders of impulse conduction, sinus node dysfunction, or recent myocardial infarction (29).

VIII. AMIODARONE FOR PHARMACOLOGICAL CARDIOVERSION

Intravenous administration of amiodarone for conversion of AF has been evaluated in several studies. According to a recent meta-analysis, there are six placebo-controlled randomized studies involving 595 patients (30). This analysis demonstrates that amiodarone is superior in reestablishing sinus rhythm 6 to 8 hr after the start of therapy (56% sinus rhythm in the amiodarone group compared to 43% in the placebo group) and at 24 hr (82 vs. 56%). Of note, all six studies used different dosing schedules for amiodarone, which makes direct comparison somewhat difficult. Several aspects of this analysis deserve comment. For instance, the high rate of sinus rhythm conversion in the placebo patients indicates that the majority of patients enrolled in these studies had suffered from paroxysmal recent-onset AF. Of even greater importance is the inefficacy of amiodarone in cardioverting AF rapidly as indicated by the low rate of sinus rhythm within the first hour (17 vs. 11% in the placebo group).

At least seven additional studies comprising 587 patients have compared the efficacy of amiodarone to that of class IC drugs (30). Class IC drugs were more effective than amiodarone in converting AF when analyzed for the first 2 hr after start of therapy, for the first 3 to 5 hr, and for the first 6 to 8 hr. At 24 hr, however, no significant difference persisted between the various

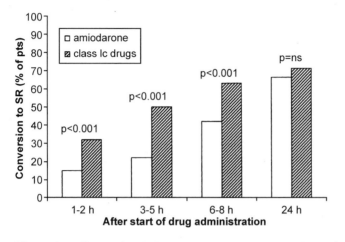

Figure 3 Efficacy of amiodarone and class IC antiarrhythmic drugs in reversing AF according to the time after the start of drug administration. Note the significantly shorter time interval to AF conversion after class IC drug administration. (Modified from Ref. 30.)

drugs (66% sinus rhythm in the amiodarone group vs. 71% in the class IC group) (Fig. 3). Similarly, the incidence and quality of side effects were comparable except for the occurrence of atrial flutter with 1:1 AV conduction, which was observed in 3 patients on flecainide but not in any of the amiodarone-treated patients.

Taken together, therefore, amiodarone appears to be less effective than class IC drugs for the pharmacological cardioversion of AF. Particularly if one aims at rapid restoration of sinus rhythm, the complex pharmacokinetic and pharmacodynamic profile of amiodarone seems to be responsible for its somewhat delayed onset of action. On the other hand, amiodarone may be more effective for the prevention of AF recurrences (31,32). As already indicated, an important advantage of amiodarone is the lack of proarrhythmic and negative inotropic effect, which makes this compound particularly interesting in patients with impaired LV function.

IX. DL-SOTALOL FOR PHARMACOLOGICAL CARDIOVERSION

DL-sotalol is a class III antiarrhythmic drug with additional nonselective beta-blocking effects (33). The compound exhibits significant so-called reverse use dependence, which implies only little prolongation of repolarization at high heart rates and more profound prolongation at low rates. Accordingly, sotalol is of very limited usefulness for the acute cardioversion of AF, particularly with oral administration (34). Similarly, intravenous sotalol has been shown to be less effective than flecainide or ibutilide for reversion of AF (21,35).

X. NEW CLASS III AGENTS FOR PHARMACOLOGICAL CARDIOVERSION

A. Dofetilide

The efficacy of dofetilide for pharmacological cardioversion is limited. In several studies (36,37), the conversion rates to normal sinus rhythm ranged between 15 and 29%, in part depending on the dose used. The compound is available only for oral use. Owing to a significant risk for proarrhythmic reactions (torsades de pointes tachycardia), the drug can be used only in-hospital, with mandatory continuous ECG monitoring. Partially as a result of this requirement, dofetilide is not marketed in all countries.

B. Ibutilide

Ibutilide, available only for intravenous administration, is a new class III antiarrhythmic agent that prolongs repolarization, mainly by enhancing the slow inward sodium current and blocking the rapid component of the delayed rectifier potassium current (38). The compound has recently been released for pharmacological conversion of AF and atrial flutter in the United States. Ibutilide has been subjected to evaluation in several prospective controlled trials. In comparison to placebo, ibutilide had higher conversion rates (28 to 31% compared to 0 to 2%) (39–42). Of note, there was a short time to conversion of only 27 to 33 min. In two actively controlled studies, ibutilide was superior to procainamide (conversion rates of 51 compared to 21%) and to intravenous sotalol (conversion rates 44 vs. 11%) (35,42). Oral et al. showed that electrical transthoracical cardioversion of AF is facilitated by ibutilide pretreatment (43). The only concern with this drug is the potentially high incidence of torsades de pointes tachycardias, which have been reported in up to 8% of treatment attempts. This hazard requires close ECG monitoring during and after drug administration.

C. Tedisamil

Tedisamil sesquifumarate is a soluble salt of tedisamil, a drug initially developed as a bradycardic agent, which slowed heart rate without direct effects on the cardiac beta receptor (44). Tedisamil blocks a variety of potassium currents, such as the transient outward current (I_{to}), the ATP-sensitive outward current (I_{KATP}) the sustained potassium outward current (I_{so}), the inward rectifier currents (I_{Kr}, I_{Ks}), and the chloride channel (TKA-I_{Cl}). At high concentrations, the sodium channel (I_{Na}) is also blocked (44). Accordingly, the drug is a complex antifibrillatory agent. After extensive experimental studies with this compound, tedisamil is currently under investigation for acute termination of AF and atrial flutter (45).

XI. ANTICOAGULATION BEFORE AND AFTER PHARMACOLOGICAL CONVERSION

The most devastating complication of AF is atrial thrombus formation with subsequent embolization, particularly stroke. In general, oral anticoagulation reduces the risk of stroke in AF patients by ~ 60% (46). Recent guidelines for the management of AF recommend anticoagulation for 3 to 4 weeks prior to cardioversion for patients with AF of unknown duration or of >48-hr duration (47). The guidelines also indicate that LA thrombus and systemic embolization have been documented in patients with AF of shorter duration, but the need for anticoagulation in such patients remains less clear (47). Accordingly, it is common clinical practice not to anticoagulate patients with AF of shorter than 48-hr duration. If the precise duration of AF cannot be determined, transesophageal echocardiography can be used to exclude the presence of atrial thrombi prior to cardioversion therapy (48,49). In such patients, atrial contractile dysfunction, so-called atrial stunning, can still be observed for some time after successful cardioversion (50), so that thrombus formation within the mechanically inactive atria is possible and anticoagulation after cardioversion may be warranted.

XII. CLINICAL RECOMMENDATIONS

Based on the evidence derived from prospective controlled studies, pharmacological cardioversion may be attempted in patients with recent-onset paroxysmal AF. The highest success rates have been observed in AF of less than 48-hr duration. In patients with longer-lasting, persistent episodes of AF, electrical cardioversion is the treatment of choice. For chemical cardioversion, class IC drugs appear to have the highest success rates. Class III drugs are somewhat less effective, but ibutilide in particular seems to have a rapid onset of action. Careful consideration of (1) the underlying structural heart disease and (2) the duration of AF is mandatory in all cases. All antiarrhythmic drugs have the potential to cause serious side effects, which makes careful patient surveillance obligatory during and after drug administration.

REFERENCES

1. Feinberg W, Blackshear JL, Laupacis A, et al. Prevalence, age distribution, and gender of patients with atrial fibrillation: analysis and implications. Arch Intern Med 1995; 155:469–473.
2. Sopher SM, Camm AJ. Atrial fibrillation: maintenance of sinus rhythm versus rate control. Am J Cardiol 1996; 77:24A–37A.
3. Nattel S. New ideas about atrial fibrillation 50 years on. Nature 2002; 415:219–226.
4. Allessie MA, Bonke FI, Schopman FJ. Circus movement in rabbit atrial muscle as a mechanism of tachycardia: III. The "leading circle" concept: a new model of circus movement in cardiac tissue without the involvement of an anatomical obstacle. Circ Res 1977; 41:9–18.
5. Yue L, Feng J, Gaspo R, et al. Ionic remodeling underlying action potential changes in a canine model of atrial fibrillation. Circ Res 1997; 81:512–525.
6. Bosch RF, Scherer CR, Rub N, et al. Molecular mechanisms of early electrical remodeling: transcriptional downregulation of ion channel subunits reduces $I(Ca,L)$ and $I(to)$ in rapid atrial pacing in rabbits. J Am Coll Cardiol 2003; 41:858–869.
7. Nattel S, Singh BN. Evolution, mechanisms, and classification of antiarrhythmic drugs: focus on class III action. Am J Cardiol 1999; 84:11R–19R.
8. Li D, Melnyk P, Feng J, et al. Effects of experimental heart failure on atrial cellular and ionic electrophysiology. Circulation 2000; 101:2631–2638.
9. Li D, Benardeau A, Nattel S. Contrasting efficacy of dofetilide in differing experimental models of atrial fibrillation. Circulation 2000; 102:104–112.
10. Wang J, Bourne GW, Wang Z, et al. Comparative mechanisms of antiarrhythmic drug action in experimental atrial fibrillation. Importance of use-dependent effects on refractoriness. Circulation 1993; 88:1030–1044.
11. Suttorp MJ, Kingma JH, Lie AH, et al. Intravenous flecainide versus verapamil for acute conversion of paroxysmal atrial fibrillation or flutter to sinus rhythm. Am J Cardiol 1989; 63:693–696.
12. Capucci A, Boriani G, Botto GL, et al. Conversion of recent-onset atrial fibrillation by a single oral loading dose of propafenone or flecainide. Am J Cardiol 1994; 74:503–505.
13. Jalife J, Berenfeld O, Mansour M. Mother rotors and fibrillatory conduction: a mechanism of atrial fibrillation. Cardiovasc Res 2002; 54:204–216.
14. Kneller J, Leon J, Nattel S. How do class 1 antiarrhythmic drugs terminate atrial fibrillation? A quantitative analysis based on a realistic ionic model [abstr]. Circulation 2001; 104:5.
15. Wijffels MC, Dorland R, Mast F, et al. Widening of the excitable gap during pharmacological cardioversion of atrial fibrillation in the goat: effects of

cibenzoline, hydroquinidine, flecainide, and D-sotalol. Circulation 2000; 102: 260–267.

16. Kawase A, Ikeda T, Nakazawa K, et al. Widening of the excitable gap and enlargement of the core of reentry during atrial fibrillation with a pure sodium channel blocker in canine atria. Circulation 2003; 107:905–910.

17. Coplen SE, Antman EM, Berlin JA, et al. Efficacy and safety of quinidine therapy for maintenance of sinus rhythm after cardioversion. A meta-analysis of randomized trials. Circulation 1990; 82:1106–1116.

18. Echt DS, Liebson PR, Mitchell LB, et al. Mortality and morbidity in patients receiving encainide, flecainide, or placebo. The cardiac arrhythmia suppression trial. N Engl J Med 1991; 324:781–788.

19. Fenster PE, Comess KA, Marsh R, et al. Conversion of atrial fibrillation to sinus rhythm by acute intravenous procainamide infusion. Am Heart J 1983; 106:501–504.

20. Fresco C, Proclemer A, for the PAFIT 2 Investigators. Management of recent onset atrial fibrillation. Eur Heart J 1996; 17:41–47.

21. Reisinger J, Gatterer E, Heinze G, et al. Prospective comparison of flecainide versus sotalol for immediate cardioversion of atrial fibrillation. Am J Cardiol 1998; 81:1450–1454.

22. Murdock CJ, Kyles AE, Yeung-Lai-Wah JA, et al. Atrial flutter in patients treated for atrial fibrillation with propafenone. Am J Cardiol 1990; 66:755–757.

23. Biffi M, Boriani G, Bronzetti G, et al. Electrophysiological effects of flecainide and propafenone on atrial fibrillation cycle and relation with arrhythmia termination. Heart 1999; 82:176–182.

24. Alp NJ, Bell JA, Shahi M. Randomised double blind trial of oral versus intravenous flecainide for the cardioversion of acute atrial fibrillation. Heart 2000; 84:37–40.

25. Stroobandt R, Stiels B, Hoebrechts R. Propafenone for conversion and prophylaxis of atrial fibrillation. Propafenone Atrial Fibrillation Trial Investigators. Am J Cardiol 1997; 79:418–423.

26. Botto GL, Bonini W, Broffoni T, et al. Conversion of recent onset atrial fibrillation with single loading oral dose of propafenone: is in-hospital admission absolutely necessary? Pacing Clin Electrophysiol 1996; 19:1939–1943.

27. Boriani G, Biffi M, Capucci A, et al. Oral propafenone to convert recent-onset atrial fibrillation in patients with and without underlying heart disease. A randomized, controlled trial. Ann Intern Med 1997; 126:621–625.

28. Bianconi L, Mennuni M, Lukic V, et al. Effects of oral propafenone administration before electrical cardioversion of chronic atrial fibrillation: a placebo-controlled study. J Am Coll Cardiol 1996; 28:700–706.

29. Khan IA. Single oral loading dose of propafenone for pharmacological cardioversion of recent-onset atrial fibrillation. J Am Coll Cardiol 2001; 37:542–547.

30. Chevalier P, Durand-Dubief A, Burri H, et al. Amiodarone versus placebo and classic drugs for cardioversion of recent-onset atrial fibrillation: a meta-analysis. J Am Coll Cardiol 2003; 41:255–262.

31. The AFFIRM First Antiarrhythmic Drug Substudy Investigators. Maintenance of sinus rhythm in patients with atrial fibrillation. J Am Coll Cardiol 2003; 42:20–29.
32. Roy D, Talajic M, Dorian P, et al. Amiodarone to prevent recurrence of atrial fibrillation. N Engl J Med 2000; 342:913–920.
33. Hohnloser SH, Woosley RL. Sotalol. N Engl J Med 1994; 331:31–38.
34. Hohnloser SH, van de Loo A, Baedeker F. Efficacy and proarrhythmic hazards of pharmacologic cardioversion of atrial fibrillation: prospective comparison of sotalol versus quinidine. J Am Coll Cardiol 1995; 26:852–858.
35. Vos MA, Golitsyn SR, Stangl K, et al. Superiority of ibutilide (a new class III agent) over DL-sotalol in converting atrial flutter and atrial fibrillation. The Ibutilide/Sotalol Comparator Study Group. Heart 1998; 79:568–575.
36. Falk RH, Pollak A, Singh SN, et al. Intravenous dofetilide, a class III antiarrhythmic agent, for the termination of sustained atrial fibrillation or flutter. J Am Coll Cardiol 1997; 29:385–390.
37. Norgaard BL, Watchell K, Christensen PD, et al. Efficacy and safety of intravenously administered dofetilide in acute termination of atrial fibrillation and flutter: a multicenter, randomized, double-blind, placebo controlled trial. Am Heart J 1999; 137:1062–1069.
38. Murray KT. Ibutilide. Circulation 1998; 97:493–497.
39. Ellenbogen KA, Stambler BS, Wood MA, et al. Efficacy of intravenous ibutilide for rapid termination of atrial fibrillation and atrial flutter: a dose-response study. J Am Coll Cardiol 1996; 28:130–136.
40. Stambler BS, Wood MA, Ellenbogen KA, et al. Efficacy and safety of repeated intravenous doses of ibutilide for rapid conversion of atrial flutter or fibrillation. Circulation 1996; 94:1613–1621.
41. Abi-Mansour P, Carberry PA, McCowan RJ, et al. Conversion efficacy and safety of repeated doses of ibutilide in patients with atrial flutter and atrial fibrillation. Study Investigators. Am Heart J 1998; 136:632–642.
42. Volgman AS, Carberry PA, Stambler B, et al. Conversion efficacy and safety of intravenous ibutilide compared with intravenous procainamide in patients with atrial flutter or fibrillation. J Am Coll Cardiol 1998; 31:1414–1419.
43. Oral H, Souza JJ, Michaud GF, et al. Facilitating transthoracic cardioversion of atrial fibrillation with ibutilide pretreatment. N Engl J Med 1999; 340:1849–1854.
44. Dorian P. Antiarrhythmic drug therapy of atrial fibrillation: focus on new agents. J Cardiovasc Pharmacol Ther 2003; 8(suppl I):S27–S31.
45. Singh BN. Atrial fibrillation: Epidemiologic considerations and rationale for conversion and maintenance of sinus rhythm. J Cardiovasc Pharmacol Ther 2003; 8(suppl I):S13–S26.
46. Hart RG, Benavente O, McBride R, et al. Antithrombotic therapy to prevent stroke in patients with atrial fibrillation: a meta-analysis. Ann Intern Med 1999; 131:492–501.
47. Fuster V, Ryden LE, Asinger RW, et al. ACC/AHA/ESC guidelines for the management of patients with atrial fibrillation: executive summary. J Am Coll Cardiol 2001; 38:1231–1266.

48. Klein AL, Grimm RA, Murray RD, et al. Use of transesophageal echo-cardiography to guide cardioversion in patients with atrial fibrillation. N Engl J Med 2001; 344:1411–1420.

49. Manning WJ, Silverman DI, Katz SE, et al. Impaired left atrial mechanical function after cardioversion: relation to the duration of atrial fibrillation. J Am Coll Cardiol 1994; 23:1535–1540.

50. Jahangir A, Munger TM, Packer DL, Crijns HJGM. Atrial fibrillation. In: Podrid PJ, Kowey PR, eds. Cardiac Arrhythmias. Philadelphia: Lippincott Williams & Wilkins, 2001:457–500.

10
Maintenance of Normal Sinus Rhythm with Antiarrhythmic Drugs

James A. Reiffel
Columbia University College of Physicians and Surgeons and New York Presbyterian Hospital, New York, New York, U.S.A.

There are several therapeutic applications for antiarrhythmic drugs (AADs) in patients with atrial fibrillation (AF). AAD may be used (1) to produce cardioversion, (2) to facilitate direct current (DC) cardioversion by reducing defibrillation thresholds (class III AADs), (3) to prevent immediate or early reversion (IRAF and ERAF, respectively) after cardioversion during post-conversion remodeling (short-term therapy), (4) to maintain normal sinus rhythm (NSR) during chronic therapy, and (5) to facilitate conversion of fibrillation to flutter (class IA and IC AADs and amiodarone), which may then be amenable to termination or prevention with antitachycardia pacing or ablative techniques. *The major focus of this chapter is the use of AADs to maintain NSR over the long term in patients with paroxysmal AF (PAF) or after conversion in patients with persistent AF.* It should be noted, however, that the algorithmic approach to selecting AAD for short-term therapy (weeks to 1 to 3 months) should be the same as that detailed herein for long-term (chronic) therapy.

When AADs are considered for the maintenance of NSR, many additional issues must be addressed. These include, among others, (1) whether, why, and when to use an AAD; (2) which drug to use; (3) where and how to initiate it; (4) what dosing regimen to consider; (5) how to judge efficacy; (6) specific safety precautions that may be necessary for the agent chosen (or how to minimize risk); and (7) what follow-up regimen will be necessary. Under which drug to use, one must also address whether a specific drug or drug class is preferred over others as the initial drug or next choice;

195

which, if any, agents must be avoided; and whether to require a proprietary agent vs. allowing formulation substitution. Each of these considerations is be reviewed in this chapter, with a strong focus on clinical practice applicability of the information provided. Supportive clinical trial data are cited when appropriate to provide the reader with background reference material.

I. WHETHER, WHY, AND WHEN TO USE AN AAD

In the aftermath of the now completed trials comparing the strategies of rate vs. rhythm control for the management of AF (see Chap. 5), which all failed to show any survival benefit with a strategy of rhythm control, the most definitive current reason for maintaining NSR is symptom relief or, more specifically, to reduce symptoms associated with AF that persist despite adequate ventricular rate control (see Chap. 6) and appropriate anticoagulation (see Chap. 7). In this respect, it is important to recognize that, in its untreated state, AF may present with a wide variety of symptoms, either singly or in combination, or may be asymptomatic.

When AF is symptomatic, the symptoms may result from the typically rapid ventricular response (the rate) in the absence of atrioventricular (AV) nodal dysfunction, from the irregular ventricular response, from the loss of effective atrial contractions and AV synchrony, and/or from emboli. In my experience, rate-related symptoms commonly include rapid palpitations, dizziness, dyspnea, and/or chest pain or other ischemic equivalents. Palpitations may also be the result of the irregular ventricular response, but this can be appreciated with certainty only by a reevaluation of symptoms following achievement of rate control (see Chap. 6). Similarly, dyspnea may result from either the effects of a rapid rate and/or from the hemodynamic effects of loss of atrial contraction/AV synchrony. The latter is most commonly in play when there is a structural heart disease alteration of left ventricular (LV) compliance or function. Thus, dyspnea, too, requires reevaluation following achievement of rate control. Fatigue and "lack of normal pep" are also common complaints in patients with AF. In my experience, it is rare for these symptoms to resolve with rate control; thus establishment and maintenance of NSR is typically required for their resolution. Implicit in these observations, therefore, is that for some symptoms, such as fatigue, one can tell early on in an encounter with an AF patient that a rhythm-control strategy will likely be needed to restore a meaningful quality of life, whereas for many, if not most symptoms, rate control should be pursued as the initial strategy, followed by a reevaluation of symptom status before a decision to pursue or not to pursue the restoration/maintenance of NSR can be definitively made. In this regard, it is important to note that the 2001 guidelines of the American College of

Cardiology/American Heart Association/European Society of Cardiology (ACC/AHA/ESC) for the management of AF (1) recommend that, AADs should usually be employed only in the patient who has not achieved an adequate quality of life (QoL) following rate control and anticoagulation (if appropriate). Similarly, the guidelines suggest that for most patients with persistent AF, AADs not be employed after cardioversion (see Chap. 8) of their initial episode unless markers for a high likelihood of recurrence and/or the specific symptom presentation dictate their use. Rather, the frequency and tolerance of recurrences should dictate the therapeutic path to follow. If episodes are infrequent and reasonably tolerated even when recurrent, intermittent cardioversion, particularly if pharmacological (see Chap. 9), is usually preferable to daily AAD administration. Despite these guidelines, there may be situational considerations where any recurrence may be deemed undesirable (as with the guidelines of the Federal Aviation Administration for pilots) such that AAD may be employed following the first episode regardless of the symptom status. The same might be considered true for patients who have severe symptoms (such as syncope with AF in the setting of a hypertrophic obstructive cardiomyopathy) or significant contraindications to anticoagulant therapies (although convincing proof that maintaining NSR actually reduces embolic events remains lacking). For patients with AF who are asymptomatic (or minimally symptomatic) during their episodes, there has been no demonstrated benefit to the prevention of AF with AAD and they should not be used, though rate control (to prevent tachycardia-induced cardiomyopathy) and appropriate anticoagulation are still necessary.

II. DRUG CHOICE, DRUG ADMINISTRATION, AND DETERMINATION OF EFFICACY

When a therapeutic strategy of attempting to maintain NSR has been chosen, a treatment selection process must then be activated. Such a process must reflect considerations of the various clinically important features each potential treatment (pharmacological or nonpharmacological) possesses. For AAD, these include expected efficacy rates, pharmacokinetic and pharmacodynamic properties and interactions, and potential untoward events. The latter require recognition of the type and severity of any underlying structural heart disease that may be present, recognition of any alterations in metabolism and clearance that may exist in the patient at hand, and recognition of any other proarrhythmic precipitants (see below) that may be present.

As regards efficacy, the clinician must always remember that none of our current drugs are perfect for maintaining NSR. The same appears true for those now in clinical trials. For an AAD to be effective therapy for AF, it must interact beneficially with the electrophysiological mechanisms generating and/or maintaining the patient's AF. In some, suppression of automatic foci serving as triggers may be effective. In others, interruption of potential reentrant pathways is necessary. In yet others, eliminating conditions that facilitate AF (see below) is helpful. Accordingly, AADs may prevent AF by a variety of mechanisms (Table 1). Since AF may be initiated and/or maintained by different mechanisms in different patients, it should be immediately obvious that no single AAD should or could be uniformly effective.

In theory, any drug that prolongs refractoriness in the atria, whether by sodium-channel inhibition or impairment of repolarizing currents, could be effective for AF prevention, as prolongation of refractoriness might eliminate the excitable gap that usually exists in reentrant circuits. In patients in whom atrial ectopy or automatic tachyarrhythmias induce AF, drugs that suppress automaticity may also prevent the development of recurrent AF. The latter may be necessary in patients without structural heart disease, in whom AF is often triggered by rapidly firing foci from the pulmonary veins, although clinical efficacy comparisons among drugs have not yet been reported specifically for this population of patients. Consequently, in those patients in whom AF can be shown to repeatedly be precipitated by an atrial automatic rhythm, the efficacy balance among AADs should shift towards

Table 1 Mechanisms by Which Antiarrhythmic Drugs May Prevent Atrial Fibrillation

Suppression of initiating ectopy whether
Automatic
Reentrant
Triggered
Prevention of tachyarrhythmias that might degenerate into atrial fibrillation, such as
Atrial flutter
PSVT[a]
Suppression of early retrograde conduction via, or reentry within, accessory pathways
Alter atrial substrate to prevent establishment of reentry via
Prolongation of refractoriness
Inhibition of conduction
Vagolytic or sympatholytic effects to prevent autonomic nervous system facilitation of atrial fibrillation via
Bradycardia mechanisms
Ectopy
Shortened refractoriness

[a] Paroxysmal supraventricular tachycardia.

class I agents or amiodarone and away from pure class III AAD, as the latter has no significant effects on automatic depolarizing currents. Such a consideration may at least partly underlie the observation that in the trials that led the U.S. Food and Drug Administration (FDA) to approve dofetilide for the treatment of AF, efficacy was demonstrated for the reduction of recurrent persistent AF (for which approval was received) but not for the reduction of recurrent PAF (for which approval was not received). Unfortunately, we often cannot tell whether a triggering arrhythmia is automatic in its mechanism; furthermore, dose limitations may preclude uniform achievement of the electrophysiological alterations necessary to achieve efficacy, regardless of whether the focus is on a reentrant or an automatic mechanism.

The selection of an AAD for the prevention of recurrent AF should involve a consideration not only of the electrophysiologic and autonomic properties possessed by the drug but also of the probable contributing factors to AF in the specific patient, if recognized, and the risk and inconvenience inherent in the therapeutic choice being considered. Additionally, because the electrophysiological effects of AADs can be reversed by the administration of catecholamines (2), the effectiveness of an AAD may be altered by the agent being used for rate control. Accordingly, beta blockers and perhaps verapamil (via its reduction of norepinephrine at ganglionic nerve terminals) may prevent the catecholeamine reversal of AAD effect, which can occur during periods of exercise or stress. In contrast, digitalis and diltiazem will not. Thus AAD efficacy may be different in the presence of beta blockers and perhaps verapamil than in the presence of digitalis or diltiazem.

For patients with recurrent AF and no reversible underlying disorder, recurrences remain likely despite AAD therapy. In almost all series of AAD trials for AF, approximately 40% to 60% of patients will have a recurrence during a follow-up of 6 to 36 months (3–40). Thus efficacy cannot be realistically defined as the complete absence of recurrent AF. Rather, efficacy has to be defined as the reduction in the frequency, duration, and severity of AF events so as to result in a satisfactory improvement in the patient's QoL. Moreover, AADs should be chosen so as to maximize patient compliance (convenient regimens, tolerable cost, low discontinuation rates) and minimize serious risk (organ toxicity and proarrhythmia).

When possible, a mechanistic approach to AAD therapy for AF is useful (Table 2). In this regard, for patients in whom AF appears to be triggered by periods of high vagal tone, such as those with postprandial or nocturnal PAF, a vagolytic approach to therapy has been useful in my experience. For example, I have now followed several dozen patients in whom a belladonna derivative at bedtime (alone or combined with an AAD) or a bedtime dose of disopyramide (without daytime doses) substantially reduces clinical events, freeing the patient from the costs, risks, and

Table 2 Mechanistic Approach to the Treatment of Atrial Fibrillation

Vagolytic—in patients with features of vagally induced AF, such as
  Nocturnal AF
  Postprandial/postbending AF
Sympatholytic—in patients with features of catecholeamine-induced AF, such as
  Stress-induced AF
  Exercise-induced AF
Avoidance of stimulant-induced AF (determined by patient history) including
  Alcohol
  Red wine (in particular)
  Caffeine
  Chocolate
  Monosodium glutamate
Anti-inflammatory therapy for pericarditis-mediated AF, such as
  Post CABG[a]
Treatment of identified hyperthyroidism or hypothyroidism

[a] Coronary artery bypass grafting.

nuisance effects of additional daytime medication. In others, whose events appear to be triggered by exercise, stress, or caffeine, beta blockers may be useful for AF prevention rather than just for rate control. In other circumstances, a setting-specific algorithm is most useful. Classical in this regard is AF that occurs in the first month or two following cardiac surgery. In most circumstances this is not a chronic arrhythmic disorder and it has somewhat specific drug recommendations (see Chap. 13). However, for most AF circumstances, a mechanistic or situation-specific approach to AAD selection is not feasible; therefore, a more generalized, empirical, and safety-driven algorithmic approach is now recommended (1,41,42), guided by the type and severity of underlying structural heart disease that may be present. Such algorithms have been primarily based on avoidance of organ toxicity and ventricular proarrhythmic events.

III. SPECIFIC DRUGS, DRUG CLASSES, AND EFFICACY

The class IA and IC agents and sotalol, dofetilide, azimilide, and amiodarone have all been shown to have efficacy for prevention of AF that is greater than that of placebo (3–40) (Table 3). Representative placebo-controlled studies have shown efficacy rates for placebo that have varied from 32% to 42% at 6 months and from 15% to 36% at 12 months, while efficacy rates with these AADs have varied from 45% to 79% at 6 months and from 31% to 54% at 12

Table 3 Comparative Placebo vs. Antiarrhythmic Drug Efficacy for AF

Investigator	Drugs	Number of patients	Study duration	Efficacy	p Value
Boisel (5)	Quinidine	24	6 months	79%	<0.01
	Placebo	24		42%	
Sodermark (6)	Quinidine	101	12 months	52%	<0.001
	Placebo	75		35%	
Hillestad (7)	Quinidine	48	12 months	31%	<0.05
	Placebo	52		15%	
Lloyd (9)	Quinidine	28	6 months	67%	NS
	Placebo	25		32%	
Lloyd (9)	Disopyramide	29	6 months	45%	NS
	Placebo	25		32%	
Karlson (12)	Disopyramide	44	12 months	54%	<0.01
	Placebo	40		30%	
Stroobandt (39)	Propafenone	102	6 months	67%	<0.01
	Placebo	25		35%	
Van Gelder (16)	Flecainide	36	12 months	47%	NS
	Placebo	37		36%	
Bendett (37)	Sotalol	62	12 months	47%	<0.01
	Placebo	69		29%	
Singh (35)	Dofetilide	100	12 months	66%	<0.001
	Placebo	106		21%	

months in the same studies (5–7,9,12,16,35–40) (Table 3). Although the specific efficacy rates. vary among series, it is likely that the differences in absolute efficacy rates largely reflect interseries differences among patients—e.g., underlying heart disease, type of AF presentation, AF duration, prior drug resistance, actions of the concomitant rate-control agent if any (see above), and so on. Support for this contention comes from the various active drug-comparison trials, also been published (3,4,9–11,13,14,17,20,25,43–48), in which the efficacy rates between or among the drugs being compared have usually been similar within a series but different from series to series (Table 4). While some data, such as those of Zarembski et al. (17) and the widely cited CTAF trial (43), suggests that amiodarone in particular maybe more effective than other available AADs for the prevention of AF, this has not uniformly been the observation (10,20,44). In CTAF, amiodarone was compared in a randomized trial to propafenone and sotalol. Efficacy at 1 year for the prevention of 10 min or more of symptomatic AF was approximately 75% for amiodarone but only approximately 45% for both propafenone and sotalol. However, as amiodarone is more effective than the other two agents in

Table 4 Comparative Antiarrhythmic Studies for Atrial Fibrillation

Investigator	Drug	Number of Patients	Study Duration	Efficacy	p Value
Jull-Moller (4)	Sotalol	98	6 months	52%	NS
	Quinidine	85		48%	
Lloyd (7)	Quinidine	28	6 months	67%	NS
	Disopyramide	29		45%	
Zehender (10)	Quinidine	11	3 months	90%	NS
	Amiodarone	12		92%	
Reimold (14)	Propafenone	50	12 months	30%	NS
	Sotalol	50		37%	
Chimenti (23)	Flecainide	97	12 months	77%	NS
	Propafenone	103		75%	
Aliot (24)	Flecainide	48	12 months	77%	NS
	Propafenone	49		76%	
Naccarelli (25)	Flecainide	122	9 months	71%	<0.001
	Quinidine	117		55%	
Bellandi (26)	Propafenone	102	12 months	70%	<0.005
	Sotalol	106		45%	
Richiardi (28)	Propafenone	102	12 months	45%	NS
	Quinidine	102		30%	
Lee (29)	Propafenone	48	3 months	87%	<0.01
	Quinidine	48		46%	
Rasmussen (11)	Flecainide	30	6 months	81%	<0.01
	Disopyramide	30		44%	
Crijns (13)	Propafenone	25	6 months	55%	NS
	Disopyramide	31		67%	
Zarembski (17)	Amiodarone	107	6 months	60%	NA
	Flecainide	163		34%	

providing rate control in AF, we must consider that some of the apparent difference may represent AF that is present but undetected by the patient. Moreover, the mean doses of both propafenone and sotalol achieved in this trial were lower than are usually recommended. Although the CTAF report suggests that the propafenone and sotalol doses were limited due to intolerance, they nonetheless stand in contrast to the doses tolerated in many other studies and to the doses recommended in the package inserts for the therapy of AF. Accordingly, if efficacy in preventing recurrent AF is similar among AADs and certainly not an order of magnitude greater for amiodarone than for other agents, then for most patients the drug selection process should be guided primarily by safety considerations. This is particularly true for arrhythmias such as AF, where recurrences are rarely life-threatening; hence neither should be its therapy. Cost, convenience, and overall drug tolerance are also distinguishing considerations. As regards tolerance, for example, quinidine has consistently been discontinued more often than flecainide or sotalol in direct active drug comparison studies (4,20,25) despite similar rates of efficacy, which largely explains why the use of quinidine has declined since the advent of class IC and III AADs.

Notably, since individual AADs are often not effective in maintaining NSR, serial AAD administration has also been examined. Crijns et al. (3) prospectively examined 127 patients with chronic AF who underwent serial drug treatment: stage I, flecainide; stage II, sotalol (or quinidine if sotalol was contraindicated); and stage III, amiodarone. At 2 years, 31% of the patients still treated with the first drug would be in sinus rhythm; using the staged approach, 63% of the patients were maintained in NSR. Unfortunately, here too the results between trials are not consistent, as observations by Antman et al. using propafenone, sotalol, and then amiodarone (49) and by the STAF investigators (45) using up to four AADs and four cardioversions were less impressive. In STAF, fewer than 25% of patients remained in NSR by 4 years.

IV. SAFETY CONSIDERATIONS IN AAD SELECTION FOR AF

Although nuisance symptoms—such as loose stools, reduced appetite, constipation, metallic taste, photosensitivity, altered skin pigment, and the like—as well as inconvenient dosing regimens are important considerations in AAD selection, the major safety considerations should include potentially lethal adverse effects. These may be grouped as organ-toxic or ventricular-proarrhythmic (see below). Additional important safety considerations that may relate to individual patients or specific cardiac disorders are the negative inotropic potential and bradyarrhythmic potential (nodal suppression, conduction block) of AADs. These clearly come into play in patients with underlying sinus node dysfunction and/or advanced conduction disease, where AAD administration may necessitate permanent pacemaker implantation before starting a class I or III AAD (in the setting of sinus node disease) or a class I drug (in patients with His-Purkinje dysfunction), or where underlying congestive symptoms or severely depressed ventricular function may preclude the use of a negatively inotropic AAD regardless of its other merits. As regards inotropy, however, note should be made of the positive inotropic effects of the pure class III AADs (e.g., dofetilide, azimilide), amiodarone, and the D-isomer of sotalol. Because of the latter, in patients with congestive symptoms too severe to tolerate a beta blocker, in contrast to just a low left ventricular ejection fraction (LVEF), are contraindications to DL-sotalol (the form available in the United States).

Organ toxicity, as distinguished from more benign nuisance effects, may be defined as noncardiac end-organ effects that have the potential for a lethal outcome. Examples include lupus erythematosus, agranulocytosis, thrombocytopenia, pulmonary fibrosis, hepatitis, and thyrotoxicosis. Although the AADs that carry risk for such toxicity do so only in the minority of exposed patients and can usually be discontinued prior to a fatality by careful follow-up (see below), unfortunate outcomes do occur. Thus, as a general rule, only those AADs with the lowest potential for an organ-toxic event should be considered as first-line agents for the therapy of AF unless proarrhythmic risk becomes a more serious concern. The currently available AADs with the lowest risk for organ toxicity include (alphabetically) disopyramide (which is often limited by other side effects), dofetilide (which is well tolerated but may be limited by multiple drug interactions, similar to the numerous drug interactions seen with amiodarone), flecainide, propafanone, and sotalol. In contrast, amiodarone, procainamide, and quinidine carry significant risk for organ toxicity. Package insert guidelines provide details about the hematological, hepatic, thyroid, and/or pulmonary follow-up necessary for the ongoing surveillance of patients taking these agents. Even with low-dose amiodarone (200 mg/day or less), the risk of pulmonary fibrosis (some cases with fatal outcome despite scheduled follow-up testing) has been shown in recent prospectively performed trials—such as CASCADE, EMIAT, and CAMIAT (46–48)—to average approximately 1.5% to 2.0% per year and has been as high as 3% to 12% (21,46).

Proarrhythmia, for purposes of this discussion, may be defined as the production of any new arrhythmia by a therapy during the treatment of a preexisting arrhythmia. For practical purposes in treating AF, however, clinicians are most concerned about proarrhythmic events taking the form of a hemodynamically destabilizing or lethal ventricular tachyarrhythmia induced by an AAD. Ventricular fibrillation (VF), a rapid polymorphic ventricular tachycardia (VT) such as torsades de pointes (TdP), or sustained monomorphic VT would all be relevant examples. Importantly, in considering the production of proarrhythmia, several interacting conditions come into play and—unlike the case with organ toxicity—the risk is not simply a property of the drug. Rather, proarrhythmia represents the effect of interactions between a drug's electrophysiological actions, underlying structural or functional ventricular disorders, and additional modulating factors such as heart rate, electrolyte status, gender, and concomitant therapies (50,51). Typically these are best understood in the context of specific drugs given in the presence of specific underlying structural heart disease states (Table 5).

Class IC AADs cause conduction slowing through potent sodium-channel blockade as their most prominent effect. In the normal ventricle, where conduction at baseline is uniform, homogeneous conduction slowing resulting from such drugs should not produce a proarrhythmic response. However, in states where nonhomogeneous conduction exists within the myocardium—whether from anatomical disorders such as myocardial scar, fibrosis, infiltration, or inflammation or from functional impairment in gap junctions and action potential configuration, such as during ischemia—conduction slowing produced by class IC (or class IA) drugs can result in areas of normal conduction becoming slow and areas of slow conduction developing conduction block. This inhomogeneity can produce the substrate for reentry and cause sustained VT or VF, resulting in increased mortality, as was seen in the CAST and other postmyocardial infarction studies (52,53). In recent reports, all serious proarrhythmias with a class IC AAD used for AF occurred in patients with structural disease or in whom a bradyarrhythmia-mediated proarrhythmic event had been seen previously with another drug (54,55). Because the class IC AADs have not produced excess proarrhythmic mortality in the absence of structural heart disease, in contrast to their effect in the setting of structural disorders, they have been approved for the therapy of AF *only* in patients without structural heart disease. In this circumstance, hypertension without significant LV hypertrophy (LVH) is not considered structural heart disease, whereas if LVH is present, class IC AADs should be avoided. Significant LVH is often associate with fibrosis on microscopic examination and/or with subendocardial ischemia. When in doubt, the preference should go to propafenone rather than flecainide, as proarrhythmia appears to be less with propafenone.

In addition to a proarrhythmic consequence resulting from conduction slowing, proarrhythmia may result from prolongation of repolarization, as occurs with class III and IA drugs. Under these circumstances, proarrhythmia usually takes the form of TdP, which can be asymptomatic, produce dizziness or syncope, or yield VF, depending on its duration, and can occur in patients either with or without structural heart disease, though more often in the former. Because most episodes of TdP are self-terminating and may not even be long enough to produce symptoms, the actual risk of fatality from TdP is lower than the observed incidence of TdP. The risk for developing TdP is increased in the setting of bradycardia, ventricular hypertrophy, hypokalemia, and/or hypomagnesemia (and, hence during diuretic use), congenital QT prolongation or QT prolongation produced by concomitant drugs, or with excessive AAD levels (56). Ventricular hypertrophy can promote TdP because hypertrophied myocytes develop prolonged action potential duration, with

Table 5 Drug–Disease Proarrhythmic Interactions

Ventricular structure	Altered electrophysiology	Probable risk for proarrhythmia[a]
Normal	None	IA, dofetilide > sotalol > IC ≥ amiodarone
LVH	Increased action potential duration and after depolarizations	IA, dofetilide > sotalol > flecanide > propafenone > amiodarone
Without QRS or strain		
With strain		
With wide QRS	Add ischemia	IC > IA > dofetilide,sotalol > amiodarone
	Add reduced cell contact	IC > IA > dofetilide,sotalol > amiodarone
IHD	Ischemic changes (scar-related and functional)	IC ≫ IA > dofetilide,sotalol > amiodarone
Infiltrate, fibrotic	Poor cell contact	IC ≫ IA≥dofetilide,sotalol > amiodarone
Severe dilated cardiomyopathy	Poor cell contact, increased action potential duration	IC ≫ IA≥dofetilide,sotalol > amiodarone

Key: IHD, ischemic heart disease; LVH, left ventricular hypertrophy.
[a] Hemodynamically significant or life-threatening.

altered outward potassium currents similar to those produced by class IA or III AADs and consequently additive to them when these agents are employed. Additionally, the incidence of drug-induced TdP is almost twofold higher in women than in men (56). In patients with supraventricular tachyarrhythmias and no major risk markers for TdP, such as those enrolled in clinical drug trials, the TdP incidence appears to be in the range of 0.3% to 3% (56–60). It is lower with amiodarone than with sotalol or the "pure" class III AADs dofetilide and azimilide. Because drug-related TdP is increased with brady-cardia or following a pause, it may be more apt to be seen if drug-induced bradycardia is also present and at or following AF termination rather than during the faster rates present during AF. It is for this reason that it is usually advised to start class IA or III AADs under in-hospital observation when AF. is present, whereas this recommendation is not consistently made when the patient is in NSR at the time the drug is begun (see below). Because dofetilide and sotalol are renally excreted, the risk for TdP is also increased if the dose is not adjusted for renal function in addition to the QT-interval response (see the detailed dose-adjustment instructions in the package inserts for these two agents).

In patients with structural disorders that preclude the use of class I AADs (see above), class III AADs should be considered when treatment is needed. In contrast to the results seen in CAST and the potential risk of class III agents for TdP, there has been no increased mortality in careful, well-conducted, placebo-controlled studies with DL-sotalol following myocardial infarction (MI) (the Julian study) (59), dofetilide in patients with heart failure of ischemic or nonischemic origin (the DIAMOND trial) (60), azimilide in high risk post-MI patients (the ALIVE trial) (61), or amiodarone in post-MI or heart failure trials (47,48,62,63). In such studies, patients with excessive factors for TdP risk are excluded or the factors are corrected prior to drug administration. This lesson is important for clinical practice, lest the incidence of TdP be excessive in an individual practitioner's experience.

V. ALGORITHMIC GUIDELINES FOR AAD SELECTION IN THE AF PATIENT

The above issues, taken together, have led several investigators and expert panels to recommend a safety-based algorithmic approaches for the selection of an AAD when such drugs are needed to treat AF patients (1,41,42). The similarities between them have been remarkable. The latest, developed jointly by the ACC, AHA, and ESC in conjunction with the North American Society of Pacing and Electrophysiology (1) now represents sanctioned management guidelines for the AF patient. Although any algorithm can be only a starting point many individual patient considerations might modify its application (Table 6), an algorithm provides at least an initial guide that focuses on the important considerations regarding organ toxicity and proarrhythmic potential that which must be overriding initial determinants in AAD selection. Highlights of this algorithm follow. The reader is referred to the ACC/AHA/ESC position paper for further background, details, and discussion.

A. Patients Without Structural Heart Disease

First-line agents are flecainide, propafenone, or sotalol. None of these three agents are organ-toxic. Sotalol has the convenience of both rate and rhythm control in a single agent and poses only a small risk of TdP in the normal heart if appropriate precautions are taken, whereas flecainide and propafenone are not proarrhythmic in the normal heart but do require the addition of a rate-control agent. Other AADs have been considered less desirable choices because of issues of organ toxicity, proarrhythmic potential, or intolerance or because of limited experience (i.e., dofetilide).

B. Patients With Hypertension

In the absence of LVH >1.4 cm (1), propafenone or flecainide are the drugs of choice, with propafenone being preferable in my opinion. Any LVH increases the risk concern of sotalol and other class III AADs, making them second-line choices. If LVH >1.4 cm exists, amiodarone becomes the agent of choice, as both class I and other class III agents must be avoided.

Table 6 Patient Characteristics That May Affect Algorithms

Prior drug history
    Inefficacy
    Intolerance
Absolute/relative contraindications
Potential for concomitant drug interactions
Prior drug compliance history
Anticipated stability of underlying heart disease
Anticipated stability of hepatic/renal function
    Metabolism
    Elimination
Utility of nonantiarrhythmic actions of selected antiarrhythmic drug
Gender

C. Patients With Coronary Artery Disease

In the absence of congestive failure severe enough to preclude beta-blocker administration, sotalol is the drug of choice. Dofetilide (plus a rate-control agent) or amiodarone (because of its organ toxicity profile) are considered second-line agents. The rate-control agent cannot be verapamil, as it is contraindicated with dofetilide (and diltiazem must be used with caution). Class I AADs must be avoided. If uncertainty about the tolerance of sotalol exists as regards its beta-blocker potential, I have found that low-dose beta blockade alone can be initiated and then a switch to sotalol can be made if an equivalent degree of beta blockade has been achieved and tolerated. On a milligram-for-milligram basis, sotalol has about one-third to one-half the beta-blocker potency of propranolol or metoprolol.

D. Patients With Congestive Heart Failure (Ischemic or Nonischemic)

Dofetilide (plus a rate-control agent) and amiodarone are the only agents recommended for consideration. Class I AADs must be avoided.

E. Other Disorders

Other specific cardiac disorders have not all been directly addressed in the published algorithms, but the principles remain the same. In hypertrophic cardiomyopathy, for example, proarrhythmic concerns would suggest that amiodarone would be the drug of choice, as other class III agents would have an increased risk of TdP, as would class IA agents, and class I agents would likely also pose an increased proarrhythmic risk in the form of VT/VF. Mitral regurgitation that is mild and without either significant ventricular dilation or dysfunction would be treated as no structural heart disease, since, for purposes of AADs, structural disease is defined (see above) as an anatomical or functional disorder that interacts pathophysiologically with AAD electrophysiology to enhance proarrhythmic risk. However, for mitral regurgitation with significant ventricular dilation or with LV dysfunction, the class I agents would no longer be favored. By this definition, isolated mitral stenosis would not be considered a significant structural disorder; aortic valve stenosis would be a significant disorder only when LVH had developed, and so on.

VI. DOSING

While the dose chosen for any AAD must often be individualized—based upon patient history, size, hepatorenal function, concomitant drug therapy, and other modulating factors—there are dose ranges and regimens that are frequently required and/or advised. They include propafenone, 150 to 300 mg bid (a sustained-release preparation with somewhat different dosing is currently undergoing the approval process); flecainide, 50 to 200 mg bid; sotalol, 120 to 160 mg bid (while the starting dose is often cited as 80 mg bid, clinical trial data suggests that this dose primarily has beta-blocking actions but little if any class III effects, and it has not been superior to placebo in 6-month AF prevention in clinical studies); dofetilide, 500 µg bid; and amiodarone (off label), 100 to 200 mg/day (after a loading regimen of about half the regimen used for VT). For quinidine, the dose varies with the preparation used. For procainamide and disopyramide (off label), the doses have been extrapolated from those used for ventricular arrhythmias.

Additionally, if and/or when one or more generic versions of a proprietary AADs are or become available, the clinician will have to decide whether or not to allow formulation substitution for the branded product. Generic versions of proprietary drugs can significantly reduce the cost of medications to patients. However, generic congeners may not be clinically equivalent to proprietary drugs, despite the "bioequivalence" declarations made by the FDA when they are approved (64–66). Arrhythmia recurrence, proarrhythmic events, and death have all been reported with formulation substitution of generic antiarrhythmic agents, similar to the serious consequences that have been reviewed in the literature for other narrow therapeutic drugs/situations, such as with anticonvulsants, immunosuppressives in transplant recipients, and anticoagulants (64–66). Consequently, some expert sources strongly advise against formulation substitution with AADs, whether used for AF or for other arrhythmias (64–66).

VII. WHERE AND HOW TO INITIATE AAD THERAPY

Some debate exists as to the proper site for the initiation of an AAD for AF (67,68). Rapid detection and correction of efficacy and adverse effects (such as early proarrhythmia, bradycardia, intolerance, or drug interactions) favors inpatient initiation. Convenience and, under most circumstances, lower cost and patient preference favor outpatient initiation. Circumstances under which adverse event rates, including proarrhythmia, are expectedly low would favor outpatient initiation, as would the use of an agent whose elimination half-life is so long as to render in-hospital monitoring to steady state impractical.

Accordingly, outpatient initiation appears suitable for class IC AADs in patients without structural heart disease or underlying sinus node/conduction disorders, which is consistent with their package inserts; for selected class III agents in patients with a low risk for TdP, where data in the literature are supportive (e.g., sotalol when the patient is in NSR azimilide) (1,37,38,67,68), which may not be consistent with their package insert guidelines; and for amiodarone. There are no package insert guidelines for amiodarone for AF, as it is not approved for AF in the United States. The same holds true for procainamide, disopyramide, and moricizine, which also do not have FDA approval for the treatment of AF. Note that "outpatient" need not mean unmonitored, as transtelephonic or evolving web-based telemetric monitoring can be used to follow patients during drug initiation. With such monitoring, for example, I follow sinus rates and QT intervals during loading. Moreover, in this circumstance, I advise slower dose escalation than I would employ during inpatient initiation. "Outpatient" means "nonurgent"! Rather than using a drug's average half-life to calculate the time to steady state, before which the dose should not be increased, in the outpatient setting I advise using the drug's longest reported half-life to calculate the time to steady state.

Inpatient initiation should be considered for all patients with sinus node dysfunction or conduction disorders, significant structural heart disease, those receiving a drug whose proarrhythmia may be idiosynchratic (quinidine), and patients who are to begin an AAD while in AF in whom sinus rhythm has not been seen previously (so that underlying sinus node dysfunction as a contributing factor to AF cannot be excluded). Most published guidelines suggest that all class IA agents be initiated in the inpatient setting. The decision is straightforward for dofetilide. Its approval by the FDA mandates in-hospital initiation because all studies with this agent have been carried out only in the inpatient setting and no significant outpatient experience exists. Also, its database suggests that often the TdP seen with dofetilide requires an intervention, such as termination with intravenous $MgSO_4$ (2 g IV) in contrast to spontaneous termination. Inpatient initiation is also advised by the FDA when sotalol is used for AF. [See the Betapace AF package insert. Betapace AF is the only sotalol formulation approved for AF; branded Betapace and generic sotalol preparations are not (57,64).] The ACC/AHA/ESC guidelines (1), however, as noted earlier, suggest that sotalol can be initiated on an outpatient basis if the patient is in NSR and has no high risk markers for TdP. Recall, however, that even with in-hospital initiation, proarrhythmia may develop later during the course of therapy in association with a change in underlying disease, altered electrolyte concentrations, ischemia, a change in concomitant therapy, a change in metabolism or clearance (e.g., altered renal or hepatic function), a change in drug dose, or a change in drug formulation. Thus, inpatient initiation should not be considered conclusive as to the absence of risk for proarrhythmia when it has not been seen by the time of patient discharge home.

VIII. FOLLOW-UP PROTOCOLS

Because proarrhythmia may occur late if risk factors develop during chronic drug administration or drug clearance becomes impaired and because organ toxicity is typically an ongoing rather than just an acute risk, follow-up protocols are necessary for patients treated with AADs and should be followed faithfully. I suggest having a reminder form in each patient's chart. With the use of class I AADs, ischemia and structural ventricular disorders need to be detected early. Thus, echocardiograms and stress tests should be performed serially at intervals appropriate for the patient's age, disease risk factors, and history, which in some patients will be yearly. With dofetilide, sotalol, and flecainide, renal function needs to be periodically assessed. With all class IA or III AADs, serum potassium and magnesium need to remain in the normal range. Personally, I check chemistry 7 profiles and an ECG (for QT interval) at least every 6 months in patients on dofetilide, sotalol, and azimilide. Azimilide, if and when approved, will also require differential white blood cell counts, as will be detailed in its package insert, because of the infrequent occurrence of significant neutropenia with this agent, especially in the first 4 months. For amiodarone, I advise a follow-up protocol similar to that utilized when amiodarone is used for ventricular arrhythmias (e.g., thyroid, liver, pulmonary, and visual assessment by appropriate history and laboratory evaluation every 6 months). When the patient is cared for by more than one physician—such as an electrophysiologist, a cardiologist, and a primary care physician—communication between them is essential at the time an AAD is begun, so that each is fully aware that the patient is on the agent and a coordinated follow-up regimen can be established among them.

IX. CONCLUDING COMMENTS

Clearly, the decision to use an AAD for the therapy of AF—and the considerations required once a positive decision for such use has been made—involves complex issues. It is my hope that the material provided above will help the reader to better characterize and understand these decisions and issues so as to enhance the care they provide to their patients—both to use them in the correct patients and to use them correctly to achieve the maximum benefit for those who rely on these clinicians for their expertise and council.

REFERENCES

1. Fuster V, Ryden LE, Asinger RW, et al. Practice Guidelines, European Society of Cardiology Committee for Practice Guidelines and Policy Conferences (Committee to Develop Guidelines for the Management of Patients with Atrial Fibrillation). North American Society of Pacing and Electrophysiology. ACC/AHA/ESC Guidelines for the Management of Patients with Atrial Fibrillation: Executive Summary A Report of the American College of Cardiology/American Heart Association Task Force on Practice Guidelines and the European Society of Cardiology Committee for Practice Guidelines and Policy Conferences (Committee to Develop Guidelines for the Management of Patients with Atrial Fibrillation) Developed in Collaboration with the North American Society of Pacing and Electrophysiology. Circulation 2001; 104(17):2118–2150.

2. Sager PT, Behboodikhah M. Frequency-dependent electrophysiologic effects of D,L-sotalol and quinidine and modulation by beta-adrenergic stimulation. J Cardiovasc Electrophysiol 1996; 7:102–112.

3. Crijns HJ, Van Gelder IC, Van Gilst WH, et al. Serial antiarrhythmic drug treatment to maintain sinus rhythm after electrical cardioversion for chronic atrial fibrillation or atrial flutter. Am J Cardiol 1991; 68:335–341.

4. Juul-Moller S, Edvardsson AN, Rehnqvist-Ahlberg N. Sotalol versus quinidine for the maintenance of sinus rhythm after direct current conversion of atrial fibrillation. Circulation 1990; 82:1932–1939.

5. Boissel JP, Wolfe E, Gillet J, et al. Controlled trial of a long-acting quinidine for maintenance of sinus rhythm after conversion of sustained atrial fibrillation. Eur Heart J 1981; 2:49–55.

6. Sodermark T, Yansson B, Olson A, et al. Effect of quinidine on maintaining sinus rhythm after cardioversion of atrial fibrillation or flutter. A multicenter study from Stockholm. Br Heart J 1975; 37:486–492.

7. Hillestadt L, Bjerkerlund C, Dale J, et al. Quinidine in maintenance of sinus rhythm after electroversion of chronic atrial fibrillation. A control study. Br Heart J 1971; 33:518–521.

8. Grande P, Sonne B, Pedersen A. A controlled study of digoxin and quinidine in patients DC reverted from atrial fibrillation to sinus rhythm. Circulation 1986; 74:II-101.

9. Lloyd EA, Gersh BJ, Forman R. The efficacy of quinidine and disopyramide in the maintenance of sinus rhythm after electroversion from atrial fibrillation: a double-blind study comparing quinidine, disopyramide, and placebo. S Afr Med J 1984; 65, 367–369.

10. Zehender M, Hohnloser S, Muller B. Effects of amiodarone versus quinidine and verapamil in patients with chronic atrial fibrillation: results of a comparative study and 2-year follow up. J Am Cardiol 1992; 19:1054–1059.

11. Rasmussen K, Andersen A, Abrahamsen A, et al. Flecainide versus disopyramide in maintaining sinus rhythm following conversion of chronic atrial fibrillation. Eur Heart J 1998; 9:1–52.

12. Karlson BW, Torstensson I, Abjorn C, Jansson SO, Peterson LE. Disopyr-

amide in the maintenance of sinus rhythm after electroversion of atrial fibrillation. A placebo-controlled one-year follow up study. Eur Heart J 1988; 9:284–290.

13. Crjns HJGM, Gooselink ATM, Lie KI. Propafenone versus disopyramide for the maintenance of sinus rhythm after electrical cardioversion of atrial fibrillation: a randomized double-blind study. Cardiovasc Drugs Ther 1996; 2:145–152.

14. Reimold SC, Cantillon CO, Friedman PL, Antman EN. Propafenone versus sotalol for suppression of recurrent symptomatic atrial fibrillation. Am J Cardiol 1993; 71:558–563.

15. Antman EM, Beamer AD, Cantillon C, McGowan N, Goldman L, Friedman P. Long-term oral propafenone therapy for suppression of refractory symptomatic atrial fibrillation and atrial flutter. J Am Coll Cardiol 1988; 12:1011–1018.

16. Van Gelder JC, Crijns HJ, Van Gilst WH, Van Wijk LM, Lie KI. Efficacy and safety of flecainide acetate in the maintenance of sinus rhythm after electrical cardioversion of chronic atrial fibrillation or atrial flutter. Am J Cardiol 1989; 64:1317–1321.

17. Zarembski DG, Nolan PE, Slack MD, Caruso AC. Treatment of resistant atrial fibrillation. A meta-analysis comparing amiodarone and flecainide. Arch Intern Med 1995; 155:1885–1891.

18. Chun SG, Sager PT, Stevenson WG, Nadamanee K, Middelkauff HR, Singh BN. Long-term efficacy of amiodarone for maintenance of normal sinus rhythm in patients with refractory atrial fibrillation or flutter. Am J Cardiol 1995; 76:47–50.

19. Gold RL, Haffajee CI, Charos G, Sloan K, Baker S, Alpert JS. Amiodarone for refractory atrial fibrillation. Am J Cardiol 1986; 57:124–127.

20. Szyszka A, Paluszkiewicz P, Baszynska H. Prophylactic treatment after electroconversion of atrial fibrillation in patients after cardiac surgery—a controlled two year follow up study. J Am Coll Cardiol 1993; 21:A-201.

21. Middlekauff HR, Wiener I, Stevenson WG. Low-dose amiodarone for atrial fibrillation. Am J Cardiol 1993; 71(suppl):75F–81F.

22. Anderson JL. Long-term safety and efficacy of flecainide in the treatment of supraventricular tachyarrhythmias: the United States experience. Am J Cardiol 1992; 70(suppl):11A–18A.

23. Chiemienti M, Cullen MT, Casadei G, for the Flecainide and Propafenone Italian Study (FAPIS) Investigators. Safety of long-term flecainide and propafenone in the management of patients with symptomatic paroxysmal atrial fibrillation: report from the flecainide and propafenone Italian study investigators. Am J Cardiol 1996; 77(suppl):60A–65A.

24. Aliot E, Denjoy I, and the Flecainide AF French Study Group. Comparison of the safety and efficacy of flecainide versus propafenone in hospital out-patients with symptomatic atrial fibrillation/flutter. Am J Cardiol 1996; 77(suppl):66A–71A.

25. Naccarelli GV, Dorian P, Hohnloser SH, Coumel P, for the Flecainide

Multicenter Atrial Fibrillation Study Group. Prospective comparison of flecainide versus quinidine for the treatment of paroxysmal atrial fibrillation/flutter. Am J Cardiol 1996; 77(suppl):53A–59A.

26. Bellandi F, Dabizzi RP, Niccoli L, Cantini F, Palchetti R. Propafenone and sotalol: long term efficacy and tolerability in the prevention of paroxysmal atrial fibrillation. A placebo-controlled double-blind study. G Ital Cardiol 1996; 26:379–390.

27. Anderson JL, Gilbert EM, Alpert BL, Henthorn RW, Waldo AL, Bhandari AK, Hawkinson RW, Prichett EL. Prevention of symptomatic recurrences of paroxysmal atrial fibrillation in patients initially tolerating antiarrhythmic therapy: a multicenter, double-blind, crossover study of flecainide and placebo. Circulation 1989; 80:1557–1570.

28. Richiardi E, Gaita F, Greco C, Gaschino G, Comb Costa G, Rosettani E, Brusc A. Propafenone versus hydroquinidine in long-term pharmacological prophylaxis of atrial fibrillation. Cardiologica 1992; 37:123–127.

29. Lee SH, Chen SA, Chiang CE, Tai CT, Wen ZC, Wang SP, Chang MS. Comparison of oral propafenone and quinidine as an initial treatment option in patients with symptomatic paroxysmal atrial fibrillation: a double-blind, randomized trial. J Intern Med 1996; 239:253–260.

30. Clementy J, Dulhoste MN, Laiter C, Denjoy I, Dos Santos P. Flecainide acetate in the prevention of paroxysmal atrial fibrillation: a nine month follow up of more than 500 patients. Am J Cardiol 1992; 79(suppl):44A–49A.

31. Sonnhag C, Kallryd A, Nylander E, Ryden L. Long term efficacy of flecainide in paroxysmal atrial fibrillation. Acta Med Scand 1988; 224:563–569.

32. Hammill SC, Wood DL, Gersh BJ, Osborn MJ, Holmes DR Jr. Propafenone for paroxysmal atrial fibrillation. Am J Cardiol 1988; 61:473–474.

33. Leclerca JF, Chouty F, Denjoy J, Coumel P, Slama R. Flecainide in quinidine resistant atrial fibrillation. Am J Cardiol 1992; 70(suppl):62A–65A.

34. Anderson JL, Platt ML, Guarnieri T, Fox TL, Maser MJ, Prichet EL. Flecainide acetate for paroxysmal supraventricular tachycardias. Am J Cardiol 1994; 74:578–584.

35. Singh SN, Zoble RG, Yellen L, et al. Efficacy and safety of oral dofetilide; in converting to and maintaining sinus rhythm in patients with chronic atrial fibrillation/flutter: the symptomatic atrial fibrillation investigative research on dofetilide (SAFIRE-D) study. Circulation 2000; 102:2385–2390.

36. Greenbaum R, Campbell TJ, Channer KS, et al. Conversion of atrial fibrillation and maintenance of sinus rhythm by dofetilide. the EMERALD (European and Australian Multicenter Evaluative Research of Atrial Fibrillation Dofetilide) study [abstr]. Circulation 1998; 98(suppl I):1–633.

37. Benditt DG, Williams HH, Jin J, et al. Maintenance of sinus rhythm with oral D,L-sotalol in patients with symptomatic atrial fibrillation and/or atrial flutter. Am J Cardiol 1999; 84:270–277.

38. Pritchett EL, Page RL, Connolly SJ, Marcello SR, Schnell DJ, Wilkinson WE. Antiarrhythmic effects of azimilide in atrial fibrillation: efficacy and dose-response. J Am Coll Cardiol 2000; 36:794–802.

39. Stroobandt R, Stiels B, Hoebrechts R, et al. Propafenone for conversion and prophylaxis of atrial fibrillation. Am J Cardiol 1997; 79:418–423.

40. Wanless RS, Anderson K, Joy M, et al. Multicenter comparative study of the efficacy and safety of sotalol in the prophylactic treatment of patients with paroxysmal supraventricular tachyarrhythmias. Am Heart J 1997; 133:441–446.

41. Reiffel JA. Selecting an antiarrhythmic agent for atrial fibrillation should be a patient-specific data-driven decision. Am J Cardiol 1998; 82:72N–81N.

42. Reiffel JA, Camm AJ, Haffajee CJ, et al. International consensus roundtable on atrial fibrillation. Cardiol Rev 2000; 12(suppl):1–19.

43. Roy D, Talajic M, Dorian P, et al. Amiodarone to prevent recurrence of atrial fibrillation. N Eng J Med 2000; 342:913–920.

44. Leenhardt A, Thomas O, Coumel P. Pharmacological treatment of atrial fibrillation. Arch Malad Coeur Vaisseaux 1997; 90:41–46.

45. Louis A, Cleland JG, Crabbe S, Ford S, Thackray S, Houghton T, Clark A. CAPRICORN, COPERNICUS, MIRACLE, STAF, RITZ-2, RECOVER and RENAISSANCE and cachexia and cholesterol in heart failure. Eur J Heart Fail 2001; 9:381–387.

46. The CASCADE Investigators. Randomized antiarrhythmic drug therapy in survivors of cardiac arrest (the CASCADE study). Am J Cardiol 1993; 72:280–287.

47. Julian DG, Camm AJ, Frangia G, Janse MJ, Munoz A, Schwartz PJ, Simon P. Randomized trial of effect of amiodarone on mortality in patients with left ventricular dysfunction after recent myocardial infarction(EMIAT). Lancet 1997; 349:667–674.

48. Cairns JA, Connolly SJ, Roberts R, Gent M. Randomized trial of outcome after myocardial infarction in patients with frequent or repetitive ventricular premature depolarization (CAMIAT). Lancet 1997; 349:675–682.

49. Antman EM, Beamer AD, Cantillon C, et al. Therapy of refractory symptomatic atrial fibrillation and atrial flutter; a staged care approach with new antiarrhythmic drugs. J Am Coll Cardiol 1990; 15:698–707.

50. Reiffel JA, Correira J. "In the absence of structural heart disease…" what is it and why does it matter as regards antiarrhythmic drug therapy? Am Heart J 1994; 128:626–629.

51. Reiffel JA. The impact of structural heart disease on the selection of class III antiarrhythmics for atrial fibrillation and flutter. Am Heart J 1998; 135:551–556.

52. The CAST Investigators. Preliminary report: effect of encainide and flecainide on mortality in a randomized trial of arrhythmia suppression after myocardial infarction [special report]. N Engl J Med 1989; 32:406–412.

53. Teo KK, Yusus S, Furberg CD. Effects of prophylactic antiarrhythmic drug therapy in acute myocardial infarction: an overview of results from randomized controlled trials. JAMA 1993; 270:1589–1595.

54. Prystowsky EN. Inpatient versus outpatient initiation of antiarrhythmic drug therapy for patients with supraventricular tachycardia. Clin Cardiol 1994; 98: II-7–II-10.

55. Hughes MM, Trohman RG, Simmons TW, Castle LW, Wilkoff BL, Morant VA, Maloney JD. Flecainide therapy in patients treated for supraventricular tachycardia with near normal left ventricular function. Am Heart J 1992; 123:408–412.

56. Reiffel JA, Appel G. Importance of QT interval determination and renal function assessment during antiarrhythmic drug therapy. J Cardiovasc Pharmacol Ther 2001; 6:111–119.

57. Reiffel JA. Is it rationale, reasonable or excessive, and consistently applied? One view of the increasing FDA emphasis on safety first for the release and use of antiarrhythmic drugs for supraventricular arrhythmias. J Cardiovasc Pharmacol Ther 2001; 6:333–339.

58. Kassotis J, Costeas C, Blitzer M, Reiffel JA. Rhythm management in atrial fibrillation with a primary emphasis on pharmacologic—part 3. Pacing Clin Electrophysiol 1998; 21:1133–1145.

59. Julian DG, Prescott RJ, Jackson FS, Szekely P. Controlled trial of sotalol for one year after myocardial infarction. Lancet 1982; 1:1142–1147.

60. Torp-Pedersen C, Moller M, Bloch-Thomsen PE, et al. Dofetilide in patients with congestive heart failure and left ventricular dysfunction. N Engl J Med 1999; 341:857–865.

61. The ALIVE Trial Investigators. The ALIVE Trial. Presented at the Annual Scientific sessions of the American College of Cardiology, 2002.

62. Doval HC, Nul DR, Grancelli HO, Varini SD, Soifer S, Corrado G, Dubner S, Scapin O, Perrone SV. Randomized trial of low-dose amiodarone in severe congestive heart failure. Lancet 1994; 344:493–498.

63. Singh SN, Fletcher RD, Fisher SG, Singh BN, Lewis HD, Deedwania P, Massie BM, Colling C, Lazzeri D. Amiodarone in patients with congestive heart failure and asymptomatic ventricular arrhythmia. N Engl J Med 1995; 333:77–82.

64. Reiffel JA. Drug choices in the treatment of atrial fibrillation. Am J Cardiol 2000; 85:12D–19D.

65. Reiffel JA. Issues in the use of generic antiarrhythmic drugs. Curr Opin Cardiol 2001; 16:23–29.

66. Reiffel JA. Formulation substitution and other pharmacokinetic variability: underappreciated variables affecting antiarrhythmic efficacy and safety in clinical practice. Am J Cardiol 2000; 85:46D–52D.

67. Reiffel JA. Inpatient versus outpatient antiarrhythmic drug initiation: safety and cost-effectiveness issues. Curr Opin Cardiol 2000; 15:7–11.

68. Marcus FI. Risks of initiating therapy with sotalol for treatment of atrial fibrillation. J Am Coll Cardiol 1998; 32:177–180.

11
Device Therapy for Atrial Fibrillation

Lai Chow Kok
*Medical College of Virginia, Virginia Commonwealth University
and Hunter Holmes McGuire, Veterans Affairs Medical Center,
Richmond, Virginia, U.S.A.*

Paul A. Levine
*St. Jude Medical Cardiac Rhythm Management Division, Sylmar
and Loma Linda University, School of Medicine, Loma Linda,
California, U.S.A.*

Kenneth A. Ellenbogen
*Medical College of Virginia, Virginia Commonwealth University,
Richmond, Virginia, U.S.A.*

I. INTRODUCTION

Atrial fibrillation (AF) is by far the most common significant cardiac arrhythmia, affecting an estimated 4 million people worldwide. Its incidence may be increasing, and its prevalence increases as the population ages. Its hemodynamic consequences include decreased cardiac output, increased sympathetic nervous system activation, increased risk of thromboembolic complications, and abnormal rate response to exercise. The treatment of AF with antiarrhythmic drug therapy has been disappointing due to a low rate of efficacy and potentially life-threatening side effects (1,2). The health care costs associated with management of this arrhythmia are staggering. AF accounts for over one-third of all hospital days and patient discharges where arrhythmia is coded as the principal diagnosis. The estimated cost of management of patients with AF in the United States alone is over $1 billion.

New insights into the underlying pathophysiology of AF have fueled enthusiasm for developing potentially curative nonpharmacological therapies, including catheter ablation and cardiac pacing. Rapid advances in our understanding of AF and new developments in computer/software technology over the last decade have provided physicians with the opportunity to utilize pacemakers as therapeutic tools for the treatment of AF in patients. The role of devices in AF therapy has evolved from conventional bradycardia pacing in sick sinus syndrome (SSS) and for patients with a slow ventricular response in chronic AF or following atrioventricular (AV) junctional ablation to atrial pacing for AF prevention and antitachycardia pacing or atrial defibrillation for AF termination.

The ultimate goals of AF therapy are to maintain a stable atrial rhythm and/or minimize the consequences of AF, which include prevention of thromboembolic events, prevention of tachycardia-induced cardiomyopathy, and relief of symptoms. Additionally, the therapy must be cost-effective while not resulting in increased mortality or morbidity.

II. ATRIAL PACING FOR AF PREVENTION

A variety of experimental studies in different animal models have shown that AF is due to the presence of either multiple reentrant wavelets or a dominant single reentrant wavelet (3). In order for AF to be established, appropriate triggers (premature atrial complexes, or PACs) are required for initiation, and appropriate atrial substrate (inhomogeneous atrial refractoriness for facilitation of reentrant wavelets) is needed for AF to be maintained. Preventive pacing algorithms have been designed to suppress AF triggers, and new pacing lead designs may alter the underlying atrial substrate by allowing for pacing access to multiple or alternative atrial sites.

A. Suppression of Triggers

The exact role of PACs in AF initiation is still a matter of debate, although several investigators have observed that PACs triggering AF tend to have shorter coupling intervals and to be more likely to arise from the posterior left atrium, especially in or around the pulmonary veins (4,5). PAC suppression can be achieved by either permanently elevating the lower pacing rate or by dynamic overdrive pacing.

The results of fixed-rate atrial pacing on AF prevention have been mixed. In a small trial, AF was eliminated in 14 of 22 patients over a 30-day period when the atrial pacing rate was programmed to 10 beats per minute (bpm) faster than the mean heart rate (6). In another study, overdrive pacing did not offer any advantage for AF suppression over rate-responsive pacing with a base rate of 60 bpm in patients with sick sinus syndrome, even though a significant increase in total duration of atrial pacing was achieved with the overdrive pacing algorithm (7). The PA[3] investigators reported similar outcomes in a series of 97 drug-refractory AF patients who were randomized to DDI with a lower rate of 30 bpm (DDI 30) or DDIR with lower rate of 70 bpm (DDIR 70) prior to planned AV junctional ablation (8). Patients in this study had three or more episodes of symptomatic AF in a year, were refractory or intolerant to medical therapy, and were being considered for AV junctional ablation. Diagnostic data were collected after a 2-week stabilization period to allow for lead maturation and stabilization of antiarrhythmic therapy. After 3 months of atrial pacing, the atrium was found to be paced $67 \pm 31\%$ of the time in patients randomized to DDIR 70 compared to no atrial pacing in patients with DDI 30. While atrial pacing significantly reduced the burden of PACs from baseline (3.8 to 0.5/hr, $p < 0.01$), it had no effect on AF prevention. The time to first episode of AF recurrence was identical between atrial pacing and no pacing (1.9 days; 95% CI 0.8 to 4.6, vs. 4.2 days; 95% CI 1.8 to 9.5, $p = $ NS). In fact, pacing may have been deleterious as a lower AF burden was observed in patients randomized to no pacing (0.24 vs. 0.67 hr/day, $p = 0.08$). Eleven patients in this study who crossed over to the pacing arm were found to have earlier AF recurrence after pacing compared to no pacing, and the total AF burden in these 11 patients was significantly greater during atrial pacing. Sixty-seven patients who subsequently underwent AV junctional ablation participated in the second phase of the PA[3] trial (9). Following ablation, they were randomized to DDDR pacing or VDD pacing in a crossover study design with 6 months of pacing in each arm. The trial was designed to study the potential benefits in the prevention of AF of atrial pacing over atrial sensing while maintaining AV synchronization. The outcome of the second phase was identical to the first phase. There was no difference in the time to first AF episode between DDDR pacing and VDD pacing (0.37 vs. 0.5 days, $p = $ NS). The AF burden increased over time in both groups, with 6.93 hr/day of AF reported in the DDDR group and 6.30 hr/day in the VDD group at the 6-month follow-up. At the end of 1 year, 43% of patients developed permanent AF. Atrial pacing did not prevent progression to chronic AF in this group of patients with symptomatic paroxysmal AF and no primary bradycardia indications for pacing.

The dynamic atrial overdrive pacing algorithm introduced by St. Jude Medical (Sylmar, CA), labeled AF Suppression, achieves a similar effect of ensuring constant atrial capture without having to program an elevated lower base pacing rate. The hypothesized advantage of these algorithms is to minimize pauses following ectopic atrial beats, suppress atrial ectopy, and reduce dispersion of refractoriness by maintaining control of rate and rhythm while also avoiding a fixed high pacing rate, which can be uncomfortable for patients and possibly induce a tachycardia and consequent cardiomyopathy. This algorithm works by incrementally increasing the paced rate upon detection of intrinsic atrial events until no further atrial sensed events occur.

Pacing is maintained for a programmable duration before it is decreased again in steps, until the intrinsic rate appears or a lower pacing rate or sensor rate is reached (Fig. 1). Again, sensing of atrial events will result in an increase of the atrial pacing rate. Other device manufacturers have incorporated similar algorithms into their devices; specific details of individual algorithms are best found in the device manuals. A partial list of algorithms that have been incorporated into a variety of devices is given in Table 1.

The Atrial Preference Pacing algorithm (Medtronic, Minneapolis, MN) monitors the P-P interval and shortens the atrial escape interval by a programmable value that is fixed over the allowed rate range, while the AF Suppression algorithm (previously known as Dynamic Atrial Overdrive, or DAO) increases atrial paced rate variably, depending on the functional rate at the time, for a programmable duration of time based on detection of intrinsic atrial activity. These algorithms have been especially well studied. The overall mean heart rate was not significantly increased when these algorithms were used and, more importantly, the algorithms were well tolerated by patients (10,11). The AF Suppression algorithm was developed to allow for the normal circadian variation in cardiac rhythm while still providing overdrive pacing using the intrinsic atrial rhythm as a guide for the overdrive rate. If the rhythm were totally under the control of the pacemaker (sensor-based), the rate could still fluctuate in a manner similar to circadian variation using the dynamic adjustment of the resting rate based on relative sensor activity. Algorithmic increases in the atrial paced rate would be based on a relative increase in native atrial activity, which could be either sinus or atrial premature beat (APBs) (12). To minimize frequent fluctuations, at least two native events had to be

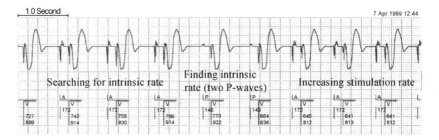

Figure 1 ECG demonstrating the dynamic atrial overdrive (DAO) suppression algorithm in a patient with a biventricular device. The annotated event markers and electronic calipers document the behavior of the algorithm. This strip is recorded at a paper speed of 50 mm/sec. On the first three beats of this tracing, there is AV pacing at a short AV delay (to provide resynchronization therapy), with progressive lengthening of the V-V cycle length. This is followed by two native atrial beats (sensed) at a higher rate, resulting in an increase in the atrial paced rate within the programmed parameters.

Table 1 Pacing Algorithms to Prevent Atrial Fibrillation

Overdrive sinus rhythm algorithms
    Atrial Fibrillation Suppression (formerly Dynamic Atrial Overdrive, or DAO),
      (St. Jude Medical)
    Atrial Preference Pacing (Medtronic)
    Atrial Pacing Preference (Guidant)
    Sinus Rhythm Overdrive (Ela-Sorin)
    DDD+ (Biotronik)
    Pace Conditioning (Vitatron)
Pacing to prevent AT reinitiation
    Post-Mode-Switch Overdrive Pacing (Medtronic)
Overdrive algorithms post-PACs
    Acceleration on PAC (Ela-Sorin)
    PAC Suppression (Vitatron)
Pacing to prevent pauses
    Atrial Rate Stabilization (Medtronic)
    Post–Extrasystolic Pause Suppression (Ela-Sorin)

detected within a 16-cycle window. An increase in atrial ectopy is often demonstrated preceding the development of paroxysms of atrial fibrillation.

The effectiveness of the AF Suppression algorithm was subjected to a prospective multicenter randomized trial comparing the effects of the algorithm added to standard DDDR pacemaker to that of a standard DDDR pacemaker (12). All subjects required pacing support for a primary bradycardia indication and had documented recurrent episodes of paroxysmal AF prior to device implantation. A total of 399 patients were enrolled in the study, which was completed in December 2000. The results were submitted to the U.S. Food and Drug Administration (FDA) with approval for commercial device release in late 2001. The trial endpoint was symptomatic AF burden defined as days of electrocardiography (ECG)-documented episodes of AF. The definition was very conservative in that any episode of documented AF lasting longer than 20 sec and occurring during a given day was considered as "1 day of AF." A 20-sec episode was effectively equal to hours of AF for the purpose of defining AF burden. This would bias the results against the algorithm demonstrating a benefit. All patients carried a transtelephonic monitor for ECG documentation of symptomatic episodes. The results were analyzed using an intention-to-treat design, with the DAO group shown to have a 25% reduction in AF burden compared to the group with the algorithm disabled (Fig. 2). When the patients with no AF episodes during the first 30 days following pacemaker implantation were excluded from both groups, the group with the AF Suppression algorithm enabled had a 35%

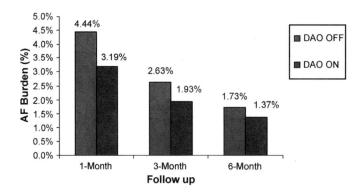

Figure 2 Results of the ADOPT-A protocol. This study enrolled 399 patients to 6 months of DDDR pacing with a base rate of 60 bpm with the DAO algorithm off and then 6 months to a base rate of 60 bpm with DAO algorithm on. A progressive improvement in both groups of AF patients was seen over time, but the patients with the suppression algorithm on had a lower symptomatic AF burden.

reduction in AF burden compared to the group with the algorithm disabled. The subset analysis effectively eliminated patients in whom standard DDDR pacing alone was likely to be effective for AF prevention. Forty-five percent of patients demonstrated a benefit from standard DDDR pacing without the need for any special algorithm. The remaining patients presumably had a more advanced stage of disease. In addition to the initial benefit associated with pacing, a remodeling effect of pacing was also seen in both groups, with a progressive reduction in episodes of AF at 1, 3, and 6 months of follow-up. However, the relative additional benefit of AF Suppression persisted at each of these interim points.

The diagnostic event counters are integral to the assessment of the efficacy of these devices to prevent AF. One must be reasonably certain that the event counter diagnostics are appropriate and not reporting inappropriate numbers of automatic mode switching (AMS) episodes due to far-field R-wave oversensing, failing to detect the atrial fibrillatory signals, and hence not mode switching or experiencing signal dropout that may be causing the system to exit and reenter mode switching for the same arrhythmic event, thus falsely increasing the number of presumed AF episodes. Other characteristic information also measured during these trials includes the duration of each episode, the atrial rate that triggered the episode, and the total percentage of time the device functioned in a non-atrial-tracking pacing mode. This information must be analyzed to determine the effectiveness of these algorithms (Figs. 3 and 4).

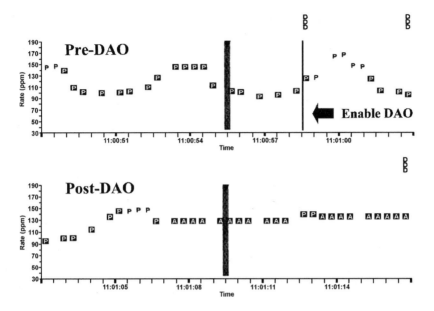

Figure 3 Event record demonstrating pre- and postinitiation of DAO algorithm. A series of two event-record printouts show the marked rate fluctuation before DAO is enabled. The vertical line on the top rhythm is the point of enabling DAO. There is a short period of time during which the system is setting itself, monitoring the rhythm before it starts to increment the rate. In addition, since the atrial rate was a sensed rate, the increment in atrial paced rate started at the base or sensor-driven rate. With each rate increment in accord with the programmed parameter, the system determined whether there were still sensed beats or if atrial pacing was present. As shown on the bottom printout, there is rate stabilization that continues in accord with the overdrive cycle. Before this ends, there are two cycles of PV pacing at a slightly higher rate, and the atrial paced rate is again increased in accord with the DAO algorithm.

In contrast, in a short-term follow-up study of the Atrial Pacing Preference Pacing algorithm, there was no beneficial effect of overdrive pacing on the overall incidence of AF in 31 patients with paroxysmal AF (12). In a small series of 15 patients with sick sinus syndrome, the overdrive pacing algorithm (DDDR + consistent atrial overdrive pacing) was shown to significantly reduce the frequency of PACs, but it did not alter the number of mode-switching episodes (47 ± 90 vs. 42 ± 87, DDDR vs. DDDR + consistent atrial pacing, $p > 0.05$) (11). A similar reduction in the number of PACs was demonstrated in a larger series of 61 patients, but no overall effect on reduction of symptomatic paroxysmal AF episodes was seen (14).

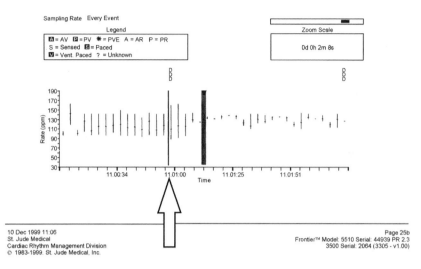

Figure 4 Event record documentation of enabling of AF-suppression algorithm. This event record shows how the DDDR pacing system in a biventricular device works. The intrinsic rhythm demonstrates a marked sinus arrhythmia; activation of the DAO algorithm occurs at the arrow. Within a few seconds the rhythm stabilizes with a marked reduction in the degree of rate fluctuation.

B. Effect on Atrial Substrate Suppression of Compensatory Pause

PACs may also initiate AF by altering the underlying atrial substrate to support re-entry. The short–long cycles caused by postextrasystolic pauses following PACs may increase dispersion of atrial refractoriness, making it conducive to the maintenance of reentrant wavelets (13). Pacing algorithms that respond to spontaneous PACs have been designed to maintain homogeneous refractoriness. The pacing response to a PAC can be a single paced beat, a series of paced beats coupled with autoadaptive decay, or pacing rate acceleration for a programmable duration. A pacing algorithm utilizing a series of paced beats in response to PACs was studied in 70 patients with a history of frequent atrial ectopy (14). The algorithm was tested in a crossover study design involving alternating 2 hr of programming the algorithm "on" and "off" for 24 hr. This pacing algorithm had no effect on the overall PAC burden (by pacemaker counters or Holter analysis) or overall AF episodes. Only patients with frequent AF (>5 episodes/24 hr) experienced a lower AF burden with this pacing algorithm. Furthermore, this algorithm was frequently inactivated by salvos of PACs in more than 75% episodes. This would suggest that while the algorithm may be effective in the event of a PAC, it is not able to prevent short bursts of PACs, which are more likely to induce AF. Additionally, while some algorithms may be effective at decreasing the number of PACs, experience with the hope that these algorithms might also decrease the number of episodes of AF has been disappointing.

Pacemakers that incorporate separate algorithms for PAC suppression to maintain homogenous atrial refractoriness have been designed and tested. The Atrial Therapy Efficacy and Safety Trial (ATTEST) evaluated the role of AT500 (Medtronic, Minneapolis, MN) pacemakers that incorporated three different pacing algorithms (Atrial Preference Pacing, Atrial Rate Stabilization, and Post Mode Switching Overdrive) in AF prevention (15). The study enrolled 368 patients with standard bradycardia indications and a history of AF (with at least one documented episode of AF in the last 3 months) to receive the AT500 pacemakers. Patients were randomized to have the algorithms programmed "on" or "off." Over 75% of the study population had a history of paroxysmal AF. At the end of 3 months, there was no difference between the two groups with regard to median AT (atrial tachycardia)/AF burden (4.2 hr/month "on" vs. 1.1 hr/month "off," $p = 0.20$) and frequency of AT/AF (1.3 episodes per month "on" vs. 1.2 episodes per month "off," $p = 0.65$). The number of symptomatic episodes of AT/AF was similar in patients with the algorithm "on" or "off." A retrospective analysis of multiple patient subgroups was unable to identify any baseline patient characteristics or the use of any antiarrhythmic drugs that predicted a responder subgroup. This study suggests that the specific AF-prevention and tachycardia termination algorithms did not reduce the frequency or burden of AF over the short term.

The PIPAF (16) study utilized the ELA Chorum 7334 pacemaker with multiple algorithms (sinus rhythm overdrive, postextrasystolic pause suppression, and acceleration on PACs) to prospectively evaluate 38 patients in a prospective crossover design being paced with or without the algorithms enabled for a period of 3 months in each mode. The endpoints were number of episodes per week (6.0 vs. 5.9) and cumulative duration (12.0 vs. 11.7 hr). There was no difference between the two groups.

There have been a number of studies evaluating the Post-Mode Switch Overdrive Pacing (PMOP) algorithm in helping to stabilize the atrium after spontaneous termination of atrial fibrillation. Israel et al. (17) showed that PMOP appeared to be arrhythmogenic, with an increased immediate or early recurrence of the atrial tachyarrhythmia with the algorithm ($p = 0.006$) when the PMOP rate was programmed to 80 bpm. When the rate was programmed to 120 ppm (18)—on the assumption that after a tachyarrhythmia, the rate of 80 bpm may have been too low—no benefit could be demonstrated. A third study, by Adler et al. (19), involving 136 patients, evaluated the PMOP rate of 80 and reported a statistically significant benefit ($p = 0.02$) during the overdrive period. These investigators continued to monitor these patients and demonstrated that within 1 hr of arrhythmia termination, AT or AF had commonly recurred, and the incidence of atrial arrhythmias was similar in both groups.

C. Reducing Dispersion of Refractoriness—Multisite Pacing

Patients with paroxysmal AF can have profound intra- and interatrial conduction delay, as evidenced by broader P waves on the surface ECG (20,21). This conduction delay increases the dispersion of atrial refractoriness, favoring AF induction (22,23). Pacing may correct the conduction delay, reduce dispersion of refractoriness, and improve atrial homogeneity. These goals can be achieved by simultaneous pacing from more than one site (multisite or dual-site pacing) to allow synchronization of left and right atrial activation or pacing from a unique location such as Bachmann's bundle or the interatrial septum.

Dual-site pacing has been shown to be effective in preventing AF by reducing conduction delay (20). D'Allones et al. demonstrated a significant reduction of the P wave duration (from 187 ± 29 ms to 106 ± 14 ms, $p = 0.0001$) by pacing simultaneously from the high right atrial and distal coronary sinus in patients with a P-wave duration >120 ms (24). They reported a 64% success rate for maintenance of sinus rhythm in 86 patients with intra-atrial delay after a mean follow-up of 33 months. An initial concern of dual-site pacing was raised with a report of a high dislodgement rate of the coronary sinus lead, but this issue has been resolved with the development of a specifically designed lead for the coronary sinus (Medtronic SP 2188) (25). Saksena et al. proposed a different method of reducing total atrial activation time by the placement of a screw-in pacing lead near the os of the coronary sinus instead of in the distal coronary sinus. An advantage of this method is the ease of both implantation and extraction while using conventional active fixation leads. The initial experience reported by these investigators appeared promising (26). They showed that dual-site pacing significantly increased the duration of the AF free interval in a series of 15 patients with AF and bradycardia, although no difference in the AF free interval was observed between single-site vs. dual-site pacing. Pacing therapy, regardless of the number of sites, also reduced the number of reported symptomatic episodes and the number of antiarrhythmic drugs compared to prior to pacemaker implantation. A subsequent report on 30 patients with longer follow-up duration again demonstrated better AF control with pacing regardless of pacing site (high right atrium vs. coronary sinus os) (27).

To provide a more definitive answer, a group of investigators initiated a multicenter study to examine the effectiveness of dual-site pacing therapy in AF prevention (28). The study randomized 118 patients with symptomatic AF and bradycardia to one of three pacing modes (overdrive high-right-atrial pacing; dual-site atrial pacing; or support pacing at a lower rate of 50 bpm or in VDI pacing mode) using a crossover trial design. The study found no significant difference in the time between dual- and single-site pacing (RR 0.835, $p = 0.175$) for freedom from symptomatic AF during a mean follow-up of 12.1 ± 6.9 months. In patients who developed recurrent AF, the median time to AF recurrence was 1.77 months for dual-site pacing, 0.62 months for high-right-atrial pacing, and 0.44 months for support pacing ($p < 0.09$, dual-vs. high-right-atrial pacing; $p < 0.05$, dual vs. support pacing; $p > 0.7$, high-right-atrial vs. support pacing). Patients reported better quality-of-life scores when randomized to overdrive high-right-atrial pacing or dual-site pacing compared to the support mode, but no difference was observed between the first two pacing modalities. The study did not show superiority of dual-site pacing over high-right-atrial pacing with regard to the use of antiarrhythmic drugs or frequency of AF episodes. Dual-site pacing was found to be more effective in suppressing AF when compared to high-right-atrial pacing in the presence of concomitant class I or III antiarrhythmic agents, but the number of patients in this analysis was too small to provide any firm conclusions. While this study had demonstrated the safety and feasibility of dual-site atrial pacing, it did not provide convincing evidence for the role of multisite pacing in AF prevention, particularly in AF patients with bradycardia. PAF patients with a prolonged P wave (≥ 90 to 120 ms) may benefit from dual-site pacing, as suggested by a nonrandomized study (12), but this will need further confirmation from large prospective randomized trials.

The role of dual-site pacing in patients with paroxysmal AF without a conventional bradycardia indication for pacing was also examined (29). Lau et al. randomized 22 patients with recurrent AF on sotalol in a crossover study design to 12 weeks of either pacing with sotalol or sotalol alone. All patients received pacemakers with the Continuous Atrial Pacing algorithm to ensure a higher percent of atrial pacing. The study showed that dual-site pacing reduced the frequency of PACs and prolonged the time to first symptomatic AF episode, but it had no effect on the frequency of AF. Both arms had the same number of patients with AF recurrence. This result has been confirmed by other studies of similar size involving the same patient population (30–32). These studies seem to suggest that dual-site pacing has, at best, modest efficacy in reducing the overall AF burden, and that the complexity of the additional pacing leads may relegate this pacing mode to patients with frequent symptomatic AF who have failed a combination of antiarrhythmic and ablation therapies (Table 2).

Table 2 Clinical Trials of Dual- and Alternative-Site Pacing for AF Suppression

Study	N	Patient population	Study design	Endpoint	Follow-up	Results
NIPP-AF (27)	22	No bradycardia + PAF (≥2 episodes in 3 months) All patients on sotalol	Multicenter prospective randomized crossover trial of DAP vs. sotalol with 12 weeks for each phase.	Time to first symptomatic AF	40 weeks	DAP vs. sotalol 50 ± 30 vs. 15 ± 17 days ($p < 0.01$). No. of pts with AF recurrence with DAP vs. sotalol 16 vs. 16 ($p =$ ns)
Levy et al. (29)	20	No bradycardia + drug refractory PAF (≥3 episodes in 1 week)	Single-center prospective randomized DAP vs. RAA pacing crossover study 1 month for each phase	1. No. PAF episodes 2. Duration of PAF (days) 3. AF burden (total % of time in 1 month)	1 month	RAA vs. DAP pacing 1. 77 ± 98 vs. 52 ± 78 ($p =$ ns); 2. 4.8 ± 5.4 days vs. 6.3 ± 9.8 days ($p =$ ns) 3. 14 ± 16% vs. 19 ± 30% ($p =$ ns)
Leclercq et al. (26)	83	Drug-refractory PAF (≥2 episodes in 6 months)	Single-center prospective nonrandomized DAP (30 pts; all with P wave ≥ 120 ms) RAA (53 pts; 21 pts with P wave ≥ 120 ms)	Time to PAF or permanent AF (AF lasting >3 months)	18 ± 15 months	Pts with P wave ≥ 120 ms: PAF incidence DAP vs. RAA, 30 vs. 71% ($p < 0.01$) Permanent AF DAP vs. RAA, 3 vs. 38% ($p < 0.01$) Pts with P wave < 120 ms: PAF incidence DAP vs. RAA, 30 vs. 28% ($p =$ ns) Permanent AF incidence DAP vs. RAA, 3 vs. 12% ($p =$ ns)

Study	N	Patient population	Study design	Endpoint	Follow-up	Results
D'Allones et al. (21)	86	Drug refractory PAF P wave ≥ 120 ms	Single center prospective nonrandomized	Sinus rhythm	Mean 33 months (6–109)	At follow-up, 64% (55 pts) in sinus rhythm, of which 33% (27 pts) with ≥1 AF recurrence Drug therapy in the 55 pts reduced compared to baseline from 1.7 ± 0.5 drugs/pt to 1.4 ± 0.6 drugs/pt, ($p = 0.011$)
DAPPAF (25)	118	Bradycardia + PAF (≥2 episodes in 3 months) 46 patients on class I or III	Multicenter prospective randomized crossover DAP vs. RAA vs. support pacing. 6 months in each phase	Time to first symptomatic AF	12.1 ± 6.9 months	Freedom from symptomatic AF DAP vs. RAA, RR = 0.835 ($p = 0.175$) DAP vs. support, RR = 0.715 ($p = 0.073$) RAA vs. support, RR = 0.709 ($p = 0.188$)
Mirza et al. (28)	19	No bradycardia + drug-refractory PAF	Single-center prospective randomized crossover RAA vs. CS vs. DAP (70 ms interatrial delay) vs. DAP (16 ms interatrial). 3 months in each phase	No. of AF episodes	15 months	Mean no AF episodes/ month compared to baseline of 16/month RAA: 10.5 ($p = 0.003$) CS: 9.3 ($p = 0.015$) DAP 70: 7.3 ($p = 0.0007$) DAP 16: 7.2 ($p = 0.0007$)
Bailin et al. (37)	120	Bradycardia + PAF	Multicenter prospective randomized trial of RAA vs. BB pacing	Time to chronic AF (2 consecutive ECG with AF 2 months apart)	1 year	Freedom from chronic AF at 1 year BB vs. RAA pacing, 75 vs. 47% ($p < 0.05$)

Table 2 Continued

Study	N	Patient population	Study design	Endpoint	Follow-up	Results
Padeletti et al. (45)	46	Bradycardia + PAF ($\geq$2 episodes of AF in 3 months)	Multicenter prospective randomized RAA vs. CS pacing for 6 months. Each arm randomized to CAP-off and CAP-on programming.	1. Time to first AF (days) 2. Symptomatic AF episodes/month 3. PAF burden (min/day)	6 months	CS vs. RAA pacing 1. CAP-on 6.7 vs. 6.7, p = ns; CAP-off 9.6 vs. 6.8, p = ns 2. CAP-on 0.2 $\pm$ 0.5 vs. 1.9 $\pm$ 3.8, p < 0.05; CAP-off 0.2 $\pm$ 0.5 vs. 2.1 $\pm$ 4.2, p < 0.05 3. CAP-on 41 $\pm$ 72 vs. 193 $\pm$ 266, p < 0.05; CAP-off 47 $\pm$ 84 vs. 140 $\pm$ 217, p < 0.05
DeVoogt et al. (46)	170	Bradycardia and PAF	Multicenter prospective randomized trial of RAA vs. IAS pacing for 3 months. Each arm randomized to AF Suppression on or off. Also involved a separate control group of 85 who did not have PAF.	1. AF burden (min/day) 2. Quality of life	3 months	RAA: off vs. on—76 min vs. 38.9 min, p = 0.033 IAS: off vs. on—74.1 min vs. 22.0 min, p = 0.027 IAS on AA meds: off vs. on—78.1 vs. 19.9 min, p = 0.013 Control: off vs. on—0.5 vs. 0.6, p = ns

Key: BB, Bachmann's bundle; CAP, consistent atrial pacing; CS, coronary sinus; DAP, dual-site atrial pacing; RAA, right atrial appendage; min, minutes; RR, relative risk; PAF, paroxysmal atrial fibrillation; Pt, patient, IAS; interatrial septal pacing.

D. Atrial Pacing Following Cardiac Surgery

Atrial fibrillation is a common problem following cardiac bypass surgery and valve replacement/repair. The incidence of this complication varies from 10% to 40% depending on multiple factors, including patient age. While the results of permanent biatrial pacing for AF prevention have been mixed, the results of temporary biatrial pacing for postoperative AF prevention following coronary artery bypass surgery were more consistent. AF is a common arrhythmia following bypass surgery and is often associated with prolonged hospitalization and increased hospital cost (33). The strategy of preoperative use of antiarrhythmic drugs for AF prevention is limited to patients undergoing elective cardiac surgery (34,35).

Routine epicardial pacing lead placement following cardiac surgery provides an opportunity to study the role of pacing in the prevention of postoperative AF. Two recently published studies have shown that biatrial pacing lowered the incidence of postoperative AF (36,37). A meta-analysis also showed that biatrial pacing reduced the incidence of postoperative AF and shortened hospital stay (38). In the meta-analysis, overdrive biatrial pacing was associated with a risk reduction of developing AF of 2.6 (CI 1.4 to 4.8), while fixed high-rate biatrial pacing was associated with a risk reduction of 2.5 (CI 1.3 to 5.1). For comparison, overdrive right atrial pacing was associated with a risk reduction of only 1.8 (CI 1.1 to 2.7). Blommaert and colleagues (39) demonstrated a significant reduction in the incidence of paroxysmal AF in postoperative open heart patients with single-site pacing in conjunction with Medtronic's continuous atrial pacing algorithm. The incidence of postoperative AF was reduced from 27% in the control group to 10% in the active pacing group ($p = 0.036$). While there are lessons to be learned from post-open heart surgery patients, the mechanism and substrate for their arrhythmias are likely to differ from those of patients whose arrhythmias occur spontaneously.

Fan et al. found that pacing decreased the mean P-wave duration irrespective of the pacing sites, although biatrial pacing showed the greatest reduction in P-wave dispersion compared to left or right atrial pacing ($42 \pm 8\%$ vs. $13 \pm 6\%$ for left atrial pacing, $p < 0.05$; $10 \pm 9\%$ for right atrial pacing, $p < 0.05$) (40). In their study, there was no difference in the baseline mean P-wave duration or P-wave dispersion between patients who developed postoperative AF and those who did not, but patients who maintained sinus rhythm postoperatively were found to have a significant reduction in P-wave duration and P-wave dispersion with biatrial pacing compared to their baseline. This observation suggests that failure to reduce dispersion of atrial refractoriness with pacing led to the development of postoperative AF. This observation may explain the less than satisfactory outcome of the dual-site atrial pacing studies discussed earlier.

E. Reducing Dispersion of Refractoriness—Alternative-Site Atrial Pacing

Another method of shortening the total atrial activation time is by pacing the atrium from selected sites. At present, it is generally accepted that routes of preferential interatrial conduction exist and that pacing at these sites will preexcite the left atrium. Pacing at Bachmann's bundle is sometimes referred to as interatrial septal pacing; it is the largest anatomical interatrial communication and probably accounts for the majority of interatrial conduction. The structure is a band of tissue that extends from the right of the superior vena cava transversally to the anterior wall of the left atrium and up to the left atrial appendage (Fig. 5). This alternative pacing site had been shown to be effective in AF prevention (Table 2). The incidence of chronic AF at 1 year was lowered with Bachmann's bundle pacing compared to atrial appendage pacing (47 vs. 75%, $p < 0.05$), and most patients who progressed to chronic AF did so within the first 4 months following device implantation (41). All 120 patients in this study had paroxysmal AF and about one-third had previously undergone AV-nodal ablation. Pacing in this region resulted in shorter P-wave duration compared to sinus rhythm or right atrial appendage pacing. Pacing from this site has been shown to reduce P-wave duration to the same extent as dual-site (high right atrial and coronary sinus os) pacing (41). Bachmann's bundle pacing has also been shown to reduce the window of AF inducibility in the animal model, and this may be another mechanism whereby the incidence of AF can be reduced (42).

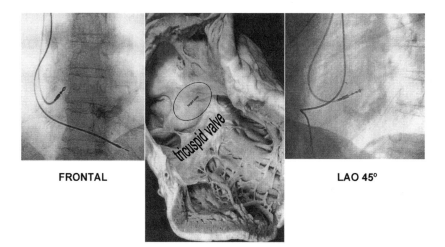

FRONTAL   **LAO 45°**

Figure 5 Pathological and radiological demonstration of interatrial septal pacing (Bachmann's bundle pacing).

The low interatrial septum, near the triangle of Koch, is another alternative pacing site that has been studied (43). A recent necropsy study on the human heart has demonstrated consistent myocardial connections between the right and left atrium along the coronary sinus, especially proximally (44). In a series of 46 patients, pacing at the low interatrial septum was found to be more effective than atrial appendage pacing in reducing AF burden, although either site reduced the AF frequency when compared to the preimplantation frequency (45). Again, P-wave duration during pacing at the low interatrial septum was significantly reduced compared to sinus rhythm. These studies suggest that, over an intermediate period of time, pacing at these selected sites may prevent or slow progression of AF, and that leads positioned at these sites appear to be as stable and safe as at the conventional atrial appendage position.

A prospective study comparing pacing sites with and without St. Jude Medical's AF Suppression algorithm was presented at the Late Breaking Clinical Trials session at NASPE 2003. This was the Overdrive Atrial Septum Stimulation (OASES) in patients with paroxysmal atrial fibrillation and a standard indication for pacing (46,47). A total of 170 patients participated in the trial. In addition, there were 85 more patients who were paced for standard indications without a history of paroxysmal AF. This group served as a control for adverse symptoms associated with the algorithm and appropriateness of the internal diagnostics in the pacemaker. The atrial lead was placed in either the right atrial appendage ($n = 85$) or the low interatrial septum ($n = 85$) and patients were randomized to the AF Suppression algorithm being enabled or disabled for consecutive 3-month periods. AF burden was defined as the number of minutes in atrial fibrillation per day. For the Right Atrial Appendage group, the AF Suppression algorithm reduced the burden from 76.0 to 38.9 min/day ($p = 0.033$). In the atrial septal paced group, the burden decreased from 74.1 min/day with the algorithm off to 22.0 min/day with the AF Suppression algorithm enabled ($p = 0.027$). A subset analysis was performed on those patients being paced from the interatrial septum who were concomitantly being treated with antiarrhythmic agents, and this demonstrated a further improvement (burden reduced from 78.1 to 19.9 min/day, $p = 0.013$). This later observation supports the conclusion that device therapy, perhaps with special algorithms and unique site-specific locations, will be most effective when it is part of a hybrid approach to the management of these patients.

III. ATRIAL PACING FOR AF TERMINATION

Antitachycardia pacing (ATP) is a reliable mode of therapy in arrhythmias with a large excitable gap such as atrial flutter or slower organized ATs. On the other hand, AF with shorter excitable gap and the lack of a single reentrant pathway does not lend itself to easy pace termination. Recent animal studies have shown that by timing the delivery of pacing, the success of AF termination can be improved (48). There are several potential advantages to incorporating ATP into devices for the management of AF. Atrial flutter and AF frequently coexist in the same patient and, not uncommonly, atrial flutter can degenerate into AF. Delivery of ATP while the patient is in atrial flutter or an even slower organized atrial tachycardia may prevent AF initiation. Alternatively, AF may be converted to atrial flutter with antiarrhythmic agents, and the availability of ATP would allow for termination of atrial flutter.

Atrial ATP is now available in some implantable cardioverter/defibrillators (ICDs) and pacemakers. The effectiveness of ATP in reducing atrial tachyarrhythmias (AT/AF) was examined in patients who received Medtronic 7250 Jewel AF dual-chamber ICD. This study enrolled 269 patients receiving ICDs with at least two prior episodes of AF or ATs in the year preceding implant (50). Patients were randomized to 3-month periods of ATP on or ATP off with crossover. ATP algorithm for AT/AF termination in this study were atrial burst-plus (atrial burst followed by two extrastimuli), atrial ramp (atrial autodecremental ramp), and atrial 50-Hz burst pacing up to 3 sec (Fig. 6). Atrial burst 50-Hz pacing successfully converted 24% of the 121 AF episodes identified in 52 patients. The burden of AT/AF was reduced during periods with therapies on, but the actual reduction of AF burden with ATP could not be determined, as no distinction was made between AF and other atrial tachycardias in the analysis. A larger study, by Adler et al., involving 537 patients implanted with the same ICDs showed that ATP (50-Hz burst) was successful in converting 30% of 880 AF episodes in 101 patients (50). The relatively lower success rate of pace termination is attributable to the shorter excitable gap present in AF, as evidenced by the indirect relationship between successful outcome and underlying cycle length of the AT/AF. The success of ATP for termination of AT/AF was 29% if the cycle length $\leq$ 190 ms but 65% when cycle length $>$ 320 ms (50). It was also observed that ATP had a higher success rate (34 vs. 10%, $p < 0.01$) if it was delivered within the first 10 min of AF onset. Prompt AF detection and delivery of ATP may prevent electrical remodeling after AF onset and promote sinus rhythm. Similar ATP efficacy of 54% for AT/AF termination was reported in the ATTEST study, which utilized the same atrial termination algorithms in patients who received pacemakers (15). However, no further analysis in outcome of ATP in AF alone was provided in this study and the definition of AF, analogous to ventricular fibrillation (VF) in the ICDs, is physician dependent. If the rate is sufficiently low, this may be a rapid but still organized AT.

In the analysis performed by Gillis et al. on the Gem III AT database, the device correctly identified AT or AF in 96% of 728 episodes. This device

DEMONSTRATION ONLY - AT/AF Episode #3 Report

ICD Model: GEM III AT 7276   Serial Number: PKE200210R   Date of Visit: Nov 27, 2000

Episode #3 - AT   Chart speed: 25.0 mm/sec

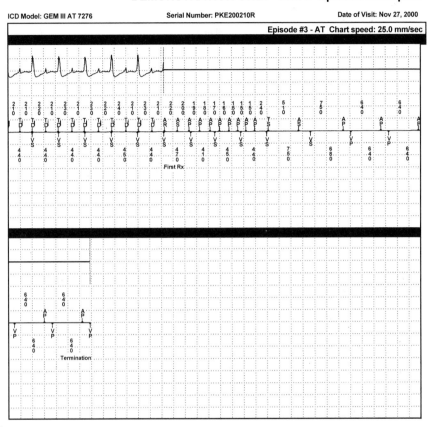

Figure 6 Stored interrogation from a Medtronic Gem III AT 7276 showing termination of a rapid atrial tachycardia by autodecremental ramp pacing. Tracings shown from top to bottom are stored composite EGM (Atip to HVB), A–A interval (ms), marker annotation channel, V–V interval (ms).

delivered 50-Hz burst pacing, atrial ramp, or burst-plus pacing. The percentage of episodes that were successfully terminated was adjusted for multiple episodes per patient. Atrial ATP (ramp or burst-plus) terminated 40% of episodes classified as AT, while the device terminated only 26% of the episodes classified as AF (Fig. 7). In contrast to prior studies, 50-Hz burst pacing terminated only 12 of 109 episodes of AT (12% adjusted) and 65 of 240 episodes of AF (25% adjusted). If efficacy was defined as termination within 20 sec of delivery of pacing therapy, ATP therapies terminated 32% (adjusted, 139 of 383 episodes) episodes of AT, and 15% of AF (adjusted, 34 of 240

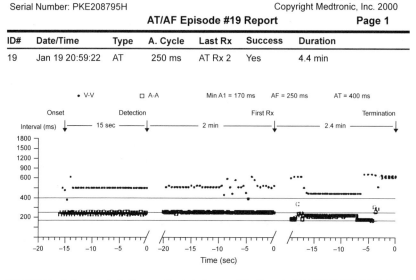

Jan 24, 2002 16:10:12

Figure 7 Interrogated diagnostic data from a Medtronic GEM III AT 7276 showing detection of a rapid AT terminated after the delivery of the second therapy.

episodes). For 50-Hz burst pacing using a definition of termination within 20 sec, AT was terminated in 4% of episodes and AF in 15% of episodes. These observations suggest that prior studies reporting a higher efficacy rate for pace termination of AF with 50-Hz burst pacing probably included patients who had spontaneous terminations of AT/AF and rapid atrial flutter classified by the device as AF. The efficacy of ATP for termination of AT was correlated with atrial cycle length. There is little information in these studies as to the recurrence of atrial tachyarrhythmias after termination. In a study by Adler and associates (19) evaluating the impact of Post-Mode Switch Overdrive Pacing (PMOP) on atrial stability after termination of an atrial tachyarrhythmia, the PMOP algorithm was initially effective, but within 1 hr the incidence of recurrence was the same in both groups. Additionally, ventricular proarrhythmia secondary to atrial ATP was not observed.

A note of caution was raised by Schmitt et al. (51) with respect to using the internal diagnostics in the pacemaker as the arbiter of successful termination. One must be certain that the system is functioning properly, so that when the markers or diagnostics report that an output pulse was delivered, it is successfully captured, and also that all appropriate events are detected. They described a case in which the system reported termination of AF by the

ATP algorithms in the AT500. Of 17 episodes of atrial fibrillation, 15 (90%) were reported by the system as being successfully terminated; but on careful review, the atrial output pulses were ineffective and the device claimed termination inappropriately. This experience is consistent with studies from the late 1990s demonstrating an inability to pace-terminate "true" AF from either single or multiple sites using rapid pacing (52,53).

In another study, Israel et al. identified a subgroup of patients who received anti-AT pacing devices for AF and were found to have regular, slow AT that were pace-terminated by their devices. In these patients, it is likely that AF organizes over time into an AT that can be pace-terminated. The device classifies the arrhythmia based upon its rate at initial detection. The electrogram (EGM) storage capability of these devices showed that patients with AF frequently also have atrial arrhythmias where atrial EGMs show various types of organization. In their analysis, atrial EGMs were classified as type I (monomorphic, discrete signals separated by an isoelectric line with a minimal cycle length > 200 ms), type II (meets neither type I or type II definition), and type III (polymorphic or nondiscrete signals, no isoelectric baseline, with minimal cycle length < 200 ms). At the time of arrhythmia onset, 182 episodes of AT were classified as types II and III, and 51 of 182 episodes organized into type I AT. The antitachycardia pacing success rate for type I arrhythmias was much higher than the success rate for types II and III. With multivariate analysis, no clinical factors—including age, antiarrhythmic drug therapy, left atrial diameter, and LV function—showed a significant correlation with ATP success.

An added benefit of incorporating atrial ATP therapy and atrial preventive algorithms in an ICD is that AF may increase the risks of spontaneous ventricular tachycardia (VT) or ventricular fibrillation (VF) in ICD patients. Retrospective analysis has shown that 8.6% of all VT/VF episodes were initiated or preceded by an episode of AT or AF ("dual tachycardia"), and this was present in 20.3% of 537 ICD patients (54). AT/AF was successfully terminated during ventricular therapy (ATP or shock) for VT/VF in 40% of the dual tachycardia episodes. The median interdetection interval for the subsequent VT/VF was 108 hr when AT/AF was successfully terminated, compared to 15 min if AT/AF persisted after ventricular therapy ($p < 0.001$). This finding suggests that successful AF termination with ATP may delay the onset of spontaneous VT or VF.

IV. CONVENTIONAL PACING IN AF PATIENTS

AF is a common clinical manifestation of sick sinus syndrome (SSS), and patients with SSS often require pacing for conventional bradycardia indication. Earlier uncontrolled studies found that VVI pacing was deleterious to ventricular function and was associated with higher incidence of AF (55–58). It has been suggested that ventricular pacing may promote AF by atrial stretching from transient high atrial pressure as a result of asynchronous atrial contraction from retrograde VA conduction during VVI pacing. The choice of pacing modality in patients with SSS is important if the incidence of AF is to be minimized; this clinical issue has been the subject of several recently published prospective randomized clinical trials.

Andersen et al. were the first to establish the effectiveness of atrial pacing over ventricular pacing in reducing AF incidence in SSS patients. They randomized 225 patients with SSS to either single-chamber atrial or single-chamber ventricular pacing (59). A significant reduction in thromboembolic events was reported in patients randomized to atrial pacing (6 patients in atrial group vs. 20 patients in ventricular group, $p = 0.008$) during the initial mean follow-up of 3.3 years. Patients randomized to atrial pacing had a lower incidence of AF compared to those on ventricular pacing (13.6 vs. 23.5%, $p = 0.12$). The beneficial effect of AF reduction was seen only after 2 years of randomization and persisted with longer follow-up (23.6 vs. 34.8%, $p = 0.012$). Furthermore, improved survival was demonstrated in the atrial pacing group when follow-up was extended to 8 years (RR 0.66, $p = 0.045$) (60). A more modest effect on AF incidence was reported in a larger study involving 407 patients, the Pacemaker Selection in the Elderly (PASE) trial (61). All patients received DDD pacemakers and then were randomly programmed to VVIR or DDDR. There was no difference in the overall AF incidence between the VVIR and DDDR mode (19 vs. 17%, $p = 0.80$) after a mean follow-up of 1.5 years, although a higher AF incidence was observed in the subgroup of SSS patients randomized to single-chamber ventricular pacing (28 vs. 19%, $p = 0.06$). No difference in AF incidence was found in the subgroup of patients with AV block. The lack of statistical difference in overall AF incidence may be attributed to high crossover rates from VVIR to DDDR pacing (26%) due to pacemaker syndrome.

In order to minimize the high crossover rates observed in PASE, whereby all patients in that trial received dual-chamber pacemakers and were randomized to either single-programming or dual-chamber programming, the Canadian Trial of Physiologic Pacing (CTOPP) study randomized patients to either physiological (dual-chamber) pacemakers or ventricular-based (single-chamber) pacemakers (62). This was the first large-scale multicenter prospective randomized trial that compared the effects of physiological pacing and ventricular pacing modes on overall cardiovascular death and stroke. A total of 2569 patients were enrolled in the study; after a mean follow-up of 3.5 years, patients randomized to physiological pacing were found to have a lower incidence of AF (annual rate of 5.3 vs. 6.6%, $p = 0.05$). There was no significant difference in the primary outcome of stroke or cardiovascular death (4.9 vs. 5.5%, $p = 0.33$) between the two pacing modes. Failure to demonstrate a significantly lower AF incidence with physiological pacing may be attributed to the fact that less than half of the patients in the study had sinus-node dysfunction. In another report, the investigators reported a relative reduction of 27% for progression to chronic AF with physiological pacing, from 3.8% to 2.8% per year, $p = 0.0016$ (63).

To avoid the confounding variable of AV conduction disease on the outcome of AF and pacing, the MOST (Mode Selection Trial in Sinus-Node Dysfunction) trial enrolled only SSS patients. A total of 2010 patients with SSS were randomized to ventricular or dual-chamber pacing (64). The effect of pacing mode on AF incidence was almost immediate and obvious within the first 12 months of follow-up. Overall AF incidence was lowered with dual-chamber pacing (HR 0.79, $p = 0.008$), and fewer patients progressed to chronic AF with dual-chamber pacing (15.2 vs. 26.7%, $p < 0.001$). Patients with no prior history of AF receiving dual-chamber pacemakers had a lower incidence of AF after randomization, compared to those on ventricular pacing (HR 0.50, $p = 0.001$). A smaller reduction in AF incidence was observed in the dual-chamber group if they had prior history of AF (HR 0.86, $p = 0.12$). Patients receiving dual-chamber pacing also reported small but measurable improvements in quality of life over the study period. However, this trial showed no difference in outcome with respect to hospitalization for heart failure, death, or nonfatal stroke (primary endpoints) between dual-chamber and ventricular pacing.

None of the large prospective multicenter pacemaker trials have shown the dramatic benefit of reduced AF incidence as well as lowered stroke rate and mortality initially reported by Andersen et al. (59,60). A possible explanation for this observation is that the majority of patients in the Andersen study underwent atrial pacing (e.g., receiving AAI pacemakers), while patients in the large multicenter clinical trials received dual-chamber pacemakers. Continuous right ventricular pacing with resulting left bundle-branch-block morphology and asynchronous ventricular activation is increasingly being recognized as arrhythmogenic. This effect may have blunted the benefits of atrial pacing. In addition, there was an increased utilization of warfarin anticoagulation in the more recent large multicenter trials than in the Andersen study.

Sweeney et al. (65b) retrospectively analyzed the adverse effects of ventricular pacing on atrial fibrillation among patients with a normal baseline QRS duration who participated in the MOST trial (Mode Selection Trial). This was a prospective randomized trial of DDDR pacing compared to VVIR pacing, with a 6-year follow-up. The risk of AF increased linearly with the cumulative percentage of ventricular pacing for both the DDDR and VVIR groups. The risk of AF increased by 1% for each 1% increase in percent ventricular pacing, up to 85% in DDDR patients; it increased by 0.7% for each 1% increase in cumulative percent ventricular pacing up to 80% for VVIR pacing. Increased risk of AF associated with increased ventricular pacing persisted even when statistical models were adjusted for known baseline variables predictive of the risk of developing AF. Nonetheless, all these studies do suggest that atrial-based pacing is the preferred mode for prevention of AF in patients with SSS. By programming a longer AV delay to ensure intrinsic AV conduction, the incidence of AF may be even further lowered in this patient population.

A. AV Junctional Ablation

In some AF patients, achieving adequate rate control is difficult despite maximal doses of AV nodal blocking agents. The strategy of AV junctional ablation and pacing (or "ablate and pace") may be appropriate in this circumstance. This strategy has been shown to result in significant improvements in symptoms and quality of life compared to medical therapy, especially in patients with chronic AF and heart failure (65). Furthermore, several studies have noted significant improvement in functional class, exercise tolerance, and ejection fraction following AV junctional ablation and pacing (66). In patients with paroxysmal AF, dual-chamber pacemakers with mode-switching capability are implanted in an effort to maintain AV synchrony during sinus rhythm following ablation. Automatic mode switching prevents rapid ventricular tracking when patients develop AF and have AV block. The device can be reprogrammed to VVIR when AF becomes persistent or chronic. There has been concern about an increased mortality from polymorphic VT directly related to the ablation procedure. Programming a higher baseline pacing rate for the first 2 months after AV junctional ablation can minimize this complication (67). The ablate-and-pace strategy may gain wider acceptance now, as result from the AFFIRM trial did not show any mortality benefit for the rhythm-control over the rate-control arm in patients with a recent onset of AF (68). The outcome of patients undergoing ablate-and-pace therapy may improve further with pacing from alternative sites, such as the right ventricular (RV) outflow tract, the RV septum, the His bundle, and the left ventricle. Furthermore, long-term follow-up has shown this strategy to be cost-effective, particularly in symptomatic drug-refractory patients (69).

B. Newer Pacing and Therapeutic Algorithms

The irregularity of ventricular depolarization during AF has been associated with poorer cardiac performance and increased activation of the sympathetic nervous system. Ventricular rate-stabilization algorithms have been developed by various device manufacturers to regularize the R–R interval during AF in attempts to improve patient symptoms. This can be achieved by increasing the ventricular pacing rate during AF without a significant increase in mean paced heart rate, and these algorithms have been shown to suppress the R–R intervals at shorter cycle lengths and to regularize the rate. For example, the ventricular response pacing (VRP algorithm, Medtronic) alters the pacing rate by increasing it by 1 to 2 bpm after a sensed ventricular event and decreasing it by 0 to 1 bpm after a paced ventricular event (Fig. 8). The algorithm was tested in a patient group with paroxysmal AF and another group with persistent AF. The algorithm reduced the percentage of fast beats during AF, with a significant increase in the percent of ventricular pacing without affecting the mean heart rate. The impact on patient symptoms and quality of life was small, and only patients with persistent AF had an improved AF-related symptom questionnaire. These algorithms may be particularly useful for patients with biventricular pacemakers and chronic AF, as they result in a significant increase in ventricular pacing. A similar impact on rate stability was demonstrated in a group of patients with chronic AF and intact AV-nodal conduction by pacing at a faster base rate (70).

While the stand-alone atrial defibrillator has been shown to be effective, its role in AF management is still limited. Initial concerns about the potential for atrial shocks to induce ventricular fibrillation appear to have been unfounded. When shocks are delivered with appropriate R-wave synchronization and avoidance of shock delivery following a short R–R interval, the result appears to be absence of proarrhythmia. The current limitations to the more widespread utilization of these devices has been the discomfort associated with low-energy shocks and the failure to achieve a lower AF threshold

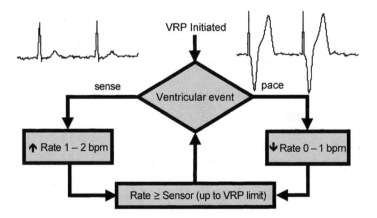

Figure 8 Schematic diagram of Medtronic rate-stabilization algorithm.

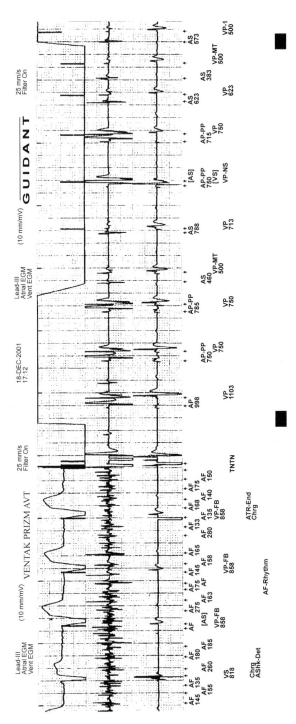
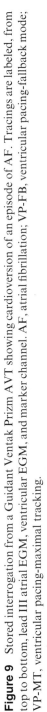

Figure 9 Stored interrogation from a Guidant Ventak Prizm AVT showing cardioversion of an episode of AF. Tracings are labeled, from top to bottom, lead III atrial EGM, ventricular EGM, and marker channel. AF, atrial fibrillation; VP-FB, ventricular pacing-fallback mode; VP-MT, ventricular pacing-maximal tracking.

with present waveforms and lead designs. The necessity for sedation prior to shock delivery makes the easy applicability of shock therapy difficult. Additionally, many patients, over time, develop more problems with immediate or early recurrence of AF following the delivery of shock therapy.

On the other hand, delivery of synchronized shock therapy for AF termination has been incorporated into the newer ICDs (Fig. 9). This therapy feature can be programmed to deliver shocks controlled by the patient or after a set length of time. The backup ICD therapy for ventricular fibrillation obviates the safety concerns of stand-alone atrial defibrillators. With these newer devices, most patients receive standard atrial leads, so that atrial DFTs tend to be much higher than in patients who received atrial defibrillators that include atrial coils to lower the atrial DFT. In clinical trials, cardioversion efficacy was 90%. Additional studies will have to be performed to determine its unique role in management of AF and its acceptance among ICD patients with atrial arrhythmias.

V. CONCLUSION

There are more therapeutic options now available for AF, particularly for patients with recurrent symptomatic AF episodes. The studies on the role of device therapy for AF have been promising thus far but have yet to achieve any of the goals of AF management with respect to primary therapy. Based on large, randomized clinical trials, patients with SSS should receive atrial-based pacing devices. Moderate-size randomized studies have shown minimal benefit of multisite pacing in AF prevention, even when combined with antiarrhythmic agents. However, alternative-site pacing, such as septal pacing (high or low), may be more advantageous, as it achieves similar results in terms of AF reduction and with less hardware. The role of ATP in AF prevention is still in its infancy and will need further studies to determine its role in conjunction with antiarrhythmic agents. Furthermore, the role of radiofrequency ablation of pulmonary veins and other sites of AF initiation has been evolving and may be offered to more patients in the future. This approach may be more acceptable to patients and may gain wider acceptance than device therapy for some groups of AF patients. In any event, there is still a large role for pacemaker therapy in the management of AF, especially in patients who cannot benefit from "curative" ablation or surgery procedures or those who have failed these procedures, particularly elderly patients who typically do not undergo them. In addition, there is an even larger base of patients who require pacing therapy for a multiplicity of standard indications and who may develop AF at a future date. Having a device implanted with preventive algorithms would provide the clinician and the patient with another therapeutic modality should this be needed at a future date. Based on our current understanding, careful selection of pacing sites and pacing algorithms may help in further reducing AF episodes in patients receiving devices.

While device therapy may be effective in stabilizing the atrium in many patients, at the present time it remains adjunctive therapy for paroxysmal AF. It constitutes one component of a hybrid approach involving pharmacological agents, devices, and ablation procedures. Further therapies may evolve over time as our understanding of AF on the basic cellular level continues to grow.

REFERENCES

1. Pritchett ELC, McCarthy EA, Wilkinson WE. Propafenone treatment of symptomatic paroxysmal supraventricular arrhythmias: a randomized, placebo-controlled, crossover trial in patients tolerating oral therapy. Ann Intern Med 1991; 114:539–544.
2. Roy D, Talajic M, Dorian P, Connolly S, Eisenberg MJ, et al. Amiodarone to prevent recurrence of atrial fibrillation. Canadian Trial of Atrial Fibrillation Investigators. N Engl J Med 2000; 342:913–920.
3. Jalife J, Berenfeld O, Skanes A, Mandapati R. Mechanisms of atrial fibrillation: Mother's rotors or multiple daughter wavelets or both? J Cardiovasc Electrophysiol 1998; 9:S2–S12.
4. Capucci A, Santarelli A, Boriani G, Magnani B. Atrial premature beats coupling interval determines lone paroxysmal atrial fibrillation onset. Int J Cardiol 1992; 36:87–93.
5. Bennett MA, Pentecost BL. The pattern of onset and spontaneous cessation of atrial fibrillation in man. Circulation 1970; 41:981–988.
6. Garrigue S, Barold SS, Cazequ S, et al. Prevention of atrial arrhythmias during DDD pacing by atrial overdrive. PACE 1998; 21:250–255.
7. Levy T, Walker S, Rex S, Paul V. Does atrial overdrive pacing prevent paroxysmal atrial fibrillation in paced patients? Int J Cardiol 2000; 75:91–97.
8. Gillis AM, Wyse G, Connolly SJ, Dubuc M, Philippon F, Yee R, et al. Atrial pacing periablation for prevention of paroxysmal atrial fibrillation. Circulation 1999; 99:2553–2558.
9. Gillis AM, Connoly SJ, Lacombe P, Philippon F, Dubuc M, et al., for the Atrial Pacing Peri-Ablation for Paroxysmal Atrial Fibrillation (PA³) Study Investigators. Randomized crossover comparison of DDDR versus VDD pacing after atrioventricular junction ablation for prevention of atrial fibrillation. Circulation 2000; 102:736–741.
10. Funck RC, Adamec R, Lurje L, Capucci A, Ritter P, Shekan D, et al. Atrial overdriving is beneficial in patients with atrial arrhythmias. First results of the PROVE study. PACE 2000; 23:1891–1893.
11. Lam CTF, Lau CP, Leung SK, Tse HF, Lee KLF, Tang MO, et al. Efficacy

and tolerability of continuous overdrive atrial pacing in atrial fibrillation. Europace 2000; 2:286–291.

12. Carlson MD, Ip J, Messenger J, Beau S, Kalbfleisch S, et al. A new pacemaker algorithm for the treatment of atrial fibrillation: results of the Atrial Dynamic Overdrive Pacing Trial (ADOPT). J Am Coll Cardiol 2003; 20:627–633.

13. Han J, Millet D, Chizzonitti B, Moe GK. Temporal dispersion of recovery of excitability in atrium and ventricle as a function of heart rate. Am Heart J 1966; 71:481–487.

14. Murgatroyd FD, Nitzsche R, Slade AK, Limousin M, Rosset N, Camm AJ, et al. A new pacing algorithm for overdrive suppression of atrial fibrillation. PACE 1994; 17:1966–1973.

15. Lee MA, Weachter R, Pollak S, Kremers MS, Naik AM, et al., for the ATTEST Investigators. The effect of atrial pacing therapies on atrial tachyarrhythmia burden and frequency. J Am Coll Cardiol 2003; 41:1926–1932.

16. Mansourati J, Bernay C, Marcon JL, deRoy L, Hidden-Lucet F, et al. Assessment of pacing algorithms in prevention of atrial fibrillation [abstr]. J Am Coll Cardiol 2002; 39:84A.

17. Israel CW, Gronefeld G, Ehrlich JR, Li YG, Hohnloser SH. Impact of a dedicated pacing algorithm for prevention of early relapses of atrial tachy-arrhythmias after successful atrial antiachycardia pacing [abstr]. Circulation 2001; 104:II-345.

18. Israel CW, Groenefeld G, Ehrlich J, Li YG, Hohnloser SH. Prevention of immediate reinitiation of atrial tachyarrhythmias by high-rate atrial overdrive pacing: results from a prospective randomized cross-over trial [abstr]. Circulation 2002; 106:II-624.

19. Adler S, Ziegler P, Koehler J, Holbrook R, Hettrick DA. Post mode switch overdrive pacing algorithm reduces atrial tachyarrhythmia recurrence in patients with bradycardia and atrial tachyarrhythmias [abstr]. Circulation 2001; 104:II-624.

20. Daubert C, Mabo PH, Berder V, Gras D, Leclerq C. Atrial tachyarrhythmias associated with high degree interatrial conduction block: prevention by permanent atrial, resynchronisation. Eur J Cardiac Pacing Electrophysiol 1994; 1:35–44.

21. Bayes de Luna A, Cladellas M, Oter R, et al. Interatrial conduction block and retrograde activation of the left atrium and paroxysmal supraventricular tachyarrhythmia. Eur Heart J 1988; 9:1112–1118.

22. Liu L, Nattel S. Differing sympathetic and vagal effects on atrial fibrillation in dogs: role of refractoriness heterogeneity. Am J Physiol 1997; 273:H805–H816.

23. Misier AR, Opthof T, van Hemel NM, et al. Increased "dispersion" of refractoriness in patients with idiopathic atrial fibrillation. J Am Coll Cardiol 1992; 19:1531–1535.

24. D'Allonnes GR, Pavin D, Leclercq C, Ecke JE, Jauvert G, Mabo P, et al. Long-term effects of biatrial synchronous pacing to prevent drug-refractory atrial tachyarrhythmia: a nine-year experience. J Cardiovasc Electrophysiol 2000; 11:1081–1091.

25. Daubert C, LeClerq C, Le Bretonm H, Gras D, Pavin D, et al. Permanent left atrial pacing with a specifically designed coronary sinus lead. PACE 1997; 20:2755–2764.

26. Saksena S, Prakash A, Hill M, Krol RB, Munsif AN, Mathew PP, et al. Prevention of recurrent atrial fibrillation with chronic dual-site right atrial pacing. J Am Coll Cardiol 1996; 28(3):687–694.

27. Delfault P, Saksena S, Prakash A, Krol RB. Long-term outcome of patients with drug-refractory atrial flutter and fibrillation after single- and dual-site right atrial pacing for arrhythmia prevention. J Am Coll Cardiol 1998; 32:1900–1908.

28. Saksena S, Prakash A, Ziegler P, Hummel JD, Friedman P, Plumb VJ, et al., for the DAPPAF Investigators. Improved suppression of recurrent atrial fibrillation with dual-site right atrial pacing and antiarrhythmic drug therapy. J Am Coll Cardiol 2002; 40:1140–1150.

29. Leclercq JF, De Sisti A, Fiorello P, Halimi F, Manot S, et al. Is dual site better than single site atrial pacing in the prevention of atrial fibrillation? PACE 2000; 23(12):2101–2107.

30. Lau CP, Tse HF, Yu CM, Teo WS, Kam R, Ng KS, et al. Dual-site atrial pacing for atrial fibrillation in patients without bradycardia. Am J Cardiol 2001; 88:371–375.

31. Mirza I, James S, Holt P. Biatrial pacing for paroxysmal atrial fibrillation. A randomized prospective study into the suppression of paroxysmal atrial fibrillation using biatrial pacing. J Am Coll Cardiol 2002; 40:457–463.

32. Levy T, Walker S, Rex S, Rochelle J, Paul V. No incremental benefit of multisite atrial pacing compared with right atrial pacing in patients with drug refractory paroxysmal atrial fibrillation. Heart 2001; 85:48–52.

33. Creswell LL, Scheuessler RB, Rosenbloom M, Cox JL. Hazards of postoperative atrial arrhythmias. Ann Thorac Surg 1993; 56:539–549.

34. Almassi GH, Schowalter T, Nicolosi AC, Aggarwal A, Moritz TE, Henderson WG, et al. Atrial fibrillation after cardiac surgery: a major morbid event? Ann Surg 1997; 276:300–306.

35. Gomes JA, Ip J, Santoni-Rigui R, Mehta D, Ergin A, Lansman S, et al. Oral D,L sotalol reduces the incidence of postoperative atrial fibrillation in coronary artery bypass surgery patients: a randomized, double-blinded, placebo-controlled study. J Am Coll Cardiol 1999; 34:334–339.

36. Daoud EG, Strickberger SA, Man KC, Goyal R, Deeb GM, Bolling SF, et al. Preoperative amiodarone as prophylaxis against atrial fibrillation after heart surgery. N Engl J Med 1997; 337:1785–1791.

37. Dauod EG, Dabir R, Archambeau M, Morady F, Strickberger SA. Randomized, double-blind trial of simultaneous right and left atrial epicardial pacing for prevention of post-open heart surgery atrial fibrillation. Circulation 2000; 102:761–765.

38. Crystal E, Connolly SJ, Sleik K, Ginger TJ, Yusuf S. Interventions on prevention of postoperative atrial fibrillation in patients undergoing heart surgery. A meta-analysis. Circulation 2002; 106:75–80.

39. Blommaert D, Gonzalez M, Mucumbitsi J, Gurne O, Evrard P, et al. Effective prevention of atrial fibrillation by continuous atrial overdrive pacing after coronary artery bypass surgery. J Am Coll Cardiol 2000; 35:1411–1415.

40. Fan K, Lee KL, Chiu CSW, Lee JWT, He GW, et al. Effects of biatrial pacing in prevention of postoperative atrial fibrillation after coronary artery bypass surgery. Circulation 2000; 102:761–765.

41. Bailin SJ, Adler S, Giudici M. Prevention of chronic atrial fibrillation by pacing in the region of Bachmann's bundle: results of a multicenter randomized trial. J Cardiovasc Electrophysiol 2001; 12:912–917.

42. Gozolits S, Fischer G, Berger T, Hanser F, Abou-Harb M, et al. Global P wave duration on the 65-lead ECG: single-site and dual-site pacing in the structurally normal human atrium. J Cardiovasc Electrophysiol 2002; 13:1240–1245.

43. Duytschaever M, Danse P, Eysbouts S, Allesie M. Is there an optimal pacing site to prevent atrial fibrillation? An experimental study in the chronically instrumented goat. J Cardiovasc Electrophysiol 2002; 13:1264–1271.

44. Chauvin M, Shah DC, Haissaguerre M, Marcellin L, Brechenmacher C. The anatomic basis of connections between the coronary sinus musculature and the left atrium in humans. Circulation 2000; 101:647–652.

45. Padeletti L, Pieragnoli P, Ciapetti C, Colella A, Musilli N, Porciani MC, et al. Randomized crossover comparison of right atrial appendage pacing versus interatrial septum pacing for prevention of paroxysmal atrial fibrillation in patients with sinus bradycardia. Am Heart J 2001; 142:1047–1055.

46. De Voogt WG, De Vusser P, Lau CP, van den Bos A, Koistenen J, et al. OASES trial: Overdrive Atrial SEptum Stimulation in patients with paroxysmal atrial fibrillation and class I and 2 pacemaker indication, Late Breaking Clinical Trials, NASPE, May 17, 2003.

47. De Voogt WG, Van den Bos A, De Vusser P, Monti A, Sinikka YM, et al. Dynamic atrial overdrive pacing from the atrial septum reduces AF burden further [abstr]. PACE 2003; 25:714.

48. Everett TE, Akar JG, Kok LC, Moorman JR, Haines DE. Use of global atrial fibrillation organization to optimize the success of burst pace termination. J Am Coll Cardiol 2002; 40(10):1831.

49. Friedman PA, Dijkman B, Warman EN, Xia A, Mehra R, Stanton MS, et al., for the Worldwide Jewel AF Investigators. Atrial therapies reduce atrial arrhythmia burden in defibrillator patients. Circulation 2001; 104:1023–1028.

50. Adler SW, Wolpert C, Warman EN, Musley SK, Koehler JL, Euler DE, for the Worldwide Jewel AF Investigators. Efficacy of pacing therapies for treating atrial tachyarrhythmias in patients with ventricular arrhythmias receiving a dual-chamber implantable cardioverter defibrillator. Circulation 2001; 104:887–892.

51. Schmitt C, Ndrepepa G, Weyerbrock S, Kolb C, Zrener B. Pseudotermination of intermittent atrial fibrillation by a pacemaker algorithm: antitachycardia pacing without capture miscounted as successful termination of fibrillation episodes. PACE 2001; 24:1824–1826.

52. Giorgberidzae I, Saksena S, Mongeon L, et al. Effects of high frequency atrial pacing in atypical atrial flutter and atrial fibrillation. J Intervent Card Electrophysiol 1997; 1:111–123.

53. Paladino W, Bahu M, Knight BP, et al. Failure of single and multi-site high-frequency atrial pacing to terminate atrial fibrillation. Am J Cardiol 1997; 80:226–227.

54. Stein KS, Euler DE, Mehra R, Seidhl K, Slotwiner DJ, et al., for the Jewel AF Worldwide Investigators. Do atrial tachyarrhythmias beget ventricular tachyarrhythmias in defibrillator recipients? J Am Coll Cardiol 2002; 40:335–340.

55. Rosenqvist M, Brandt J, Schüller HI. Long-term pacing in sinus node disease: effects of stimulation mode on cardiovascular morbidity and mortality. Am Heart J 1988; 116:16–22.

56. Santini M, Alexidou G, Ansalone G, Cacciatore G, Cini R, Turitto G. Relation of prognosis in sick sinus syndrome to age, conduction defects and modes of permanent cardiac pacing. Am J Cardiol 1990; 65:729–735.

57. Hesselson AB, Parsonnet V, Bernstein AD, Bonavita GJ. Deleterious effects of long-term single-chamber ventricular pacing in patients with sick sinus syndrome: the hidden benefits of dual-chamber pacing. J Am Coll Cardiol 1992; 19:1542–1549.

58. Sgarbossa EB, Pinske SL, Maloney JD, Simmons TW, Wilkoff BL, Castle LW, et al. Chronic atrial fibrillation and stroke in paced patients with sick sinus syndrome: relevance of clinical characteristics and pacing modalities. Circulation 1993; 88:1045–1053.

59. Andersen HR, Thuesen L, Bagger JP, Vesterlund T, Thomsen PE. Prospective randomized trial of atrial versus ventricular pacing in sick-sinus syndrome. Lancet 1994; 344:1523–1528.

60. Andersen HR, Nielsen JC, Thomsen PEB, Theusen L, Mortensen PT, Vesterlund T, et al. Long-term follow-up of patients from a randomized trial of atrial versus ventricular pacing for sick sinus syndrome. Lancet 1997; 350:1210–1216.

61. Lamas GA, Orav J, Stambler BS, Ellenbogen KA, Sgarbossa EB, Huang SKS, et al., for the Pacemaker Selection in the Elderly Investigators. Quality of life and clinical outcomes in elderly patients treated with ventricular pacing as compared with dual-chamber pacing. N Engl J Med 1998; 338:1097–1104.

62. Conolly SJ, Kerr CR, Gent M, Roberts RS, Yusuf S, Gillis AM, et al. Effects of physiologic pacing versus ventricular pacing on the risk of stroke and death due to cardiovascular events. Canadian Trial of Physiologic Pacing Investigators. N Engl J Med 2000; 342:1385–1391.

63. Skanes AC, Krahn AD, Yee R, Klein GJ, Connolly SJ, Kerr CR, et al., for the CTOPP Investigators. Progression to chronic atrial fibrillation after pacing: the Canadian Trial of Physiologic Pacing. J Am Coll Cardiol 2001; 38:167–172.

64. Lamas GA, Lee KL, Sweeney MO, Silverman R, Leon A, Yee R, et al., for the Mode Selection Trial in Sinus-Node Dysfunction. Ventricular pacing of dual-chamber pacing for sinus-node dysfunction. N Engl J Med 2002; 346:1854–1862.

65. Brignole M, Menozzi C, Gianfranchi L, Musso G, Mureddu R, Bottoni N, et al. Assessment of atrioventricular junction ablation and VVIR pacemaker versus pharmacological treatment in patients with heart failure and chronic atrial fibrillation: a randomized, controlled study. Circulation 1998; 98:953–960.

65b. Sweeney MO, Hellkamp AS, Ellenbogen KA, Greenspon AJ, McAnulty J, Freedman R, Lee KL, Lamas GA. Adverse effect of ventricular pacing on heart failure and atrial fibrillation among patients with normal baseline QRS duration in a clinical trial of pacemaker therapy for sinus node dysfunction. Circulation 2003; 107:2932–2937.

66. Wood MA, Brown-Mahoney C, Kay GN, Ellenbogen KA. Clinical outcomes after ablation and pacing therapy for atrial fibrillation. A meta-analysis. Circulation 2000; 101:1138–1144.

67. Geelen P, Brugada J, Andries E, Brugada P. Ventricular fibrillation and sudden death after radiofrequency catheter ablation of the atrioventricular junction. Pacing Clin Electrophysiol 1997; 20:343–348.

68. Wyse DG, Waldo AL, DiMarco JP, Domanski MJ, Rosenberg Y, Schron EB, et al.—The Atrial Fibrillation Follow-up Investigation of Rhythm Management (AFFIRM) Investigators. A comparison of rate control and rhythm control in patients with atrial fibrillation. N Engl J Med 2002; 347:1825–1833.

69. Jensen S, Bergfeldt L, Rosenqvist M. Long-term follow-up of patients treated by radiofrequency ablation of the atrioventricular junction. PACE 1995; 18:1614–1690.

70. Chudzik M, Wranica JK, Ruta J, Lenszewski P, et al. Rate stabilization in pacemaker patients with atrial fibrillation, influence of the ventricular pacing [abstr]. Europace 2001; 2:A95.

12
Catheter Ablation of Atrial Fibrillation

Shih-An Chen and Ching-Tai Tai
National Yang-Ming University and Taipei Veterans General Hospital, Taipei, Taiwan

I. INTRODUCTION

Atrial fibrillation (AF) contributes substantially to cardiac morbidity and mortality and is associated with an increased risk of cerebral and systemic thromboembolic events (1–3). Furthermore, AF becomes increasingly frequent with age, rising above 5% in people above age 65 (1–3). Although there is no consensus regarding the optimal treatment strategy for AF, approaches to maintaining sinus rhythm and preventing its recurrence are evolving with growing knowledge of AF mechanisms. Recently, several important studies have clearly demonstrated that the underlying mechanism of AF depends on the interplay between several factors that are categorized into substrates and triggering events (4–6).

Most paroxysmal AF is initiated by ectopic beats from a focal area that is amenable to a cure by radiofrequency catheter ablation. Persistent AF is usually maintained by an atrial substrate that accommodates multiple reentrant wavelets. Although focal triggers of AF may be found in the superior vena cava, crista terminalis, coronary sinus, vein of Marshall, interatrial septum, or left atrial posterior wall, most ectopic foci are located within the pulmonary veins (7–14). Catheter ablation of pulmonary vein and non–pulmonary vein ectopy and modification of atrial substrate is thus becoming an emerging curative therapy for AF, and this technology is still in evolution. This chapter discusses the role of pulmonary vein and non–pulmonary vein ectopy and the atrial substrate in the occurrence of AF; it also highlights current perspectives on catheter ablation for AF.

II. PULMONARY VEIN ECTOPY IN ATRIAL
FIBRILLATION (AF)

A.   Arrhythmogenic Mechanisms

How could be the pulmonary veins be arrhythmogenic? The arrhythmogenic nature of these myocardial sleeves may in part be due to their embryonic origin from the sinus venosus segment, which gives rise to the conduction system; thus this system may be subject to abnormal automaticity (15). Cheung has shown spontaneous electrical activity (pacemaker activity) in isolated pulmonary veins of the guinea pig (16). This laboratory has recently demonstrated the spontaneous depolarization of normal canine pulmonary vein (PV) cardiomyocytes and enhanced automaticity and afterdepolarizations in dogs after chronic rapid atrial pacing for 6 to 8 weeks (17,18). The Natale group further demonstrated that there are specialized conduction cells in PV tissues, and this finding suggests that PV cells have the potential for automatic depolarization (19). However, other investigators, using detailed mapping systems in experimental models, have demonstrated the important role of microreentry in PV arrhythmogenesis (20,21).

The question arises as to why PV ectopic activity becomes predominant in the genesis of AF. AF is usually associated with underlying cardiovascular diseases, such as hypertension and coronary artery disease. This stereotyped PV arrhythmogenicity may be related to left heart hemodynamics, because PV flow reflects left heart function, and the PVs are subjected to stretch from pulsatile blood flow (22). Furthermore, many investigators have demonstrated dilatation of the PV ostia in patients with paroxysmal AF (23–27). These observations suggest a role of hemodynamic factors and stretch mechanisms in the occurrence of PV ectopy, possibly followed by sustained microreentry inside PVs.

B.   Clinical Background

Intraoperative mapping studies have postulated that the left atrium acts as an electrical driving chamber for AF, showing a general tendency for reentrant circuits or ectopic beats to be present in the left atrial posterior wall (28,29). Further support was given to this theory by the successful abolition of AF in the left atrial procedure using a circumferential incision around the four PV ostia to compartmentalize the left atrium (29). However, convincing evidence that the PVs play a crucial role in the genesis of AF comes from recent clinical studies (7,8,10,11). Haissaguerre's group first studied the mechanism of spontaneous onset of AF and recognized the PVs as the triggers initiating paroxysmal AF (7,8). Focal triggers, identified as rapidly firing ectopic foci in and around the PVs, elicit a short burst of focal discharges, initiating an AF

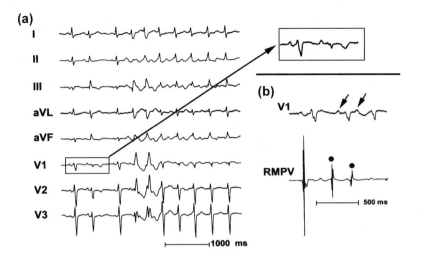

Figure 1   Panel a. The arrow in lead V1 shows a premature beat with positive P-wave polarity (biphasic P wave with negative polarity during sinus rhythm), followed by a short run of fast atrial beats with similar P-wave morphology. Panel b. The first beat was a sinus beat; the second and third beats were ectopic beats from the right superior pulmonary vein (RSPV), with a sharp and discrete PV spike potential (arrows and dots) preceding the positive P wave in V1. (From Ref. 99.)

episode that subsequently continues independently. Ablation targeting the initiating foci could eliminate PV extrasystoles, repetitive bursts of vein activity, as well as AF ("focally initiated" AF). This laboratory has also demonstrated that beta-receptor blockers, calcium channel blockers, and sodium channel blockers can suppress spontaneous ectopic beats and AF arising from the PVs (10). Moreover, several studies have demonstrated slow and/or rapid PV activation during AF or after isolation of PVs from atria, thereby suggesting PV activity may also have a role in maintaining (not just initiating) AF (7,30–34). These critical findings shed light on the important interplay between atrial substrate and PV triggers in AF pathophysiology (Fig. 1).

III. PV ABLATION

A. Focal Ablation of PVs

In the first stage of PV ablation, radiofrequency energy is delivered directly to the identified triggering foci within the PV to eliminate AF. The PV ectopy initiating an AF paroxysm is characterized by a PV potential (high-frequency spikes) preceding the left atrial potential and propagating in a distal-to-proximal PV activation sequence, then exiting from the venous ostium to the left atrium (Fig. 1). However, to precisely localize the focal trigger usually requires provocative maneuvers to facilitate the spontaneous onset of ectopic beats and AF, pulmonary angiography to explore PV anatomy, simultaneous multielectrode catheter mapping to search for the earliest ectopy initiating AF, and careful and accurate interpretation of ectopic trigger electrograms (i.e., differentiation between far-field potential and true PV potential) (35–39).

Initial attempts to focally ablate the initiating triggers were associated with good acute success rates, but a considerable number of patients required multiple procedures. At follow-up beyond 6 months, AF recurrence rates were high in spite of significant improvements in quality of life and symptoms related to AF, even in cases with recurrence (8,10,40,41). Furthermore, focal ablation within the PVs is associated with a risk of pulmonary vein stenosis (42). Thus, the limitations with focal ablation techniques have included the following: (1) inconsistent inducibility of AF; (2) a paucity of spontaneous or inducible AF episods during the procedure or no consistent firing; (3) difficult mapping if the patient were in persistent or frequently recurrent AF; (4) misinterpretation of ectopic trigger electrograms; (5) multiple triggering foci from multiple veins; (6) new foci, including latent foci in the same PV emerging at late follow-up; and (7) a high risk of PV stenosis (42). Therefore the ablation strategy has shifted to electrical isolation of pulmonary venous tissue from the left atrium itself.

B. Electrical Isolation of PVs

1. Segmental Ablation to Isolate the PVs

At the venoatrial junction, the extension of left atrial myocardium into the PVs does not cover the entire ostial circumference (43–45). Thus, electrophysiologically defined sites of preferential inputs to the PVs enable electrical disconnection to be achieved at the ostia without circumferential ablation in the majority of cases (33,34). Segmental ablation procedures can be facilitated by a specially designed multipolar circular catheter (Spiral-SC, Daig, Minnesotta, MN; or Lasso, Cordis, Sunnyvale, CA) that fits within the ostium to record the ostial PV potentials in a perimetric fashion and thus identify the earliest activation sites (the breakthrough sites from left atrium to PVs) in sinus rhythm, or during pacing of the coronary sinus, high interatrial septum, or left atrial appendage (39,46). PV potentials are usually recorded over a broad area proximally, but with greater variability. Ablation endpoints include entrance block, shown by total elimination of ostial PV vein potentials; and also exit block from PV to left atrium (if pacing inside the PVs is possible) (Figs. 2 to 4).

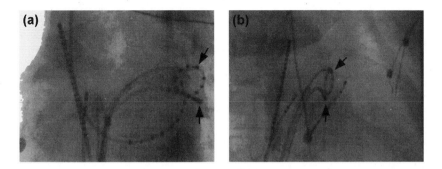

Figure 2   The upper arrowhead shows the circular catheter (spiral-SC) located in the ostium of left superior pulmonary vein; the lower arrowhead shows the ablation catheter close to the pulmonary venous ostium. Panels a and b were left and right oblique views, respectively.

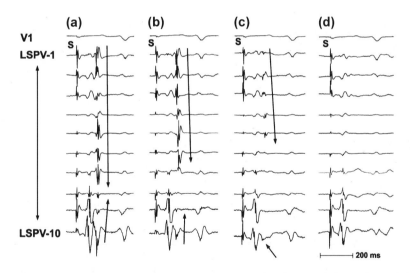

Figure 3   Panel a. One circular catheter was placed around the ostium of the left superior pulmonary vein (LSPV). The recordings showed breakthrough sites from the left atrium (LA) to the PV (during coronary sinus pacing) were on LSPV-1 and -10 (bottom side of LSPV). The activation wavefronts spread upward from LSPV-1 and -10, along both sides of the LSPV ostium, and collide on LSPV-7 and -8. Panel b. After the first application of radiofrequency (RF) energy on LSPV-10, PV potentials on LSPV-7 to -9 disappeared. Panel c. Further application of RF energy on LSPV-1 eliminated PV potential on LSPV-6. Panel d. Additional application of RF energy on LSPV-1 completely eliminated PV potentials on LSPV-1 to -5 and -10. (From Ref. 100.)

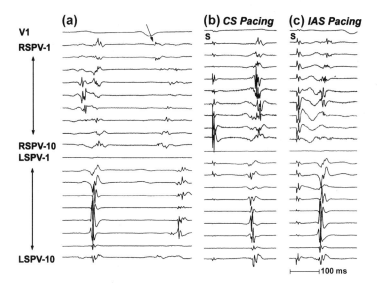

Figure 4 Simultaneous recording of electrical activity around the right superior pulmonary vein (RSPV) and left superior pulmonary vein (LSPV) by two circular catheters. During sinus rhythm and pacing from the high interatrial septum (IAS), the left atrium (LA)-to-RSPV breakthrough sites were around RSPV-4, -5, and -6 (roof of RSPV); the LA-LSPV breakthrough sites were not clear (Panels a and c). However, breakthrough sites were more concentrated on RSPV-4, -5, -7, -8, and -9 during pacing from the coronary sinus (CS) (Panel b). During ectopic beats from RSPV-1, earliest exit sites were on RSPV-1 and -9 (bottom of RSPV), and the latest exit site was on RSPV-4 (panel a).

Haissaguerre et al. ablated the ostial breakthrough sites of the identified arrhythmogenic PV using the segmental isolation technique, with an acute success rate higher than 90%; but almost half the patients had early recurrences and required repeated ablation procedures (33). Oral et al. performed segmental isolation of the left and right superior and left inferior PVs without documented arrhythmogenicity in all the PVs and only 9% of patients needed a second procedure (34). Recovery of ostial PV potentials due to a residual myocardial fascicle seemed to be a major cause in these cases; therefore careful mapping of the venous perimeter searching for a continuum between atrial-PV potential electrograms is important (47). Elimination of the ostial PV potentials also correlates better with clinical success than the acute suppression of ectopy and AF, possibly owing to isolating all potential foci in the same PV trunk (48). Additionally, the segmental ablation technique has some advantages compared to focal ablation, such as lower recurrence rate, lower incidence of ablation-induced PV stenosis, and shorter mapping and procedure times. However, variability of the PV anatomy may at times render the proper alignment of the circular catheter within the PV difficult (49,50). Also of note, there is still a high recurrence rate (nearly 30%) after the segmental ablation procedure in patients with paroxysmal AF as well as a higher recurrence rate (more than 50%) in chronic AF, which might be due to unmasked foci from the ostial edge proximal to the ablation line or atrial tissue in non-PV areas. Recently, the Natale Group used an intracardiac echo-guided technique to adjust the location of the circular catheter and monitor the microbubble during ablation. They demonstrated a lower recurrence rate compared to previous experience (51) (Table 1).

2. Circumferential Ablation

An alternative approach to isolate the PV from the left atrium is application of circumferential lesions at the venoatrial junction or atrial tissue surrounding the PVs to create a complete conduction barrier. Two techniques have been used in this strategy. One technique is the delivery of contiguous, multiple spot lesions of radiofrequency energy in a circumferential fashion outside the PV ostia, facilitated and assessed by a three-dimensional electroanatomical

Table 1 Results of Mapping-Guided Catheter Ablation for AF

	Taipei (JCE/Cir 2003)	Philadelphia (JCE 2003)	Cleveland (Cir 2003)	Milan (Cir 2003)	Bordeaux (Textbook 2004)
No. of patients	240	107	152	43	188
AF type	PAF	PAF	PAF + CAF	PAF + CAF	PAF + CAF
SHD	Yes	Yes	Yes	Yes	Yes
Targets	Non-PV/PV RA isthmus	Non-PV/PV RA isthmus	4 PV	Non-PV/PV (multiple procedures)	Non-PV/4 PV RA isthmus LA isthmus
Guidance	Fluoro	ICE, Carto	ICE	Fluoro	Fluoro
Mean follow-up	2 years	1 year	10 months	9 months	6 months
AF recurrence	34%	31%	9%	5%	18%
PV stenosis	0 (by S/S)	0 (by S/S)	0 (by S/S)	0 (by S/S)	0 (by S/S)
Major complication	1.5%	0	0	2%	3%
Mortality	0	0	0	0	0
Reference nos.	14	47, 48	51	94	87

Key: CAF, chronic atrial fibrillation; Carto, electroanatomic mapping by 3D mapping system; Fluoro, fluoroscopy; ICE, intracardiac echocardiography; MRI, magnetic resonance imaging; PAF, paroxysmal atrial fibrillation; PV, pulmonary vein; RA, right atrium; SHD, structural heart disease; S/S, symptoms/signs of significant pulmonary hypertension.

Table 2   Results of Anatomy-Guided Catheter Ablation for AF

	Milan (JACC 2003)	Maddaloni (Cir 2003)	Michigan (Cir 2004)
No. of patients	589	41	40
AF type	PAF + CAF	PAF + CAF	PAF
Structural HD	Yes	Yes	Yes
Target	LA around PV-O LA isthmus	LA around PV-O	LA around PV-O LA isthmus, posterior line
Guidance	Carto	Carto	Carto
Mean follow-up	29 months	6 months	6 months
AF recurrence	20%	20%	12%
PV stenosis	0 (by S/S)	0 (by S/S)	0 (by S/S)
Major complication	1%	5%	0
Mortality	0	0	0
Reference no.	54	93	88

Key: Carto, electroanatomic mapping by 3D mapping system; PV-O, pulmonary vein ostium; S/S, symptoms/signs of significant pulmonary hypertension.

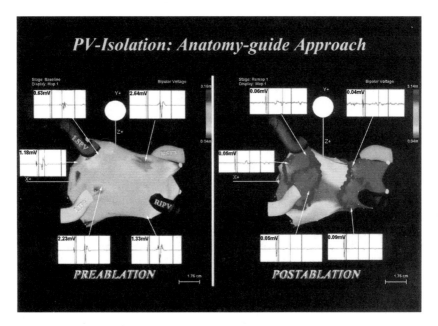

Figure 5   Circumferential ablation of left atrial tissue surrounding the four PV ostia. The electrical voltage inside the ablation line decreased significantly after ablation (Modified from Ref. 54.)

mapping system (CARTO, Biosense Webster) (52–54). Pappone et al. have reported that more than 80% of patients were free of AF without antiarrhythmic drugs after application of the circumferential lesions on atrial tissue around the four PVs. They further proposed that, in addition to PV isolation, electroanatomical remodeling of the area encompassing the PV ostia and a local denervation effect might contribute to the efficacy of the circumferential PV isolation procedure (52–54) (Table 2). The other technique used a balloon-based catheter, with an ultrasound transducer mounted near the tip in a saline-filled balloon, to create a circumferential lesion at the PV ostia (55). These studies were performed with anatomical guidance to empirically isolate three to four PVs without the need for mapping spontaneous or induced arrhythmias. However, Natale et al., using the ultrasound balloon to isolate PVs from atria, showed that only 60% of patients were free of AF without drugs at 9 months follow-up (55). Thus, inconsistent data may be derived when different ablation devices and techniques are used (Fig. 5).

IV. NON-PV ECTOPY IN AF

A. Arrhythmogenic Mechanisms

Embryological studies have demonstrated that the sinoatrial node is derived from the sinus venosus and that other remnants of the embryonic sinus venosus are present in several areas of the mammalian heart, including the musculature of the superior vena cava, coronary sinus, venous valve, and an area embedded in the proximal sulcus terminalis (56).

1. Superior Vena Cava

The proximal superior vena cava contains cardiac muscles connected to the right atrium, and atrial excitation or sinus node impulse can propagate into the superior vena cava (57–59). Superior vena cava cardiomyocytes were found to have pacemaker activity; their enhanced automaticity and after-depolarizations play a role in the arrhythmogenic potential of the superior vena cava (60). Further, this laboratory found a thin layer of myocardial tissue with more fibrotic and fatty tissue in the dorsal surface of the canine superior vena cava (61). The clinical study also showed a thin layer of myocardial tissue in the dorsal surface of the superior vena cava (15).

2. Ligament of Marshall

In 1850, Marshall first described the ligamentous fold, a vestigial tissue encompassing portions of the embryonic sinus venosus and left cardinal vein, running between the superior and inferior left PVs (62). In 1972, Scherlag et al. demonstrated electrical activity within Marshall's ligament in dogs. The two terminal ends of this atrial tract were found to have insertions into the left atrial musculature and coronary sinus (63). Doshi et al. have reported that Marshall's ligament has focal automatic activity induced by isoproterenol, and that it may contribute to the development of AF (64).

3. Coronary Sinus

In 1907, Erlanger and Blackman described a "high degree of rhythmicity" in the area near the rabbit's coronary sinus orifice (65). Coronary sinus fibers have automatic activity, therefore the sinus can be triggered into sustained, rapid rhythmic activity in the presence of norepinephrine (66).

4. Crista Terminalis

Hogan et al. found a type of specialized fiber in the canine right atrium (67). This so-called atrial plateau fiber is found consistently along the border of the crista terminalis, with inherent slow diastolic depolarization that can be enhanced by cathecholamines to the point of spontaneous discharge; it is responsible for the development of atrial ectopic foci (68).

5. Left Atrial Free Wall

Two types of sustained rhythmic activity in human atrial fibers from normal and diseased hearts have been described (69–71). One rhythm is automatic and depends on slow diastolic depolarization during phase 4; the other rhythm is triggered by delayed afterdepolarizations and occurs either spontaneously or after epinephrine superfusion (69). The myocardial cells of diseased atria are significantly hypopolarized as compared to those of normal atria (70,71). Thus, it is possible that the left atrial posterior free wall could be the site of spontaneous ectopy.

B. Clinical Background

Our laboratory first proposed the important concept of non-PV ectopy from different areas initiating paroxysmal AF (PAF) (9,13–15). Thereafter, several investigators demonstrated non-PV ectopy-initiating AF, with the incidence varying from 3.2 to 47% (7,8,10,72–74). At the present time, most PV ablation procedures are performed by isolating all PVs. Thus recurrent AF should be considered from non-PV foci if all four pulmonary veins are successfully isolated. Lin et al. demonstrated that PAF can be initiated by ectopic beats (about 28% of AF foci) originating from the non-PV areas, and the application of radiofrequency energy in the non-PV areas was effective and safe in treating PAF (15). However, less than 10% of the 240 patients had a single focus from the non-PV areas. In an earlier study, Haissaguerre et al. reported that 8.9% of patients had AF from non-PV areas, including 6.7% from the right atrium and 2.2% from the left atrial free wall (8). However, the same group reported a high (79%) incidence of non-PV foci initiating AF after PV disconnection in 160 patients with AF; these non-PV areas included the adjacent posterior wall around the PV ostium, left atrial tissue away from PV ostia, right atrium, coronary sinus, superior vena cava, and several foci (19%) that could not be localized (74). Natale et al. also reported that 18 (37.5%) of 48 chronic AF patients had right-sided foci, most of which were located near the sinus node region along the superior and midportions of the crista terminalis (72). Schmitt used biatrial mapping techniques to localize AF initiators and found that 47% of the ectopic foci were in non-PV vein areas (73). Therefore, based on these reports and the present study, non-PV ectopy is important in AF initiation.

V. NON-PV ABLATION

Our laboratory has demonstrated that the use of endocardial atrial activation sequences from the high right atrium, His bundle, and coronary sinus catheters can predict the location of AF-initiating foci (35). With the difference in the time interval between high right atrial and His bundle atrial activation obtained during sinus beats and atrial premature beats <0 msec, the accuracy for discriminating the superior vena cava and crista terminalis from PV ectopy is 100% (35). The Marchlinski and Stevenson groups have used a similar concept to define the localization of non-PV ectopy (36,37).

True activation potentials and the far-field potentials can appear in the same multipolar catheter, and the true origin of ectopy can be differentiated clearly when two multipolar catheters are simultaneously placed in the superior vena cava and right superior PV (14,15). To localize the site of ectopy and the mechanism of superior vena caval AF, three-dimensional mapping systems or a basket catheter is needed (75–77). Further, isolation of superior vena caval ectopy from atria guided by a three-dimensional mapping system or a basket catheter would be superior for focal suppression of ectopy inside the superior vena cava.

Because Marshall's ligament may have multiple insertion sites in the left atrial posterior free wall or near the PV ostium, it is difficult to differentiate Marshall's ligament ectopy from PV or left atrial posterior free wall ectopy. This laboratory has demonstrated that distal coronary sinus pacing can help differentiate Marshall's ligament potentials from PV potentials. The possibility of Marshall's ligament ectopy should be considered when so-called triple potentials are recorded around the PV ostium (13). However, the best method for differentiating Marshall's ligament ectopy from other ectopy is recording the continuous activation of Marshall's ligament from the multipolar microcatheter in Marshall's vein (12). We found a low success rate in curing Marshall's ligament ectopy initiating AF in long-term follow-up, because we did not routinely cannulate Marshall's vein and ablation sites were limited to the endocardial area (15). Hwang et al. recorded Marshall's ligament potentials from Marshall's vein to guide ablation sites, and Karitis et al. used a combined endocardial and epicardial approach to ablate Marshall's ligament ectopy initiating AF. The results showed that about 60 to 70% of patients were free of AF (78,79). Huang and Chen have sequentially delivered radiofrequency energy encircling the left superior and inferior pulmonary vein ostia and did not directly target the Marshall ligament ectopy. They were able to cure a higher proportion of patients with Marshall ligament ectopy initiating AF (80).

Although our study results demonstrated that application of radio-frequency energy in the non-PV areas may be feasible, the long-term success rate was higher in the right atrium, including superior vena cava and crista terminalis. The left atrial posterior free wall group, however, had a higher recurrence rate due to anatomical limitations and multiple ectopic foci (15). There are three possible reasons for these findings. First, electrophysiologists are more sophisticated in manipulating electrode catheters in the right than in the left atrium. Second the right atrial structures are easier to identify accurately in the right than the left atrium. Third, right-sided non-PV ectopy has a higher incidence of true focal AF (the ectopy is the driver of AF) and a lower incidence of substrate problems. Thus elimination of this ectopy is more effective in curing AF. However, the true incidence of AF recurrence is uncertain because the occurrence of AF was paroxysmal, and it is difficult to detect asymptomatic AF. Furthermore we did not routinely perform electrophysiological study in all the patients with recurrent AF. Thus we could not determine whether the recurrent AF originated from non-PV or PV foci. It is preferable to map non-PV ectopy before ablation or to try to provoke non-PV AF after isolating PVs from the left atrium (Figs. 6–10).

VI. CATHETER ABLATION OF ATRIAL SUBSTRATE

Most recently, the concept of eliminating the trigger was extended and applied to patients with established, persistent AF. Researchers employing circumferential or segmental ostial ablation for isolating PVs have reported that 20 to 60% of patients were free of chronic AF without antiarrhythmic drugs at more than 1 year of follow-up (81,82). PVs seem to play a less crucial role in

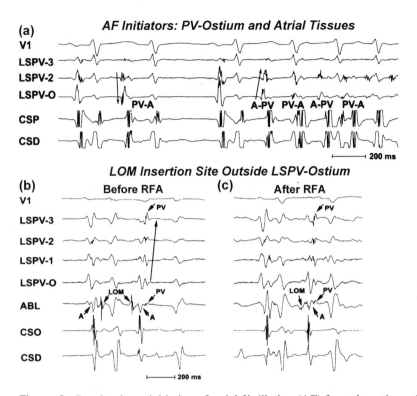

Figure 6 Panel a shows initiation of atrial fibrillation (AF) from the ostium of the pulmonary vein (PV) and left atrial posterior free wall. The first beat is a sinus beat, the second beat is a premature beat originating from LSPV-2 with conduction to the atrial tissue. The third beat is a sinus beat, and the fourth beat is an atrial premature beat originating from atrial tissue (A), with conduction to the PV. Alternating activation from the PV ostium and atrial wall was also noted. Ectopic beats from other PVs were excluded because the mapping catheters were positioned in the other three PVs for comparison with atrial ectopy. Panel b shows an ectopic beat originating from the ligament of Marshall (LOM). The LOM potential can be found in the ablation catheter, and the ablation catheter is outside the LSPV-O. Typical triple potentials (LOM-A-PV) were noted. Panel c shows diminished LOM potentials after radiofrequency ablation (RFA). LOM, ligament of Marshall; LSPV-O, ostium of left superior pulmonary vein; LSPV-1, -2, -3, the first, second, and third pair of electrodes in the LSPV; ABL, ablation catheter; CSO, ostium of coronary sinus; CSD, distal coronary sinus. (From Ref. 14.)

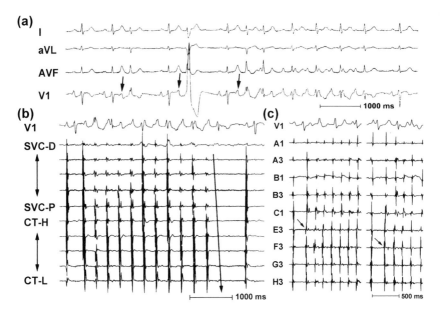

Figure 7 Initiation of AF from the superior vena cava (SVC). Panel a shows bigeminal ectopic beats (arrow) followed by initiation of tachycardia on the surface electrocardiogram (ECG). Panel b shows ectopic foci initiating tachycardia from SVC-D (distal) and conducting to SVC-P (proximal). Panel c shows ectopic beats initiating AF from SVC after isoproterenol infusion (Basket catheter recording inside SVC, with the earliest ectopic beat from E3). (From Ref. 14.)

Figure 8 Basket catheter recording inside the SVC during AF. Panel a. The first beat is a sinus beat, and the second beat is an ectopic beat from SVC-B1, C2, followed by SVC-A2 (arrowheads). Panel b. After termination of SVC-AF, reinitiation of ectopic beats from SVC-B1, C2, and A1 (arrowheads). The coupling intervals of SVC depolarizations in SVC-B1, C2, were significantly shorter than the proximal part (SVC-B4, C4); this means that there was conduction block between the distal and proximal SVC. Furthermore, the distal bipoles of the D spine (D1, D2, and D3) in the posterolateral wall do not show SVC potentials. Panel c shows another case with burst activities from the SVC, and the arrowheads show the earliest ectopic beats changed from A2, A1, and A2 to B2. Panels d and e show AF termination during segmental isolation of the proximal SVC–right atrium area, but concealed discharge from SVC is still present (black spot). A, anterior wall of SVC; D, posterolateral wall of SVC. 1, 2, 3, and 4 are the bipolar recordings from distal-to-proximal SVC. (From Ref. 14.)

AF: Multiple Migrating Foci with Conduction Block within SVC

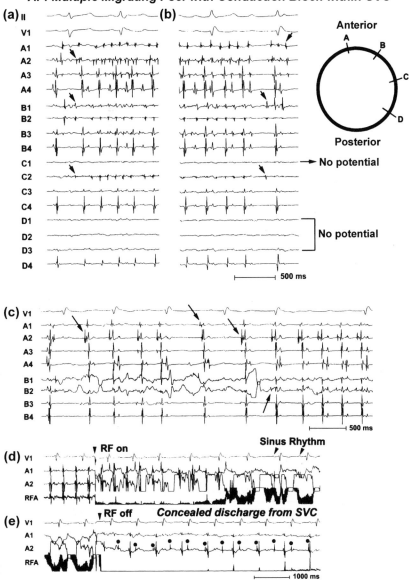

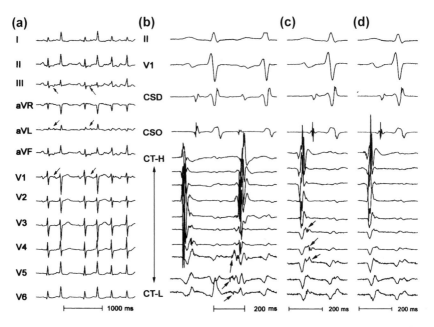

Figure 9 Panel a shows bigeminal ectopic beats (arrow), followed by initiation of AF on the 12-lead ECG. Panel b shows initiation of AF by ectopic beats originating from the low CT. Panel c shows a CT potential before ablation. Panel d shows disappearance of CT potential after ablation. HIS, His bundle; CSM, middle coronary sinus; CT-H, high crista terminalis; CT-L, low crista terminalis. (From Ref. 14.)

generating AF once AF has become persistent. However, data from recent reports of surgical isolation of PVs in patients who had mitral valve disease associated with chronic AF demonstrated that 60 to 85% patients were free of AF at more than 6 months of follow-up (83–86). The more impressive results from surgical ablation reports lend further credence to the concept that the left atrium—in particular the PVs and the area between those structures—is involved in the initiation and/or maintenance of AF. Moreover, surgical isolation of PVs can cure chronic AF, suggesting that AF-induced atrial remodeling may be reversible after elimination of the focal sources or left atrial substrate. Thus adjuvant linear ablation connecting the inferior PV to the mitral annulus or encompassing the periostial atrial tissues may be a necessary component of ablation of chronic AF. Progressive changes in the atrium's susceptibility to fibrillation once ectopy emerges is a possible cause of AF recurrence. Modification of the atrial arrhythmogenic substrate seems to be a part of curative ablation strategies for AF in cases with longer AF duration and larger atria.

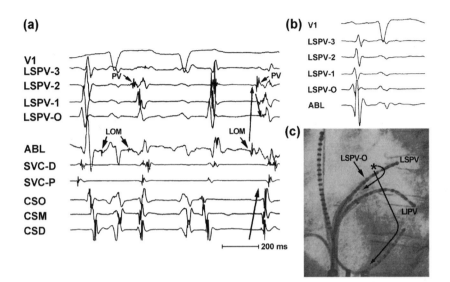

Figure 10   Panel a shows initiation of AF from the LOM. The first beat is a sinus beat, and the LOM potential can be found in the ablation catheter; the second beat is a premature beat from the LOM; the third beat is a premature beat from CSO, and the fourth beat is a premature beat from the LOM. Panel b shows disappearance of the LOM potential after ablation. Panel c shows the location of ablation catheter tip (star) and activation pattern of LOM ectopy (arrow). The LOM connects with the LSPV wall; thus the LOM ectopy conducts to LSPV-2 and to the left atrium through LSPV. LOM ectopy simultaneously conducts to CS because the LOM is connected to the CS. (From Ref. 14.)

The Bordeaux group demonstrated that the results of ablation targeting the mitral isthmus, in addition to PV electrical isolation and cavotricuspid isthmus ablation, represent a significant advance in modification of the substrate for AF, because linear conduction block can be consistently achieved in the left atrium (as with cavotricuspid isthmus ablation) (87). The Bordeaux and Michigan groups have also performed another line of lesions in the posterior wall or roof of the left atrium joining the two superior PVs; this approach with noninducibility of AF as endpoint can be expected to increase the success rate. This maneuver may increase the complications of ablation (cardiac tamponade and stroke), the potential for left atrial flutter, and the loss of left atrial transportation (87,88). Because other investigators showed similar results of catheter ablation for paroxysmal and chonic AF without adding any linear lesions in the left atrium, it is necessary to identify the patients who would truly benefit from the addition of left atrial linear ablation vs. PV electrical isolation and cavotricuspid isthmus ablation alone (51).

VII. SAFETY OF CATHETER ABLATION FOR AF

PV stenosis has emerged as an important issue in patients who undergo radiofrequency (RF) ablation of AF. Several pathophysiological responses—including thrombosis, metaplasia, proliferation, and neovascularization—may lead to PV stenosis after RF energy application around or inside the PV ostia (89). The clinical manifestations of PV stenosis are chest pain, dyspnea, cough, hemoptysis, recurrent lung infection, and pulmonary hypertension.

Although patients with PV stenosis can be asymptomatic, its severity may be related to the numbers of stenosed PVs and the degree and chronicity of PV stenosis (90,91). Follow-up methods and definitions of PV stenosis or narrowing bias the results. Yu et al. used transesophageal echocardiography to assess the effects of RF ablation on PV and found 30 to 40% of the ablated PVs had increased flow velocity (42). The incidence of PV stenosis (defined as a reduction in luminal diameter of >50%) detected by spiral computed tomography or three-dimensional magnetic resonance angiography ranged from 0 to 7% of PVs after isolation of PVs from the left atrium (26,27,90,91). Furthermore, some patients may show late progression of PV stenosis during follow-up (92). The first choice of treatment for symptomatic PV stenosis is PV angioplasty with stenting; however, restenosis is occasionally reported. Several studies have analyzed the predictors of PV stenosis, with conflicting results (90). However, the consensus is that the prevention of PV stenosis should include less energy application and the selection of ablation sites closer to the atrium.

Other major complications include cerebral emboli and cardiac perforation. The issue of anticoagulation therapy before, during, and after the ablation procedure is important but poorly studied. Continuous infusion of heparin through the long sheath is important for preventing any clot formation inside the sheath. Using an irrigated catheter with a lower power and temperature setting may be helpful in decreasing the incidence of emboli. The incidence of cardiac tamponade may be around 1 to 2%; however, it is more likely if more aggressive protocols for left atrial ablation are used. It may be caused by the transseptal puncture, improper catheter manipulation, or atrial perforation caused by application of RF energy. More experience with catheter ablation of AF would be expected to decrease the incidence of major complications. Most recently, atrial-esophageal fistulae have been reported with cases of catastrophic bleeding.

VIII. LIMITATIONS AND CONTROVERSIES

There are some important limitations and controversies regarding the efficacy of current ablation strategies.

First, the definition of "successful" AF ablation is still controversial (93,94). Stabile et al. demonstrated that complete isolation of four PVs is present in approximately 5% of patients without AF recurrence. However, Cappato indicated that complete PV isolation is necessary, since a lower AF recurrence rate was obtained (after two to three repeated procedures) following complete elimination of the connection between the atria and PV, as well as the connection between the atria and non-PV tissue (93,94). Furthermore, recent reports from other centers have shown large variations in the rates of success, recurrence, and complications, in large part because of variation in follow-up methods and periods of observation (14,47,48,51,54, 88,93–95). Large-scale randomized studies comparing different ablation approaches would be useful.

Second, currently available catheters do not accommodate the varying anatomy of the PV and pulmonary venoatrial junction (27,49,95,96). For example, most PV ostia have an oval, not a round shape; thus the circular catheter-guided ablation and balloon-isolation techniques do not fit the PVs (49). Technological improvements, including better imaging or navigation systems, and catheters and devices suitable for more delicate mapping and effective ablation may improve the results of AF ablation.

Third, energy other than standard RF may be more feasible for PV ablation (97,98). More knowledge concerning the histopathological consequences of different energy sources is necessary. Several investigators have demonstrated high efficacy and low complication rates using saline-irrigated catheters (with or without a monitoring microbubble during ablation); however, this issue is still controversial (51,87). The development of new catheter and/or different energy sources allowing creation of more demarcated circumferential lesions in left atrial tissue around PV ostia, with less energy application, will further improve the feasibility and safety of this approach.

IX. CONCLUSION

The observation that rapid focal firing of atrial myocytes within the thoracic veins and atria initiates paroxysmal AF has led to an entirely new AF ablation strategy. That is, the paradigm for AF ablation has changed dramatically from modifying the atrial substrate to eliminating the focal triggers that initiate AF. However, ablation of AF triggers as well as modification of atrial substrate may be necessary in patients with long-lasting AF or those with a significant atrial substrate problem. Due to the complex architecture of thoracic veins in relationship to the atrium and the potential risk and complexity of catheter ablation, the best candidates for AF ablation currently are symptomatic patients with frequent AF episodes that are drug-refractory. It is anticipated that continued technological improvements will facilitate the AF-curative ablation techniques and broaden the indications for ablation of AF.

ACKNOWLEDGMENTS

This chapter is supported by the following grants: NSC-92-2314-B-010-052, NSC-92-2314-B-075-117, VGH 92-238, VTY 91-P5-44, and VTY 92-P5-29.

REFERENCES

1. Feinberg WM, Blackshear JL, Laupacis A, et al. Prevalence, age distribution, and gender of patients with atrial fibrillation: analysis and implications. Arch Intern Med 1995; 155:469–473.
2. Benjamin EJ, Wolf PA, D'Agostino RB, et al. Impact of atrial fibrillation on the risk of death: the Framingham Heart Study. Circulation 1998; 98:946–952.
3. Hart RG, Halperin JL. Atrial fibrillation and stroke: concepts and controversies. Stroke 2001; 32:803–808.
4. Allessie MA, Boyden PA, Camm AJ, et al. Pathophysiology and prevention of atrial fibrillation. Circulation 2001; 103:769–777.
5. Nattel S. New ideas about atrial fibrillation 50 years on. Nature 2002; 415:219–226.
6. Peters NS, Schilling RJ, Kanagaratnam P, et al. Atrial fibrillation: strategies to control, combat, and cure. Lancet 2002; 359:593–603.
7. Jais P, Haissaguerre M, Shah DC, et al. A focal source of atrial fibrillation treated by discrete radiofrequency ablation. Circulation 1997; 95:572–576.
8. Haissaguerre M, Jais P, Shah DC, et al. Spontaneous initiation of atrial fibrillation by ectopic beats originating in the pulmonary veins. N Engl J Med 1998; 339:659–666.
9. Chen SA, Tai CT, Yu WC, et al. Right atrial focal atrial fibrillation: Electrophysiologic characteristics and radiofrequency catheter ablation. J Cardiovasc Electrophysiol 1999; 10:328–335.
10. Chen SA, Hsieh MH, Tai CT, et al. Initiation of atrial fibrillation by ectopic beats originating from the pulmonary veins: electrophysiologic characteristics, pharmacologic response, and effects of radiofrequency ablation. Circulation 1999; 100:1879–1886.
11. Hwang C, Karagueuzian HS, Chen PS. Idiopathic paroxysmal atrial fibrillation induced by a focal discharge mechanism in the left superior pulmonary vein: possible roles of the ligament of Marshall. J Cardiovasc Electrophysiol 1999; 10:636–648.
12. Tai CT, Hsieh MH, Tsai CF, et al. Differentiating the ligament of Marshall from the pulmonary vein musculature potentials in patients with paroxysmal atrial

fibrillation: electrophysiological characteristics and results of radiofrequency ablation. Pacing Clin Electrophysiol 2000; 23:1493–1501.

13. Tsai CF, Tai CT, Hsieh MH, et al. Initiation of atrial fibrillation by ectopic beats originating from the superior vena cava: electrophysiological characteristics and results of radiofrequency ablation. Circulation 2000; 102:67–74.

14. Lin WS, Tai CT, Hsieh MH, et al. Catheter ablation of paroxysmal atrial fibrillation initiated by non-pulmonary vein ectopy. Circulation 2003; 107:3176–3183.

15. Blom NA, Gittaenberger-de Groot AC, DeRuiter MC, et al. Development of the cardiac conduction tissue in human embryos using HNK-1 antigen expression: possible relevant for understanding of abnormal atrial automaticity. Circulation 1999; 99:800–806.

16. Cheung DW. Pulmonary vein as an ectopic focus in digitalis-induced arrhythmia. Nature 1981; 294:582–584.

17. Chen YJ, Chen SA, Chang MS, et al. Arrhythmogenic activity of cardiac muscle in pulmonary veins of the dog: implication for the genesis of atrial fibrillation. Cardiovasc Res 2000; 48:265–273.

18. Chen YJ, Chen SA, Chen YC, et al. Effects of rapid atrial pacing on the arrhythmogenic activity of single cardiomyocytes from pulmonary veins: implication in initiation of atrial fibrillation. Circulation 2001; 104:2849–2854.

19. Perez-Lugones A, McMahon JT, Ratliff NB, et al. Evidence of specialized conduction cells in human pulmonary veins of patients with atrial fibrillation. J Cardiovasc Electrophysiol 2003; 14:803–809.

20. Hocini M, Ho SY, Kawara T, et al. Electrical conduction in canine pulmonary veins: electrophysiological and anatomic correlation. Circulation 2002; 105:2442–2448.

21. Arora R, Verheule S, Scott L, et al. Arrhythmogenic substrate of the pulmonary veins assessed by high-resolution optical mapping. Circulation 2003; 107:1816–1821.

22. Jais P, Peng JT, Shah DC, et al. Left ventricular diastolic dysfunction in patients with so-called lone atrial fibrillation. J Cardiovasc Electrophysiol 2000; 11:623–625.

23. Lin WS, Prakash VS, Tai CT, et al. Pulmonary vein morphology in patients with paroxysmal atrial fibrillation initiated by ectopic beats originating from the pulmonary veins: implications for catheter ablation. Circulation 2000; 101:1274–1281.

24. Ho SY, Cabrera JA, Tran VH, et al. Architecture of the pulmonary veins: relevance to radiofrequency ablation. Heart 2001; 86:265–270.

25. Yamane T, Shah DC, Jais P, et al. Dilatation as a maker of pulmonary veins initiating atrial fibrillation. J Intervent Cardiovasc Electrophysiol 2002; 6:245–249.

26. Dill T, Neumann T, Ekinci O, et al. Pulmonary vein diameter reduction after radiofrequency catheter ablation for paroxysmal atrial fibrillation evaluated by contrast-enhanced three-dimensional magnetic resonance imaging. Circulation 2003; 107:845–850.

27. Kato R, Lickfett L, Meininger G, et al. Pulmonary vein anatomy in patients undergoing catheter ablation of atrial fibrillation: lessons learned by use of magnetic resonance imaging. Circulation 2003; 107:2004–2010.

28. Harada A, Sasaki K, Fukushima T, et al. Atrial activation during chronic atrial fibrillation in patients with isolated mitral valve disease. Ann Thorac Surg 1996; 61:104–111.

29. Sueda T, Nagata H, Shikata H, et al. Simple left atrial procedure for chronic atrial fibrillation associated with mitral valve disease. Ann Thorac Surg 1996; 62:1780–1796.

30. Kumagai K, Yasuda T, Tojo H, et al. Role of rapid focal activation in the maintenance of atrial fibrillation originating from the pulmonary veins. Pacing Clin Electrophysiol 2000; 23(11 Pt 2):1823–1827.

31. Haissaguerre M, Shah DC, Jais P, et al. Electrophysiological breakthroughs from the left atrium to the pulmonary veins. Circulation 2000; 102:2463–2465.

32. Oral H, Knight BP, Tada H, et al. Pulmonary vein isolation for paroxysmal and persistent atrial fibrillation. Circulation 2002; 105:1077–1081.

33. Willems S, Weiss C, Risius T, et al. Dissociated activity and pulmonary vein fibrillation following functional disconnectin: impact for the arrhythmogenesis of focal atrial fibrillation. Pacing Clin Electrophysiol 2003; 26:1363–1370.

34. Yoshihide T, Yoshito I, Atsushi T, et al. Reentrant tachycardia in pulmonary veins of patients with paroxysmal atrial fibrillation. J Cardiovasc Electrophysiol 2003; 14:927–932.

35. Lee SH, Tai CT, Lin WS, et al. Predicting the arrhythmogenic foci of atrial fibrillation before atrial transseptal procedure: implication for catheter ablation. J Cardiovasc Electrophysiol 2000; 11:750–757.

36. Soejima K, Stevenson WG, Delacretaz E, et al. Identification of left atrial origin of ectopic tachycardia during right atrial mapping: analysis of double potentials at the postermedial right atrium. J Cardiovasc Electrophysiol 2000; 11:975–980.

37. Ashar MS, Pennington J, Callans DJ, et al. Localization of arrhythmogenic triggers of atrial fibrillation. J Cardiovasc Electrophysiol 2000; 11:1300–1305.

38. Hsieh MH, Tai CT, Tsai CF, et al. Pulmonary vein electrogram characteristics in patients with focal sources of paroxysmal atrial fibrillation. J Cardiovasc Electrophysiol 2000; 11:953–959.

39. Shah DC, Haissaguerre M, Jais P, et al. Left atrial appendage activity masquerading as pulmonary vein potentials. Circulation 2002; 105:2821–2825.

40. Gerstenfeld EP, Guerra P, Sparks PB, et al. Clinical outcome after radiofrequency catheter ablation of focal atrial fibrillation triggers. J Cardiovasc Electrophysiol 2001; 12:900–908.

41. Sanders P, Morton JB, Deen VR, et al. Immediate and long-term results of radiofrequency ablation of pulmonary vein ectopy for cure of paroxysmal atrial fibrillation using a focal approach. Intern Med J 2002; 32:202–207.

42. Yu WC, Hsu TL, Tai CT, et al. Acquired pulmonary vein stenosis after radiofrequency catheter ablation of paroxysmal atrial fibrillation. J Cardiovasc Electrophysiol 2001; 12:887–892.

43. Nathan H, Eliakim M. The junction between the left atrium and the pulmonary veins. Circulation 1966; 34:412–422.
44. Saito T, Waki K, Becker AE. Left atrial myocardial extensions onto pulmonary veins in humans: anatomic observations relevant for atrial arrhythmias. J Cardiovasc Electrophysiol 2000; 11:888–894.
45. Ho SY, Sanchez-Quintana D, Cabrera JA, et al. Anatomy of the left atrium: implications for radiofrequency ablation of atrial fibrillation. J Cardiovasc Electrophysiol 1999; 10:1525–1533.
46. Chen SA, Tai CT, Lin YK, et al. A novel method using differential pacing from four atrial sites to identify breakthroughs from left atrium to pulmonary veins for pulmonary vein isolation. Pacing Clin Electrophysiol 2002; 25:II–637.
47. Gerstenfeld EP, Callans DJ, Dixit S, et al. Incidence and location of focal atrial fibrillation triggers in patients undergoing repeat pulmonary vein isolation: implications for ablation strategies. J Cardiovasc Electrophysiol 2003; 14:685–690.
48. Marchlinski Fe, Callans D, Dixit S, et al. Efficacy and safety of targeted focal ablation versus PV isolation assisted by magnetic electroanatomic mapping. J Cardiovasc Electrophysiol 2003; 14:358–365.
49. Wittkampf FH, Vonken EJ, Derksen R, et al. Pulmonary vein ostium geometry: analysis by magnetic resonance angiography. Circulation 2003; 107:21–23.
50. Mangrum JM, Mounsey JP, Kok LC, et al. Intracardiac echocardiography-guided, anatomically based radiofrequency ablation of focal atrial fibrillation originating from pulmonary veins. J Am Coll Cardiol 2002; 39:1973–1983.
51. Marrouche NF, Martin DO, Wazni O, et al. Phased-array intracardiac echocardiography monitoring during pulmonary vein isolation in patients with atrial fibrillation: impact on outcome and complications. Circulation 2003; 107:2710–2716.
52. Pappone C, Rosanio S, Oreto G, et al. Circumferential radiofrequency ablation of pulmonary vein ostia: a new anatomic approach for curing atrial fibrillation. Circulation 2000; 102:2619–2628.
53. Pappone C, Oreto G, Rosanio S, et al. Atrial electroanatomical remodeling after circumferential radiofrequency pulmonary vein ablation: efficacy of an anatomic approach in a large cohort of patients with atrial fibrillation. Circulation 2001; 104:2539–2544.
54. Pappone C, Rosanio S, Augello G, et al. Mortality, morbidity, and quality of life after circumferential pulmonary vein ablation for atrial fibrillation: outcomes from a controlled nonrandomized long-term study. J Am Coll Cardiol 2003; 42:185–197.
55. Natale A, Pisano E, Shewchik J, et al. First human experience with pulmonary vein isolation using a through-the-balloon circumferential ultrasound ablation system for recurrent atrial fibrillation. Circulation 2000; 102:1879–1882.
56. Keith A, Flack J. Anatomy (Lond) 1907; 41:172–181.
57. Spach MS, Barr RC, Jewett PH. Spread of excitation from the atrium into thoracic veins in human beings and dogs. Am J Cardiol 1972; 30:844–854.
58. Zipes DP, Knope RF. Electrical properties of the thoracic veins. Am J Cardiol 1972; 29:372–376.

59. Hashizume H, Ushiki T, Abe K. A histological study of the cardiac muscle of the human superior and inferior venae cavae. Arch Histol Cytol 1995; 58:457–464.
60. Chen YJ, Chen YC, Yeh HI, et al. Electrophysiology and arrhythmogenic activity of single cardiomyocytes from canine superior vena cava. Circulation 2002; 105:2679–2685.
61. Yeh HI, Lai YJ, Lee SH, et al. Heterogeneity of myocardial sleeve morphology and gap junctions in canine superior vena cava. Circulation 2001; 104:3152–3157.
62. Marshall J. On the development of the great anterior veins in man and mammalia: including an account of certain remnants of fetal structure found in the adult, a comparative view of these great veins in the different mammalia, and an analysis of their occasional peculiarities in the human subject. Phil Trans R Soc Lond 1850; 140:133–169.
63. Scherlag BJ, Yeh BK, Robinson MJ. Inferior interatrial pathway in the dog. Cir Res 1972; 31:18–35.
64. Doshi RN, Wu TJ, Yashima M, et al. Relation between ligament of Marshall and adrenergic atrial tachyarrhythmia. Circulation 1999; 100:876–883.
65. Erlanger J, Blackman JR. A study of relative rhythmicity and conductivity in various regions of the auricles of the mammalian heart. Am J Physiol 1907; 19:125–174.
66. Andrew LW, Paul FC. Triggered and automatic activity in the canine coronary sinus. Circ Res 1977; 41:435–445.
67. Hogan PM, Davis LD. Evidence for specialized fibers in the canine right atrium. Circ Res 1968; 23:387–396.
68. Hogan PM, Davis LD. Electrophysiological characteristics of canine atrial plateau fibers. Cir Res 1971; 28:62–73.
69. Mary-Rabine L, Hordof AJ, Danilo P Jr, et al. Mechanisms for impulse initiation in isolated human atrial fibers. Circ Res 1980; 47:267–277.
70. Gelband H, Bush HL, Rosen MR, et al. Electrophysiologic properties of isolated preparations of human atrial myocardium. Circ Res 1972; 30:293–300.
71. Ten Eick RE, Singer DH. Electrophysiological properties of diseases human atrium. Circ Res 1979; 44:545–557.
72. Natale A, Pisano E, Beheiry S, et al. Ablation of right and left atrial premature beats following cardioversion in patients with chronic atrial fibrillation refractory to antiarrhythmic drugs. Am J Cardiol 2000; 85:1372–1375.
73. Schmitt C, Ndrepepa G, Weber S, et al. Biatrial multisided mapping of atrial premature complexes triggering onset of atrial fibrillation. Am J Cardiol 2002; 89:1381–1387.
74. Shah D, Haissaguerre M, Jais P, Hocini M. Nonpulmonary vein foci: do they exist? Pacing Clin Electrophysiol 2003; 26:1631–1635.
75. Shah DC, Haissaguerre M, Jais P, et al. High-resolution mapping of tachycardia originating from the superior vena cava: evidence of electrical heterogeneity, slow conduction, and possible circus movement reentry. J Cardiovasc Electrophysiol 2002; 13:388–392.
76. Dong J, Schreieck J, Ndrepepa G, et al. Ecopic tachycardia originating from the superior vena cava. J Cardiovasc Electrophysiol 2002; 13:620–624.

77. Liu TY, Tai CT, Lee PC, et al. Novel concept of atrial tachyarrhythmias originating from the superior vena cava: insight from noncontact mapping. J Cardiovasc Electrophysiol 2003; 14:533–539.
78. Hwang C, Wu TL, Doshi RN, et al. Vein of Marshall cannulation for the analysis of electrical activity in patients with focal atrial fibrillation. Circulation 2000; 101:1503–1508.
79. Katritsis D, Ioannidis John PA, Anagnostopoulos CE, et al. Identification and catheter ablation of extracardiac and intracardic components of ligament of Marshall tissue for treatment of paroxysmal atrial fibrillation. J Cardiovasc Electrophysiol 2001; 12:750–758.
80. Hwang C, Chen PS. New insights in the anatomy of ligament of Marshall in patients with atrial fibrillation [abstr]. Pacing Clin Electrophysiol 2003; 26:962.
81. Haissaguerre M, Jais P, Shah DC, et al. Catheter ablation of chronic atrial fibrillation targeting the reinitiating triggers. J Cardiovasc Electrophysiol 2000; 11:2–10.
82. Kanagaratnam L, Tomassoni G, Schweikert R, et al. Empirical pulmonary vein isolation in patients with chronic atrial fibrillation using a three-dimensional nonfluoroscopic mapping system: long-term follow-up. Pacing Clin Electrophysiol 2001; 24:1774–1779.
83. Benussi S, Pappone C, Nascimbene S, et al. A simple way to treat chronic atrial fibrillation during mitral valve surgery: the epicardial radiofrequency approach. Eur J Cardiothorac Surg 2000; 17:524–529.
84. Sueda T, Imai K, Ishii O, et al. Efficacy of pulmonary vein isolation for the elimination of chronic atrial fibrillation in cardiac valvular surgery. Ann Thorac Surg 2001; 71:1189–1193.
85. Kalil RAK, Lima GG, Leiria TL, et al. Simple surgical isolation of pulmonary veins for treating secondary atrial fibrillation in mitral valve disease. Ann Thorac Surg 2002; 73:1169–1173.
86. Tanaka HH, Narisawa TT, Mori TT, et al. Pulmonary vein isolation for chronic atrial fibrillation associated with mitral valve disease: the mid-term results. Ann Thorac Cardiovasc Surg 2002; 8:88–91.
87. Hsu LF, Jaïs P, Sanders P, et al. Catheter ablation of pulmonary vein atrial fibrillation—segmental and limited linear ablation. In: Chen SA, Haissaguerre M, Zipes DP, eds. Thoracic Vein Arrythmias: Mechanisms and Treatment. Elmsford, NY: Blackwell, 2004:248–262.
88. Oral H, Scharf C, Chugh A, et al. Catheter ablation for paroxysmal atrial fibrillation: segmental pulmonary vein ostial ablation vs left atrial ablation. Circulation 2003; 108:2355–2360.
89. Taylor GW, Kay GN, Zheng X, et al. Pathological effects of extensive radiofrequency energy applications in the pulmonary veins in dogs. Circulation 2000; 101:1736–1742.
90. Tsao HM, Chen SA. Evaluation of pulmonary vein stenosis after catheter ablation of atrial fibrillation. Card Electrophysiol Rev 2002; 6:397–400.
91. Saad EB, Marrouche NF, Saad CP, et al. Pulmonary vein stenosis after catheter ablation of atrial fibrillation: emergence of a new clinical syndrome. Ann Intern Med 2003; 138:634–638.
92. Tsao HM, Wu MH, Tai CT, et al. Morphological changes of pulmonary vein

and left atrium after atrial fibrillation ablation: insight from long-term follow-up of magnetic resonance imaging. Heart Rhythm 2004; 1:S242 (abstract).

93. Stabile G, Turco P, Rocca VL, et al. Is pulmonary vein isolation necessary for curing atrial fibrillation? Circulation 2003; 108:657–660.

94. Cappato R, Negroni S, Pecora D, et al. Prospective assessment of late conduction recurrence across radiofrequency lesions producing electrical disconnection at the pulmonary vein ostium in patients with atrial fibrillation. Circulation 2003; 108:1599–1604.

95. Hsieh MH, Tai CT, Tsai CF, et al. Clinical outcome of very late recurrence of atrial fibrillation after catheter ablation of paroxysmal atrial fibrillation. J Cardiovasc Electrophysiol 2003; 14:598–601.

96. Tsao HM, Wu MH, Yu WC, et al. Role of right middle pulmonary vein in patients with paroxysmal atrial fibrillation. J Cardiovasc Electrophysiol 2001; 12:1353–1357.

97. Tanaka K, Satake S, Saito S, et al. A new radiofrequency thermal balloon catheter for pulmonary vein isolation. J Am Coll Cardiol 2001; 38:2079–2086.

98. Fried NM, Tsitlik A, Rent KC, et al. Laser ablation of the pulmonary veins by using a fiberoptic balloon catheter: implications for treatment of paroxysmal atrial fibrillation. Lasers Surg Med 2001; 28:197–203.

99. Brugada J, ed. Atrial fibrillation—a practical approach. 2000:47–48.

100. Cardiology International—Special issue for atrial fibrillation. 2002; Summer issue:43–45.

13
Atrial Fibrillation After Cardiac Surgery

Mina K. Chung
The Cleveland Clinic Foundation, Cleveland, Ohio, U.S.A.

Despite efforts to identify risk factors and establish effective prophylactic agents, postoperative atrial arrhythmias remain a prominent clinical problem. Atrial fibrillation (AF) is the most frequently encountered arrhythmia after cardiac surgery. This chapter addresses the epidemiology, pathogenesis, complications, prevention, and treatment of atrial arrhythmias following cardiac surgery.

I. EPIDEMIOLOGY

Atrial arrhythmias are common to all forms of major surgical procedures, although occurrence rates are greatest after cardiac surgery. Major noncardiac surgery carries a risk of supraventricular arrhythmias on the order of 3 to 4% (1). The requirement of thoracotomy for noncardiac surgical procedures increases the risk to 8 to 24% (2,3). Atrial arrhythmias have been reported to occur in 11.4 to 100% of patients after coronary artery bypass grafting (CABG) (4), with recent studies still reporting incidences of 10 to 65% (4–9) and even higher incidences (37 to 64%) after valvular surgery (5,10).

Most episodes of AF following cardiac surgery occur in the first few days, with a peak incidence on postoperative days 2 to 3 (9). A study of 1666 patients reported 4.7% of supraventricular arrhythmias occurring on the day of surgery, a peak incidence of 43.1% occurring on day 2, and only 0.4% occurring ≥9 days after surgery (7).

II. PATHOGENESIS

The mechanisms underlying nonpostoperative AF are currently believed to include focal sources, particularly arising from the ostia of the pulmonary veins (11), which initiate AF, as well as substrates, such as structural changes or electrical atrial remodeling, which promote sustained AF by supporting reentrant wavelets. The relative contributions of these foci of reentry to postoperative atrial arrhythmias have not been established. However, a case of refractory AF occurring after septal myectomy for hypertrophic obstructive cardiomyopathy reported a right superior pulmonary vein source with resolution after pulmonary vein isolation (12).

Nevertheless, multiple extrinsic and intrinsic factors have been reported that contribute to the development of AF after cardiac surgery. These include surgically induced acute atrial enlargement, hypertension or stretch; atrial ischemia and/or infarction from inadequate atrial protection from cardioplegia during bypass; trauma from cannulation or pulmonary vein venting; electrolyte abnormalities, such as hypomagnesemia; beta-blocker withdrawal; and inflammation.

Intrinsic predisposition to postoperative AF is supported by the identification of preoperative risk factors. Age-related changes in the electrophysiological properties of the atria (13), preoperative prolongation of P-wave duration (14,15) and inducibility of AF prior to cardiopulmonary bypass (16) have been associated with postoperative AF. Older age is the most consistent clinical predictor of postoperative AF (5–7,17,18). Among patients undergoing surgery for aortic stenosis, those over age 40 years had a 67% incidence of postoperative supraventricular arrhythmias, compared with an 18% incidence in patients under age 20 (13). Right atrial tissue from older patients showed diffuse spontaneous phase 4 depolarizations, local conduction disturbances, decreased resting membrane potentials with slower V_{max} of the action potential, and shorter action potential duration. Postoperative AF occurred in 1 of 10 patients undergoing cardiac surgery with normal action potentials in right atrial appendage cells, compared to 8 of 10 patients with abnormal action potentials (19). Abnormalities included depolarized resting membrane potential, a slowed action potential upstroke that could cause slowed conduction, reduced amplitude, and prolonged refractoriness. Postoperative AF has been predicted by the intraoperative inducibility of atrial fibrillation using alternating current applied to the right atrium prior to the initiation of cardiopulmonary bypass (sensitivity 94%, specificity of 41%) (16).

Excessive sympathetic or decreased parasympathetic activity may precede the onset of postoperative atrial fibrillation in some patients. In a study of 36 patients undergoing CABG, reduced heart rate complexity, higher heart rates, and more frequent atrial ectopy were observed prior to the onset of the atrial arrhythmia (20). However, RR interval heart rate variability could be lower or higher prior to onset of arrhythmias, suggesting that heightened sympathetic or vagal activation might promote atrial fibrillation in individual patients. Another study reported that onset of atrial fibrillation after CABG was preceded by an increase in the number of atrial premature complexes as well as an increase in the standard deviation of RR intervals (SDNN) and initial lower then higher low-frequency/high-frequency ratio (21). These findings were consistent with a loss of vagal tone and moderate increase in sympathetic tone prior to the onset of AF. In a study recording monophasic action potentials after surgery, 7 of 9 episodes of AF were preceded by shortening of monophasic action potential duration (22). In the two patients in whom MAP increased, beat-to-beat variability of cycle length increased, suggesting that in some patients, fluctuation in autonomic tone may be contributory. Ratios of $G_{s\ alpha}/G_{i\ alpha}$ mRNA and protein expression have also been reported to increase after CABG in patients who develop AF fibrillation and to decrease in patients without AF, supporting involvement of the adrenergic nervous system (23).

Intraoperative atrial ischemia due to inadequate cold cardioplegic arrest has also been associated with disturbed atrial conduction in animal models. Atrial conduction times have been reported to be significantly prolonged during the first 2 hr after bypass in the canine heart (24). AF that was inducible by extrastimulation was associated with increased dispersion of refractoriness and a prolongation of conduction time. The septum may be particularly prone to inadequate cooling and ischemic injury (25). In a study monitoring atrial activity from the time of administration of cardioplegia until removal of the aortic cross clamp, the mean duration of atrial activity was markedly longer among patients who developed supraventricular tachyarrhythmias than in arrhythmia-free patients (26). An interesting study was performed of heat-shock proteins, which provide protection during ischemia-reperfusion and increase postischemic cardiac functional recovery. Heat-shock proteins were measured prior to cannulation in 101 patients. Low preoperative expression of heat-shock protein was observed in the 22.3% of patients who developed postoperative atrial fibrillation (27). Of these patients, 58.3% had no detectable heat-shock proteins. In contrast, 100% of the patients who did not have postoperative AF had detectable heat shock proteins. These results suggest that the heat-shock proteins may be a measure of myocardial preconditioning that might protect against AF induced by atrial ischemia and reperfusion.

The contribution of inflammatory mechanisms to postoperative atrial arrhythmias is supported by the observation that postoperative AF is most prevalent 2 to 3 days after surgery. Atrial injury from direct ischemia or trauma might be expected to provoke AF earlier in the postoperative period. The time course of the peak incidence of AF correlates with a peaking of C-reactive protein and C-reactive protein–complement complexes (28). Pericardial effusions, likely mediated by inflammation after cardiac surgery, have been correlated with postoperative supraventricular arrhythmias (29). Systemic inflammatory response syndromes and sepsis have also been associated with postoperative AF (30).

Cellular studies have shown that patients with the greatest calcium current (I_{Ca}) have an increased incidence of postoperative AF independent of age (31). No alterations in potassium currents (I_{KI} and $I_{K,ACh}$) were reported in patients in sinus rhythm who subsequently developed postoperative AF (32). Calcium overload may be important in the initiation of postoperative AF, and patients at highest risk may have higher basal I_{Ca}. Gap junction protein connexin-40 mRNA transcript and protein have also been reported to be markedly heterogeneous and significantly higher in patients who subsequently developed AF (33). These changes were postulated to lead to a dispersion in resistive properties and conduction velocities that might promote arrhythmias.

III. CLINICAL RISK FACTORS

A. Preoperative Factors

The most consistent clinical predictor of postoperative AF after CABG is advanced age (5–8,17,18). In a multivariate analysis of 1666 patients, age was the leading correlate of postoperative AF (7). In a review of 5807 CABG patients, the risk of a postoperative supraventricular arrhythmia was 27.7% for patients ≥70 years old, compared to 3.7% for patients <40 years old (6). Advanced age was the strongest independent predictor of postoperative AF or atrial flutter.

Other reported preoperative risk factors for postoperative AF include prior atrial fibrillation (17,34) male gender (8,17), cardiomegaly (35), history of congestive heart failure (17), left atrial enlargement (35,36), SA-nodal and AV-nodal artery disease (37), peripheral vascular diseases (38), and sleep-disordered breathing (39). Right coronary artery stenosis has also been associated with postoperative atrial fibrillation (40–42) although a large study reported no association with 75% stenosis of the right coronary artery (17). Non–cardiac diseases, including chronic obstructive pulmonary disease (5,6) and chronic renal failure (6), have been associated with postoperative AF in some though not all studies (17).

Preoperative use of beta-blockers (5–7) and digoxin (5,7) have been studied, but results have been variable. Beta-blocker withdrawal in the postoperative period has been correlated with with postoperative supraventricular arrhythmias in small prospective studies (43,44). In contrast, a large prospective observational study of 2417 patients undergoing CABG with or without concurrent valvular surgery reported a lower incidence of AF in patients receiving beta-blocking agents in the preoperative period (17).

Electrophysiological parameters, including preoperative P-wave duration (14,45), P-wave signal-averaged electrocardiography (ECG) (15,46–51), and prebypass inducibility of AF using atrial stimulation (16,52) have been reported to predict postoperative AF. However, signal-averaged P-wave duration was not a significant predictor in one study when controlled for age and body weight (53). With only moderate sensitivity and specificity, these methods are not currently in widespread use.

B. Intraoperative Factors

Intraoperative factors that may contribute to the development of AF after cardiac surgery include inadequate atrial myocardial protection with atrial ischemia or infarction, acute atrial enlargement, trauma from cannulation, hypomagnesemia, longer cardiopulmonary bypass and cross-clamp times, pulmonary vein venting, and various types of cardioplegic solution related to ability to quickly cool and arrest the atria (5,17,25,54).

Various surgical approaches have been associated with AF to some degree. A lower incidence of AF has been reported after minimally invasive CABG (55,56) or valvular (57–59) surgery, though not universally. Similarly, the incidence of AF has been reported to be lower after "off-pump" procedures without cardiopulmonary bypass (60–63), but again not consistently (64–69). Studies of bicaval cannulation versus atrial cannulation have produced variable results in the CABG or valve population (17), though bicaval anastomosis appears to reduce atrial arrhythmias after orthotopic heart transplantation (70). Early small studies suggested that the use of internal mammary artery conduits may increase the risk of postoperative AF (71). However, a more recent, larger study reported a lower incidence of AF in patients receiving an internal mammary artery graft (17).

The role of electrolyte imbalances remains controversial, but lower skeletal muscle potassium concentration, higher sodium levels, hypokalemia, and hypomagnesemia have been associated with higher incidences of postoperative AF (48,54,72–74).

C. Postoperative Factors

Circulating endogenous or exogenous catecholamines can be elevated in the postoperative period, though no consistent correlation with postoperative AF has been demonstrated. Serum norepinephrine and epinephrine are elevated in the first 3 postoperative days, but with no correlation to AF and no protection by beta-blocker use following surgery (75). Somewhat surprisingly, no additional risk of supraventricular tachyarrhythmias was reported in a population given intravenous norepinephrine on a routine basis (76).

Withdrawal of beta-adrenergic blockers has been implicated as a possible mechanism predisposing to postoperative atrial arrhythmias (43,44). Beta-blockers are frequently used in the treatment of coronary artery disease and heart failure, but this therapy is frequently held in the immediate postoperative period. Heightened catecholamine sensitivity from a higher density of beta-adrenergic receptors induced by chronic beta-blocker use, along with the increase in perioperative catecholamine levels, may contribute to t he beta-blocker withdrawal syndrome if preoperative beta blockers are not continued in the postoperative period. In one study of a control group that was not treated with postoperative beta blockers, 18 of 39 patients (46%) who received beta blockers preoperatively developed atrial arrhythmias, compared to 2 of 11 patients (18%) who did not receive preoperative beta blockers, although these differences did not reach statistical significance (77).

Postoperative inflammation has been implicated as a risk for postoperative atrial arrhythmias. Studies using clinical criteria—such as pericardial rubs, ECG changes, and pleuritic chest pain—have shown no consistent correlation between postoperative pericarditis and supraventricular arrhythmias (35,78,79). Since the clinical criteria for pericarditis are neither sensitive nor specific, one study used pericardial effusion as a surrogate, finding that 63% of patients had supraventricular arrhythmias, compared to 11% without effusions (29). Of note, the presence of a pericardial effusion in this study did not correlate with clinical signs of pericarditis (pericardial rub, pain, fever).

IV. PROGNOSIS AND COMPLICATIONS

Although usually benign, postoperative AF may be associated with potential complications. These include death, systemic thromboembolism, particularly cerebrovascular accidents, hemodynamic compromise, sustained atrial fibrillation, and increased resource utilization, including length of hospital stay.

A. Atrial Thrombus Formation, Systemic Emboli, and Stroke

The clinical impact of postoperative atrial fibrillation includes a higher risk of stroke (5,8,80–82). Stroke is a potentially serious, though fortunately infrequent, consequence of CABG. The association between postoperative stroke and AF has been reported by several groups. In a study of 453 consecutive patients prospectively followed for neurological events after CABG, stroke or transient ischemic attack (TIA) occurred in 10 patients (2.2%) (80). Postoperative AF occurred in 6 of these 10 patients (60%), compared to its occurrence in 80 of 443 patients (18%) who did not have stroke or TIA ($p < 0.005$). A history of stroke or TIA and postoperative AF were identified as independent predictors of post-CABG neurological events. In a case-control study, postoperative AF occurred in 29 of 54 (54%) cases of postoperative stroke or TIA after CABG but in only 15 of 54 (28%) of controls (odds ratio for stroke with postoperative atrial fibrillation 3.0) (81). A study of 2417 patients undergoing CABG with or without valve surgery also reported that patients with major and minor neurological injury had significantly higher incidences of AF (major: 7% AF vs. 2% no AF; minor: 6 vs 2%) (17). In a study of 3855 Veterans Administration patients undergoing open cardiac surgery, stroke rate was 5.26% in patients with postoperative AF, compared to 2.95% in patients without AF ($p < 0.001$) (82). Another study of patients undergoing CABG reported a stroke incidence of 4 of 381 (1%) in patients remaining in sinus rhythm, compared to 7 of 189 (3.7%) in patients who developed postoperative AF ($p = 0.025$) (8). Postoperative AF was also an independent predictor of postoperative neurological events ($p = 0.0014$) among 1279 patients who underwent CABG and had undergone noninvasive carotid artery screening (83). Moreover, neurocognitive dysfunction is common after CABG. In a study of 308 patients, postoperative AF was associated with more neurocognitive decline 6 weeks after CABG (84). In contrast, a study of risk factors for early or delayed stroke after cardiac surgery among 2972 patients reported that AF had no impact on postoperative stroke rate unless it was accompanied by low cardiac output syndrome (85). While these and other data do not conclusively show a cause-effect relationship between brief paroxysms of AF and clinically significant systemic emboli, they heighten the concern for such complications.

B. Hemodynamic Deterioration

Hemodynamic deterioration—including hypotension, congestive heart failure, or both—may occur as a consequence of postoperative AF or its treatment. How well AF is tolerated often depends on several factors, including the ventricular rate, status of the patient's underlying ventricular function, presence of residual ischemia, and duration of the arrhythmia. The loss of atrial systole may contribute to loss of cardiac output. An increase in cardiac index from 2.7 ± 0.4 to 3.4 ± 0.1 L/min ($p < 0.05$) was observed after conversion of postoperative AF to sinus rhythm by propafenone (86).

Postoperative AF has been associated with a greater incidence of post-operative congestive heart failure, duration of intubation, and renal insufficiency (17); higher ICU readmission, perioperative myocardial infarction, persistent congestive heart failure, and reintubation (82); and higher rates of reoperation, ventilator requirement >24 hr, reintubation, ventricular arrhythmias, cardiac arrest, renal failure, infection, and pacemaker requirement (8). AF may not be entirely causative, as these associations may at least in part reflect a sicker population. Fortunately, in patients who have undergone coronary artery bypass, AF does not commonly result in severe hemodynamic compromise, and proarrhythmia from antiarrhythmic drug use is rare.

C. Prolonged Atrial Fibrillation

New AF occurring after surgery is usually transient. Most studies of patients previously free of atrial tachyarrhythmias suggest that postoperative AF rarely persists for longer than a few days, even though it is often recurrent. A low rate of recurrent AF (3.3 to 10%) is generally observed in patients after discharge from the hospital with or without antiarrhythmic drugs (87,88), although one retrospective study reported that 39% of patients had residual AF at a 6-month follow-up (89). Nevertheless, chronic AF developing de novo after cardiac surgery appears to be unusual, and long-term drug treatment for AF prevention is generally unnecessary.

D. Mortality

Some studies have reported trends toward an increase in mortality associated with postoperative AF. In a study of 570 patients undergoing CABG, overall operative mortality was 1.8% in patients maintaining sinus rhythm and 3.9% in those who developed AF ($p = 0.15$) (8). Among 462 patients who underwent noncardiothoracic surgery, the 10.2% of patients with new-onset atrial arrhythmias had higher mortality (23.4%), as did the 13% of patients with a prior history of atrial arrhythmias (mortality 8.6%), when compared to patients without atrial arrhythmias (mortality 4.3%), although most of the deaths were noncardiac and due to sepsis or cancer (90). In a VA study of 3855 patients undergoing cardiac surgery, postoperative AF was associated with higher hospital mortality (5.9% atrial fibrillation vs. 2.47% no AF), as well as 6-month mortality (9.36 vs. 4.17%), $p < 0.001$ (82). However, the increase in mortality may be related to higher comorbidities in patients developing postoperative AF.

E. Resource Utilization

Multiple studies have shown that postoperative AF prolongs hospital course and escalates expenses with hospital lengths of stay reported to be extended by 1 to 4 days and costs potentially increased by several thousand dollars per patient (5,8,17,91,92). Increased length of stay in elderly patients ≥70 years old appears largely attributable to a higher incidence of AF (93). Other recent studies have also confirmed a 1- to 5-day increase in length of stay and increases in hospital costs of several thousand dollars per patient associated with postoperative AF (5,8,91,92,94). One recent study showed AF contributing to a length of stay 1 to 1.5 days longer after cardiac surgery despite use of a clinical pathway focused on management of postoperative AF (92).

V. PROPHYLAXIS

The prevention of postoperative atrial arrhythmias has been studied using multiple pharmacological agents as well as atrial pacing. Most studies have used randomized open-label designs and relatively small numbers of patients. Such studies are summarized below and in Tables 1 through 6.

A. Digoxin

Prospective nonrandomized and randomized studies of prophylactic digoxin (Table 1) have yielded mixed results, and meta-analyses have shown no benefit (95–100). Although two of three nonrandomized trials suggested a benefit to digoxin, two of the four randomized trials failed to show a benefit, and one study showed an increase in AF with digoxin use (99). Two meta-analyses of digoxin prophylaxis trials showed no significant benefit of digoxin in preventing supraventricular arrhythmias after CABG (Table 6) (94,101). There has not been a placebo-controlled, double-blinded trial of digoxin use for postoperative AF prophylaxis.

B. Beta-Adrenergic Blockers

Multiple randomized studies have demonstrated the consistent effectiveness of beta blockers in preventing postoperative AF. Among the agents shown to be of benefit are propanolol, timolol, metoprolol, nadolol, and acebutolol (4,76–78,102–107). Table 2 summarizes randomized prospective trials of beta-blocker prophylaxis for postoperative supraventricular arrhythmias. Only four were double-blinded and placebo-controlled. One randomized trial

Table 1 Digoxin Prophylaxis Trials

Author	Year	N	Design	Digoxin regimen	% SVA		p Value
					Control	Digoxin	
Johnson (98)	1976	120	R	1–1.5 mg PO 2–3 days preop; 0.25 mg qd (pod 1)	26.0%	5.5%	<0.01
Tyras (99)	1978	140	R	1–1.5 mg PO 1 day preop; 0.25 qd (pod 1)	11.4%	27.8%	<0.05
Roffman (110)	1981	122	NR	1 mg IV (dos); 0.25 mg qd	pod 1–2 6.3% pod ≥3 22%	pod 1–2 3.7% pod ≥3 22.4%	NS NS
Csicsko (97)	1981	407[a]	NR	1mg IV (dos); 0.25 mg qd	15%	2%	<0.01
Chee (95)	1982	182	NR	0.75 mg 1 day preop; 0.25 mg qd (dos)	72% 95%[b]	5%	<0.01 <0.01
Parker (100)	1983	120	R	1–1.5 mg PO 1 day preop; 0.25 qd (pod 1)	21.4%	3.1%	<0.005
Weiner (96)	1986	98	R	0.75–1.0 mg IV (dos); 0.25 PO qd	16%	15%	NS

Key: N, number of patients; SVA, supraventricular arrhythmias; R, randomized; NR, nonrandomized; preop, preoperatively; pod, beginning postoperative day; dos, beginning or given day of surgery; NS, not significant.
[a] 270 historical controls.
[b] On digoxin preoperatively and no digoxin postoperatively.
Source: Modified from Ref. 236.

showed a negative effect of propranolol (108). However, three meta-analysis demonstrated overall significant 50 to 74% reductions in postoperative supraventricular arrhythmias with beta blockers (94,101,109).

Despite evidence supporting efficacy in the prevention of postoperative atrial arrhythmias, beta blockers had been used in only a limited manner for prophylaxis in the past, presumably because of the perception that patients would not tolerate these medications or apprehension over potential hemodynamic or pulmonary intolerance. Nevertheless, clinical use of prophylactic beta blockers does appear to be increasing. Beta blockers have been used safely, with few reported adverse effects. However, most trials excluded patients with contraindications, including significant obstructive lung disease, AV nodal block greater than first degree, and impaired left ventricular function.

C. Combined Beta-Blocker and Digoxin Prophylaxis

Several trials have studied the combined use of beta blockers and digoxin (Table 3). Two studies of digoxin plus propranolol showed significant reductions in postoperative supraventricular arrhythmias compared to treatment with digoxin alone (110,111). A meta-analysis of these two studies (Table 5) confirmed the combination of beta blockers and digoxin causing a larger reduction than beta blockers or digoxin alone, from 29.4 to 2.2%, suggesting a possible synergistic effect (94). This group subsequently performed a randomized, double-blinded trial of digoxin with acebutolol vs. digoxin and placebo in 157 patients with randomization stratified by preoperative beta-blocker use (107). There was a trend toward a lower incidence of atrial fibrillation and flutter among patients in the digoxin-plus acebutolol group (24%) compared to patients treated with digoxin alone (32%). In sum, these studies suggest that most of any benefit is likely in large part due to the beta-blocker component.

D. Calcium Channel Blockers

Studies of verapamil and diltiazem have generally yielded negative or inconclusive results. Two studies have shown oral verapamil to be ineffective in preventing AF after CABG (112,113). One study showed a trend toward a reduction in AF after lung surgery with verapamil (114). When AF did occur on verapamil, ventricular rates were slower. However, bradycardia, hypotension, and pulmonary edema were more frequent in the verapamil-treated groups.

Intravenous diltiazem may be better tolerated hemodynamically than verapamil. Intravenous diltiazem has been compared to nitroglycerin by two

Table 2 Beta-Blocker Prophylaxis Trials (Prospective Randomized Controlled Trials with ≥100 Patients)

Author	Year	N	Design	Regimen	% SVA		p Value	Comments
					Control	Drug		
Stephenson (104)	1980	223	R	Propanolol 10 mg PO q 6 hr on transfer from ICU	18%	8%	N/A	Many on preoperative beta blockers
Mohr (76)	1981	103	R	Propanolol preop, 5–10 mg PO 6 hr postop (dos)		5%		Included patients with LV dysfunction
				-Propanolol preop, none postop	40%		<0.001	
				-No propranolol preop, treated postop	27%		<0.01	
Silverman (102)	1982	100	R	Propanolol 10 mg PO q 6 hr (pod 1)	28.0%	6.0%	<0.01	All on preop beta blockers; included patients with LV dysfunction
Abel (106)	1983	100	R	Propanolol IV 1 mg × 2 pre/at CPB; 2 mg q 4 hr (dos) until able to take PO then 10 mg PO q 6 hr × 24 hr, then 20 mg PO q 6 hr to pod 6, then 10 mg PO q 6 hr × 3 days	38%	17%	<0.05	All taking preoperative propanolol. No benefit to postoperative propranolol in patients taking propranolol ≥320 mg preoperatively

Study	Year	N	Design	Regimen				Comments
Ivey (108)	1983	109	R, DB, P	Propanolol 20 mg PO q 6 hr (pod 1)	16.1%	13.2%	>0.10	All on propanolol preoperatively
Matangl (103)	1985	164	R	Propanolol 5 mg PO q 6 hr (dos)	23.0%	9.8%	0.02	All on preoperative beta blockers
Daudon (77)	1986	100	R	Acebutolol 200 mg PO bid start dose 36 hr postop	40%	0%	p < 0.001	Some on preoperative beta blockers
Vecht (4)	1986	132	R, DB, P	Timolol 5 mg PO q 12 hr (dos), 10 mg PO bid (pod 1)	19.7%	7.5%	<0.05	Most on beta blockers preoperatively
Khuri (105)	1987	141	R, DB, P	Nadolol 40 mg qd start dose (pod 1)	42%	9%	<0.001	Most on preoperative beta blockers
Ali (215)	1997	210	R	Postop resumption of preop beta blocker	38%	17%	<0.02	All on preop beta blockers; not resumed in control group
Paull (216)	1997	100	R, P	Metoprolol 50–200 mg/day based on rate	26%	24%	NS	
Connolly (217)	2003	1000	R, DB, P	Metoprolol 100–150 mg qd × 14 d or to hospital discharge	39%	31%	0.01	No significant effect on hospital length of stay or overall cost

Key: N, number of patients; D, design; R, randomized; DB, double-blinded; P, placebo-controlled; Monitoring Period, period of continuous telemetry or Holter monitoring; ECGs, electrocardiograms; dos, day of surgery; pod, postoperative day; CPB, cardiopulmonary bypass; SVA, supraventricular arrhythmias.

Source: Modified from Ref. 236.

Table 3 Combination Beta-Blocker Prophylaxis Trials (Prospective, Controlled Trials with ≥100 Patients)

Author	Year	N	Design	Control	Treatment	% SVA Control pod1–2	% SVA Control pod ≥3	% SVA Treatment pod1–2	% SVA Treatment pod ≥3	p Value
Roffman (110)	1981	172	NR	No treatment	Digoxin 1 mg IV (dos); 0.25 mg PO (pod 1)	6.3%	22%	3.7%	22.4%	NS
					Digoxin 1 mg IV (dos); 0.25 mg PO (pod 1) + propranolol 20 mg PO tid (pod 2)				2.1%	<0.005
Mills (111)	1983	179	R	No treatment	Digoxin 1mg IV (dos), 0.25mg PO (pod 1) + propranolol 10 mg PO q 6 hr (dos)	30.0%		3.4%		<0.001
Rubin (78)	1987	123	R	No treatment	Propranolol 20 mg PO q 6 hr (pod 1)	37.5%		16.2%		<0.03
					Digoxin 0.5 mg (pod 1), 0.25 mg PO qd			32.6%		NS

	Year	N	Design					
Kowey (107)	1997	157	R, DB	Digoxin 1 mg IV/PO over 24 hr, then 0.125–0.25 mg qd	Digoxin IV/PO 1 mg over 24 hr, 0.125–0.25 mg qd + acebutolol 200 mg PO/NGT q12h	32%	24%	0.11
Solomon (218)	2000	167	R	Propranolol 20 mg qid begun on admission to ICU	Propranolol 20 mg qid + Mg 18 g over 24 hr begun intraoperatively	19.5%	22.4%	0.65
Yazicioglu (219)	2002	160	R	Placebo	Digoxin 1 mg 2–3 d preop, then 0.25 mg qd + Atenolol 50 mg qd beginning 3d preop	25%	5%	0.012
					Digoxin 1 mg 2–3 d preop, then 0.25 mg qd		17.9%	NS
					Atenolol 50 mg qd beginning 3 d preop		15.4%	NS

Key: N, number of patients; SVA, supraventricular arrhythmias; R, randomized; NGT, nasogastric tube; NR, nonrandomized; DB, double blinded; pod, postoperative day; dos, day of surgery; preop, preoperatively; NS, not significant.

Source: Modified from Ref. 236.

Table 4 Randomized Class I and III Antiarrhythmic Drug Prophylaxis Trials

Author	Year	N	Design	Control	Drug regimen	% SVA Control	% SVA Drug	p Value	Comments
Class IA—Procainamide									
Laub (117)	1993	46	R, DB, P	Placebo	Procainamide 12 mg/kg IV load, 2 mg/min, then weight-adjusted PO (dos-pod 5)	38%	18%	0.2	
Gold (118)	1996	100	R, DB, P	Placebo	Procainamide PO adjusted by weight × 4 days	38%	26%	NS	38 → 13% reduction in patients with therapeutic levels ($p < 0.05$)
Class IC—Propafenone and Flecainide									
Merrick (121)	1995	207	R, DB	Atenolol 50 mg qd	Propafenone 300 mg bid	10.8%	12.4%	0.89	
Borgeat (122)	1991	30	R	Digoxin 10 ug/kg × 12 hr, then 0.24mg/24 hr	Flecainide 2 mg/kg IV load, then 0.15 mg/g/hr	47%	7%	<0.05	Thoracic surgery patients
Class III—Sotalol									
Janssen (220)	1986	130	R	Control	Sotalol IV dos (0.3 mg/kg), 80 mg PO tid (pod 1)	36.0%	2.4%	<0.01	
					Metoprolol IV (dos) 0.1 mg/kg, 50 mg PO tid (pod 1)		15.3%	<0.05	
Suttorp (128)	1990	429	R	Propranolol 10 mg q6hr	Sotalol 40 mg q 8 hr	18.8%	13.9%	NS	Trend toward less SVA in sotalol groups; fewer adverse effects in low dose groups

Reference	Year	N	Design	Control	Sotalol regimen			p	Comments
Suttorp (123)	1991	300	R, DB, P	Propranolol 20 mg q6hr; Placebo	Sotalol 80 mg q 8 hr	13.7%	0.9%	<0.005	
Nystrom (125)	1993	101	R	Placebo	Sotalol 40 mg po q 6 hr (dos-pod 6)	33%	16%	0.028	Dose reduction or discontinuation: 22% sotalol
Jacquet (130)	1994	42	R	Beta blockers	Sotalol 160 mg PO bid	29%	10%	NS	
Pfisterer (126)	1997	255	R, DB, P	Control	Sotalol IV 1 mg/kg over 2h, 0.15 mg/kg/h × 24h, then 80 mg PO q8–12h	29%	16%	0.0012	1 proarrhythmia; >90% AF within 9d; 70% of sotalol SEs after 9 days
Parikka (127)	1998	191	R	Placebo	Sotalol 80 mg bid begun 2 hr preop × 3 mos	46%	26%	<0.01	QT longer on sotalol
Gomes (124)	1999	85	R, DB, P	Metoprolol 75 mg/day	Sotalol 120 mg/day	32%	16%	0.008	2/40 (5%) hypotension, bradycardia on sotalol
Evrard (221)	2000	206	R	Placebo	Sotalol 80–120 mg bid begun 2 days preop, continued 4 d postop	38%	12.5%	<0.00001	Sotalol discontinued in 8 (7.8%) due to SEs; reduced ventricular arrhythmias/ectopy
Matsuura (222)	2001	80	R	Control	Sotalol 80 mg bid	48%	16%	<0.05	Bradycardia or hypotension in 3 sotalol pts (7.5%). Postop LOS not different.
				Age- and gender-matched control group	Sotalol 80 mg qd pod 1–14	37.5%	15%		

Table 4 Continued

Author	Year	N	Design	Control	Drug regimen	% SVA Control	% SVA Drug	p Value	Comments
Forlani (129)	2002	207	R	Control	Magnesium 1.5g qd × 6d beginning intraop pre-CPB	38%	14.8%	0.007	
					Sotalol 80 mg bid beginning pod 1		11.8%	0.002	
					Both magnesium + sotalol		1.9%	<0.0001	
Class III—Amiodarone									
Hohnloser (131)	1991	77	R, P	Placebo	Amiodarone IV 300 mg over 2 hr, 1200 mg/d × 2 d, then 900 mg/d × 2 d	21%	5%	<0.05	NSVT, HR reduced, JT prolonged by amiodarone; discontinued in 2 for QT.
Butler (132)	1993	120	R, DB, P	Placebo	Amiodarone 15 mg/kg IV over 24 hrs, 200 mg po × 5 d	20%	8%	0.07	Reduced total treated SVA, V arrhythmias, $p = 0.05$, more bradycardia with drug.
Daoud (133)	1997	124	R, DB, P	Placebo	Amiodarone PO 600 mg qd min. 7 days preop, then 200 mg qd until discharge	53%	25%	0.003	Hospitalization costs reduced in amiodarone group.

Study	Year	Design	Control	Regimen	Rx	Control	p	Comments
Redle (134)	1999	R, DB, P	Placebo	Amiodarone PO 2 g, divided 1–4 d preop; 400 mg qd × 7 days postop	33%	25%	0.30	Hospital cost no different.
Guarnieri (135)	1999	R, DB, P	Placebo	Amiodarone IV 1g/d × 2 days	47%	35%	0.01	Hospital stay not reduced.
Lee (136)	2000	R	Placebo	Amiodarone IV 150 mg, then 0.4 mg/kg/hr 3 days before and 5 days postop	34%	12%	<0.01	Ventricular rate, duration of AF, ICU length of stay reduced in amiodarone group.
Dorge (137)	2000	R	Placebo	After aortic crossclamp: Amiodarone IV 300 mg, 20 mg/kg/d × 3d	34%	24%	NS	
				Amiodarone IV 150 mg, 10 mg/kg/d × 3d		28%		
Treggiari-Venzi (143)	2000	R, DB, P	Placebo	Immediately after surgery: Amiodarone IV 900 mg/24 hr × 72 hr	27%	14%	0.14	
				Magnesium 4g/24 × 72hr		23%	0.82	
Giri (138) White (223)	2001	R, DB, P	Placebo	Amiodarone 6 g over 6 d beginning preop day 1 or 7g over 10 d beginning preop day 5	38%	22.5%	0.01	87.5% on beta blockers; CVA, VT also reduced.
Maras (139)	2001	R, DB, P	Placebo	Amiodarone 1200 mg 1 d preop, then 200 mg qd × 7 d	21.2%	19.5%	0.78	Reduced AF in patients ≥60 years old (26.7 vs 43.1%, $p = 0.05$).

Table 4 Continued

Author	Year	N	Design	Control	Drug regimen	% SVA		p Value	Comments
						Control	Drug		
Yazigi (140)	2002	200	R, DB, P	Placebo	Amiodarone 15 mg/kg oral 4 hr after ICU arrival, 7 mg/kg/d until hospital discharge	25%	12%	<0.05	
Tokmakoglu (141)	2002	241	R	No treatment	Metoprolol 100 mg po 24hr preop, digoxin 0.5 mg × 2 POD0, digoxin 0.25 mg PO + metoprolol 100 mg PO, POD to discharge	33.6%	16.8%	<0.01	
					Amiodarone IV 1200 mg/24 hr beginning with 300 mg immediately postop, then 450 mg/24h IV, 600 mg/d PO until discharge		8.3%	<0.001	
Solomon (142)	2001	102	R	Propranolol 1 mg IV q 6 hr × 48h, then 20 mg qid until discharge	Amiodarone 1g/d IV ×48 hr, then 400 mg po qd until discharge	32.7%	16%	0.05	

Key: N, number of patients; D, design; R, randomized; DB, double-blinded; P, placebo-controlled; dos, day of surgery; pod, postoperative day; SVA = supraventricular arrhythmias; NSVT = nonsustained ventricular tachycardia; V, ventricular; PO, oral; IV, intravenous; VT, ventricular tachycardia; VT, ventricular tachycardia; CVA, cerebrovascular accident; LOS, hospital length of stay; SEs, side effects.

groups. In a randomized study of 120 patients undergoing CABG (115) a 24-hr infusion of intravenous diltiazem 0.1 mg/hr reduced postoperative atrial fibrillation from 18 to 5%, compared to nitroglycerin. A small randomized study of 40 patients after CABG also reported less supraventricular tachyarrhythmia with diltiazem compared to nitroglycerin (116).

E. Antiarrhythmic Agents

Trials of class I or III antiarrhythmic drugs in the prevention of postoperative AF are summarized in Table 4.

1. Class IA Antiarrhythmic Agents

Procainamide has shown some efficacy in preventing postoperative AF after CABG. A double-blind, randomized placebo-controlled pilot trial of procainamide in 46 patients undergoing CABG reported that procainamide reduced the number of AF episodes per hour (117). In another study, the incidence of AF was significantly reduced in patients achieving therapeutic procainamide serum levels, supporting the importance of achieving therapeutic levels for efficacy with procainamide (118). Nausea was a significant side effect of therapy.

Quinidine has not been well studied for prophylaxis after surgery, and its use remains appropriately limited in view of its proarrhythmic potential, particularly in the setting of hypokalemia, which may occur commonly with diuresis after surgery. In one study, quinidine was ineffective in preventing AF after mitral valvotomy (119).

2. Class IC Antiarrhythmic Agents

The use of class IC drugs is usually limited to patients without significant ventricular dysfunction or coronary artery disease, because the Cardiac Arrhythmia Suppression Trial (CAST) showed higher mortality in post-infarction patients treated with flecainide and encainide (120). However, flecainide may be useful in patients with valvular disease, and short-term propafenone has been used by some clinicians even after CABG. *Propafenone* was reported in one study to be of similar efficacy to atenolol (121). *Flecainide* given intravenously reduced AF or atrial flutter when compared to digoxin used after thoracic surgery (122).

3. Class III Antiarrhythmic Agents

Sotalol, a class III antiarrhythmic agent with beta-blocker activity, has been effective in reducing postoperative supraventricular arrhythmias (123–127).

Table 5 Meta-analyses of Trials for The Prophylaxis of Supraventricular Arrhythmias After CABG

A. Efficacy Outcomes

Author	Date	Treatment	Total patients, N	% SVA Control	% SVA Drug	Odds ratio	95% Confidence interval	p Value
Andrews (101)	1991	Beta blocker	1549	34.0	8.7	0.28	0.21–0.36	<0.0001
		Digoxin	507	17.6	14.2	0.97	0.62–1.49	0.88
		Verapamil	432	18.2	18.2	0.91	0.57–1.46	0.69
Kowey (94)	1992	Beta blocker	1418	20.2	9.8			<0.001
		Digoxin	875	19.1	15.4			NS
		Digoxin + beta blocker	292	29.4	2.2			<0.001
Crystal (109)	2002	Beta blocker	3840	33	19	0.39	0.28–0.52	<0.00001
		Sotalol	1294	37	17	0.35	0.26–0.49	<0.00001
		Amiodarone	1384	37	22.5	0.48	0.37–0.61	<0.00001
		Pacing RA	581			0.68	0.39–1.19	
		LA	148			0.57	0.28–1.16	
		Biatrial	744			0.46	0.30–0.71	
Wurdeman (146)	2002	Sotalol	539		−21.5%[a]	0.53	0.41–0.69	<0.001
		Amiodarone	764		−14.1%[a]	0.24	0.08–0.72	<0.001
Zimmer (147)	2003	Amiodarone	1087	39.4	25.6	0.37	0.09–1.45	
		Sotalol	95	12.5	37.8	0.60	0.37–0.96	
		Procainamide	46	18.2	37.5			
		Pacing	390	22.2	33.5			

B. Other Outcomes

Author	Outcome and treatment	N	Hospital LOS or cost		Other outcomes		Significance, p Value
			Treatment difference	95% CI	Odds ratio	95% CI	
Crystal (109)	LOS						
	Beta blocker	1200	-0.66 days	-2.04-0.72			NS
	Sotalol	808	-0.40 days	-0.87-0.08			NS
	Amiodarone	944	-0.91 days	-1.59--0.24			Significant
	Overall drug	2946	-0.54 days	-0.93--0.14			Significant
	Biatrial pacing	744	-1.54 days	-2.85--0.24			Significant
	Stroke—all studies	2877			0.90	0.46-1.74	NS
Wurdeman (146)	LOS						
	Sotalol	539	-0.13 days	-0.33-0.07			NS
	Amiodarone	764	-0.18 days	-0.48-4.38			NS
Zimmer (147)	LOS—Overall	1783	-1.0 ± 0.2 days				<0.001
	Amiodarone	1087	-0.9 ± 0.3 days				0.007
	Sotalol	95	-1.0 ± 0.7 days				0.142
	Procainamide	46	2.3 ± 4.0 days				0.568
	Pacing	390	-1.1 ± 0.4 days				0.003
	Cost—all studies	998	-$1,287 ± $673				0.056
	Stroke—all studies	926			0.50	0.22-1.17	NS
	Mortality—all studies	1336			0.92	0.47-1.79	NS

Key: SVA supraventricular arrhythmias; RA, right atrial; LA, left atrial; LOS, length of stay; NS, not significant; CI, confidence interval.
[a] Weighted average rate difference between treatment and control groups.

Table 6 Postoperative Pacing Studies for Prevention of Atrial Arrhythmias After Cardiac Surgery

Author	Year	N	Atrium paced	Pacing regimen	%SVA			Comments
					C	Pace	p Value	
Gerstenfeld (156)	1999	61	RA RA + LA	100 bpm	33	29 37	>0.7	AF induced by A pacing in 3. Trend to ↓AF with pacing + beta blocker
Kurz (157)	1999	21	RA+LA	3 d AAI ↑ 10 bpm, ≤110 bpm	22	42	—	Proarrhythmia: 6/12 paced, sensing failure → AF in 5
Chung (159)	2000	100	RA	4 d AAI ↑ 10 bpm, ≤110 bpm	28.6	25.5	0.90	↑ APDs; frequent undersensing, loss of capture
Blommaert (160)	2000	96	RA	Dynamic AAI overdrive ≥80 bpm × 24 hr on POD2 (Vitatron)	27	10	0.036	59% on beta blocker; pacing and endpoints on POD 2
Greenberg (158)	2000	154	RA LA RA+LA	AAI 100–110 bpm × 72 hr	37.5	8 20 26	0.002 0.14 0.40	Overall paced 17% AF, $p < 0.005$

	Year	n	Site	Protocol			p	Comments
Fan (161)	2000	132	RA LA RA+LA	5 d ↑ 10 bpm 90–120 ppm	41.9	33.3 36.4 12.5	NS NS <0.05	56% on beta blocker
Daoud (164)	2000	118	RA RA+LA	AAT ≥5 bpm	28	32 10	0.03	Control = AAI 45 bpm
Levy (163)	2000	130	RA+LA	4 d DDD 80 bpm, atrial resynchrony algorithm (ELA)	38.5	13.8	0.001	LA at Bachmann's bundle, No postop beta blocker
Gerstenfeld (224)	2001	118	RA+LA	AAI 100 bpm × 96 hr	35	19	<0.05	All on beta blocker; benefit seen in patients age ≥70 years
Goette (162)	2002	161	RA BB	AAI 96 bpm × 5 d	42	48 37	NS	On treatment RA vs BB pacing AF incidence 50 vs 29% ($p < 0.01$)

Key: AF, atrial fibrillation; RA, right atrium; LA, left atrium; BB, Bachmann's bundle.
Source: Modified from Ref. 237.

Sotalol was more effective than beta blockers without class III activity in two of three studies comparing these agents (125,127,128). A study of magnesium and sotalol showed significant reductions in postoperative AF, suggesting a possible synergistic effect with combination use of magnesium supplementation and sotalol (129).

Sotalol's potent beta-blocking activity requires vigilance for beta blockade–associated hemodynamic and bradycardic side effects. A small study showed hemodynamically significant adverse effects requiring discontinuation in 6 of 25 patients (24%) given an intravenous load followed by oral sotalol. In this study, the incidence of supraventricular arrhythmias was not significantly reduced (130). In a study of sotalol 160 mg bid, reduction or discontinuation of sotalol was required in 11 of 50 (20%) of patients due to bradycardia, with 2 also discontinued because of hypotension (125). This dose may be excessive for some patients, particularly if other beta blockers or negatively chronotropic drugs are continued. However, another study demonstrated that oral sotalol begun 2 days prior to cardiac surgery at 80 to 120 mg bid and continued for 4 days after surgery reduced AF with good hemodynamic tolerance (124). Temporary pacing, using temporary epicardial pacing leads from surgery, was used as necessary for bradycardia. Low-dose sotalol (40 mg q 8 hr) has been reported to be better tolerated than high-dose (80 mg q 8 hr) sotalol (128). Proarrhythmia has been reported only rarely (126). Thus, sotalol appears effective, but caution is indicated to avoid the hemodynamic adverse effects associated with its beta-adrenergic blocking activity.

Amiodarone has also been studied for prophylaxis of postoperative AF, although the most cost-effective and practical dosing regimen has not been established (Table 4) (131–142). Effective regimens are noted in Table 4. Borderline or ineffective dosage regimens may have been limited by inadequate amiodarone dose loading prior to surgery or in the immediate postoperative period (134,137,139,142,143). Although the high cost of intravenous amiodarone has limited its use and cost effectiveness (144,145), the availability of competitive formulations has recently lowered its cost. Thus, intravenous and oral amiodarone is becoming a commonly used, efficacious, and cost-effective choice for prophylaxis of postoperative AF.

Meta-analyses of sotalol and amiodarone have shown that both amiodarone and sotalol were more effective than placebo in reducing postoperative atrial fibrillation and flutter after CABG (109,146,147). No differences were noted between amiodarone and sotalol for efficacy, length of stay, or adverse reactions requiring drug terminations (146).

A. Magnesium

Hypomagnesemia is common after cardiopulmonary bypass (54,148,149), and reductions in atrial arrhythmias have been reported with magnesium. The effectiveness of magnesium administration in preventing arrhythmias may depend on the achievement of adequate magnesium blood levels (54,150,151). The majority of trials have shown beneficial effects on reduction of postoperative atrial arrhythmias, although some have reported negative or borderline results using magnesium supplementation despite an increase in magnesium levels (152–154). One study reported reduction of AF with magnesium or sotalol and the largest reduction with a combination of magnesium plus sotalol (129). Magnesium given in cardioplegic solutions also appears beneficial in reducing postoperative AF (149,155).

B. Atrial Pacing

Frequent atrial ectopy after cardiac surgery has been believed to signal impending AF. In practice, this has often triggered the initiation of atrial overdrive pacing in hopes of suppressing this ectopy. The most common pacing modes used for this purpose were AAI, DVI, or DDD modes.

However, studies of right atrial pacing after cardiac surgery have not shown consistent benefits in reducing AF; pacing may even cause more frequent atrial ectopy (Table 6) (17,156–160). In a large prospective observational study of 2417 patients undergoing CABG with or without valvular surgery (17), atrial pacing—but not atrioventricular pacing—was identified as an independent predictor of postoperative AF. In one of the first randomized trials to test the hypothesis that atrial overdrive pacing would reduce the incidence of AF after cardiac surgery, atrial pacing in the AAI mode did not reduce the incidence of AF and was instead associated with an increase in atrial premature depolarizations (159). A substantial proportion of paced patients were found to have atrial undersensing, loss of capture or sinus rhythm overriding the AAI pacing producing competitive atrial pacing and premature beats. These results suggested that this mode of pacing is not beneficial in suppressing postoperative AF. Preliminary results of a follow-up study using an automatic atrial overdrive pacing algorithm likewise showed no reduction in AF.

Other published studies of single-site pacing in the right atrium (RA) for prevention of postoperative AF have also produced variable results (Table 6). A study of 61 patients treated with RA pacing at 100 bpm or no pacing reported no significant difference in the incidence of atrial arrhythmias (156). Indeed, AF was induced by atrial pacing in 3 patients. The study did suggest a trend toward decreased AF with pacing and concomitant beta-blocker therapy. Overall, 5 of 7 studies showed no significant reduction of AF with RA pacing (156,159–162).

Biatrial pacing, particularly with leads placed near Bachmann's bundle, may be more effective in preventing postoperative AF, although again, results have not uniformly shown a beneficial effect (161–164). Four of seven studies of biatrial pacing (Table 6) have reported successful reductions in AF. One notable exception is a study of biatrial pacing stopped after 21 patients due to atrial proarrhythmia (157). Patients were randomized to no pacing or AAI pacing at 10 bpm over intrinsic rhythm and ≤110 bpm. In the control arm 22% developed postoperative AF, compared to 42% of the paced group. In 6 of 12 patients paced, sensing failure occurred, leading to AF in 5 patients. A meta-analysis of pacing studies, however, did report a significant reduction in AF with biatrial pacing, whereas only nonsignificant trends toward AF reduction were seen with RA or LA single-site pacing (109). Using an AAT-triggered mode to achieve more consistent atrial pacing and dual-site atrial activation may be more effective and potentially less proarrhythmic (164). Pacing via leads placed near Bachmann's bundle also appear more effective (162,163).

C. Other Prophylactic Strategies

Miscellaneous pharmacological methods tested for prophylaxis of AF after surgery have included thyroid supplementation and anti-inflammatory therapy with steroids. A randomized, placebo-controlled trial of triiodothyronine (T3) given intravenously in 142 patients with reduced left ventricular function undergoing CABG reported a lower incidence of AF (24 vs. 46%, $p = 0.009$) (165). Methylprednisolone, studied for its effects on extubation times, incidentally produced no reduction in postoperative AF in one prospective, randomized double-blind placebo-controlled study of 60 patients who underwent CABG (166). A randomized double-blind placebo-controlled trial of dexamethasone 4 mg × 2 doses failed to reduce postoperative AF (167). However, a randomized placebo-controlled study of dexamethasone 0.6 mg/kg for reduction of postoperative shivering reported a reduction in new-onset AF (18.9 vs. 32.3%) (168).

Posterior pericardiotomy during cardiac surgery has been advocated for reduction of postoperative AF (169,170). In a randomized trial of 200 patients undergoing CABG, AF incidence was 6% in the pericardiotomy group compared to 34% in the no pericardiotomy group (169). In another randomized prospective study of 150 patients undergoing CABG, AF occurred in 9.3% of a posterior pericardiotomy–treated group and 32% in a no-posterior-pericardiotomy group (171).

D. Prophylaxis Summary and Algorithm

A summary of meta-analyses of trials for prophylaxis of supraventricular arrhythmias after CABG—including endpoints of arrhythmia reduction efficacy, length of stay, and stroke reduction—is shown in Table 5. An algorithm that may be used for prophylaxis of AF after cardiac surgery is shown in Figure 1. Patients who are eligible for beta-blocker prophylaxis may be begun on metoprolol for 5 days, monitored for occurrence of supraventricular tachyarrhythmias or side effects, and then tapered off over 3 days. Patients that can be started on a prophylactic agent preoperatively may benefit from preoperative loading with amiodarone, or the agent may be used with intravenous loading.

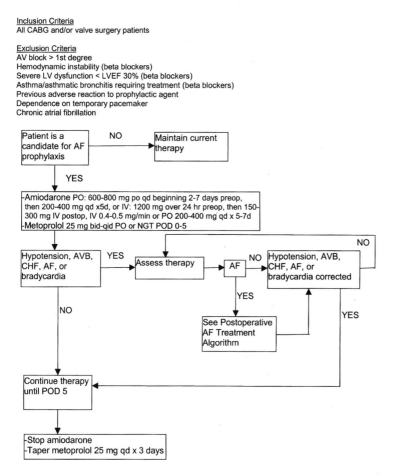

Inclusion Criteria
All CABG and/or valve surgery patients

Exclusion Criteria
AV block > 1st degree
Hemodynamic instability (beta blockers)
Severe LV dysfunction < LVEF 30% (beta blockers)
Asthma/asthmatic bronchitis requiring treatment (beta blockers)
Previous adverse reaction to prophylactic agent
Dependence on temporary pacemaker
Chronic atrial fibrillation

Figure 1 Algorithm for the prevention of atrial fibrillation after cardiac surgery. CABG, coronary artery bypass grafting; LV, left ventricle; LVEF, left ventricular ejection fraction; AF, atrial fibrillation; IV, intravenous; PO, per os (oral); NGT, nasogastric tube; POD, postoperative day; AVB, atrioventricular block; CHF, congestive heart failure. (Modified from Ref. 235.)

VI. MANAGEMENT

Treatment of postoperative AF differs little from treatment of nonpostoperative AF. Although postoperative AF is generally self-limited, symptoms, hemodynamic compromise, and concern over risk of thromboembolism often justify intervention. The onset of AF in the postoperative period is likely to be symptomatic, since it is often associated with rapid ventricular rates.

A. Rates- vs. Rhythm-Control Approaches

In patients without a prior history of AF spontaneous conversion to sinus rhythm frequently occurs without need for further therapy (172,173). Even with a rate-control approach, over 90% of patients revert to sinus rhythm 2 to 4 weeks after the onset or by their follow-up visit (173,174). In a study of a rate-control approach in 59 patients after CABG, use of digoxin with or without verapamil was associated with spontaneous conversion to sinus rhythm in 55 patients (173). By 2 to 4 weeks later, 2 of the 4 patients with continued atrial fibrillation were in sinus rhythm and 2 others in sinus rhythm had reverted to AF.

Trials of rate- vs. rhythm-control approaches to postoperative AF have to date been limited, but they support the assertion that despite early recurrences, postoperative AF appears to be self-limited in most cases, with similar recurrence rates in patients treated with rate- and rhythm-control. In a nonrandomized study of 116 patients with postoperative AF treated with class I or III antiarrhythmic drugs and rate control-drugs or rate-control drugs alone, compared to 151 patients with no AF, only 1 patient in the atrial fibrillation group was in AF at 6 weeks after discharge (175). There was a trend toward higher mortality and morbidity in the rate-control treated AF patients. In another nonrandomized study of 185 patients followed for a mean of 10 months, recurrence rates within the first month were high (32%) (176). The event rate was the same in amiodarone and nontreated patients, though it was lower in patients taking beta blockers. At the end of follow-up, AF persisted in only 1.7% of patients. In a small randomized trial of 50 patients with AF after cardiac surgery, no significant differences in time to conversion to sinus rhythm or sinus rhythm at 2 months (91% rate control, 96% rhythm control) were reported, although hospital length of stay was shorter in the rate-control strategy (mean 9 vs. 13.2 days) (174). Both groups received anticoagulation with heparin/warfarin. Another study demonstrated shorter hospital lengths with no repeat hospitalizations, bleeding complications, or thromboembolic events in the 12 of 67 patients with postoperative AF who were discharged in AF (177). Moreover, a small study of 42 patients with postsurgical AF randomized to ibutilide, propafenone, or rate control showed that while ibutilide reduced AF duration, recurrence rates were high and not significantly different between rhythm- and rate-control approaches (178).

Nevertheless, in patients with atrial arrhythmias after surgery, a rhythm-control approach is often elected to minimize symptoms, anticoagulation issues, or recovery times from surgery. A general approach to postoperative AF is described and an algorithm for treatment is shown in Figure 2.

B. Rate Control

In the absence of the need for urgent cardioversion, control of the ventricular rate becomes the primary concern during the first 24 hr. The goal is to achieve a heart rate of 70 to 100 bpm at rest. Commonly used agents include digoxin, beta blockers, and calcium channel blockers (Table 7). Intravenous or oral forms of each agent can be used, although intravenous dosing is often preferred to accelerate the onset of action. High postoperative sympathetic tone makes rate control with digoxin alone frequently ineffective. In a study comparing ventricular rate control with diltiazem vs. digoxin for AF after CABG, diltiazem achieved rate control earlier than digoxin; after 6 hr, ventricular rate control was achieved in more patients with diltiazem (85 vs. 45%) (179). After 24 hr, however, both ventricular response rates and conversion rates were similar (55% of patients on diltiazem and 65% patients on digoxin). In another study comparing intravenous diltiazem to esmolol, 66.6% of esmolol-treated patients compared to 13.3% of diltiazem-treated patients converted to sinus rhythm during the first 6 hr ($p < 0.05$), but by 24 hr 80% of the esmolol- and 66.6% of the diltiazem-treated patients had converted to sinus rhythm (not significant) (180). Monitoring for hypotension and negative inotropic effects is advised for beta blockers or calcium channel blockers.

C. Rhythm Control

1. Electrical Conversion

In patients whose atrial arrhythmia persists more than 24 hr or even less despite adequate rate control, pharmacological or electrical cardioversion can generally be attempted (181). Patients remaining in AF after an approximately 24-hr trial of drug therapy also typically undergo electrical cardioversion. Clinical instability—manifest by hypotension, ischemia, or congestive heart failure—should prompt immediate electrical cardioversion. Atrial overdrive pacing can be attempted if atrial flutter is the dominant rhythm. This can be done using temporary epicardial pacing leads placed at the time of surgery.

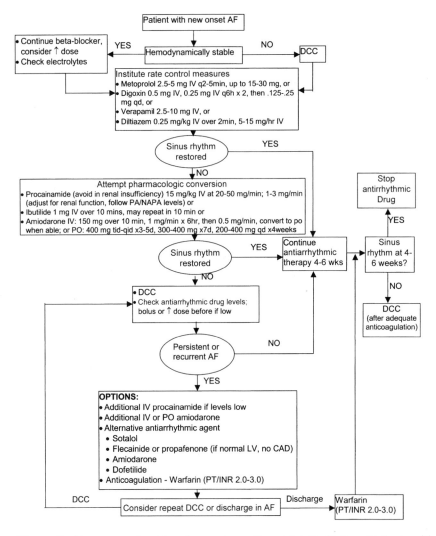

Figure 2 Treatment algorithm for postoperative atrial fibrillation. Patients with LVEF >25% and preserved renal function may be candidates for procainamide or ibutilide. Amiodarone may be the agent of choice for patients with hemodynamic instability, LVEF ≤25%, renal dysfunction, or other contraindications to procainamide. AF, atrial fibrillation; DCC, direct-current cardioversion; IV, intravenous; PO, per os (oral); PA, procainamide; NAPA, N-acetyl procainamide; LV, left ventricle; CAD, coronary artery disease. (Modified from Ref. 235.)

Table 7 Rate Control for Postoperative Atrial Arrhythmias

Agent	Loading dose	Maintenance dose	Side effects/toxicity	Comments
Digoxin	0.25–0.5 mg IV or PO, then 0.25 mg q 4–6 hr to 1 mg in 1st 24 h	0.125–0.25 mg PO or IV qd	Anorexia, nausea; AV block; ventricular arrhythmias; accumulates in renal failure	Used in CHF; vagotonic effects on the AVN; delayed onset of action; narrow therapeutic window; less effective in postop, paroxysmal AF with high adrenergic states
Beta blockers			Bronchospasm; CHF; ↓BP	Effective in heart rate control; rapid onset of action
Propranolol	1 mg IV q 2–5′ to 0.1–0.2 mg/kg	10–80 mg PO tid-qid		
Metoprolol	2.5–5 mg IV q 2–5′ to 15–30 mg	25–100 mg PO bid-tid		
Esmolol	500 ug/kg IV over·1′	50 ug/kg IV for 4′, repeat load prn and ↑ maintenance 20–50 ug/kg/min q 5–10′		Esmolol, short-acting
Calcium channel blockers				
Verapamil	2.5–10 mg IV over 2′	5–10 mg IV q 30–60′ or 40–160 mg PO tid or 120–480 mg/day, sustained release	↓BP, CHF	Rapid onset, can be used safely in COPD and DM
			↑ Digoxin level	
Diltiazem	0.25 mg/kg over 2′, repeat prn p 15′ at 0.35 mg/kg	5–15 mg/hr IV or 30–90 mg PO qid or 120–360 mg sustained release qd		Often well tolerated in low LVEF pts

Key: CHF, congestive heart failure; BP, blood pressure; AVN, atrioventricular node; AF, atrial fibrillation; COPD, chronic obstructive pulmonary disease; DM, diabetes mellitus; LVEF, left ventricular ejection fraction.
Source: Modified from Ref. 236.

Conventional cardioversion is performed as in nonpostoperative AF with monophasic or biphasic defibrillators via anteroposterior patches. A short-acting anesthetic, such as etomidate or methohexital, is administered prior to cardioversion. An R-wave synchronized shock is delivered usually at initial energies of 200 J for atrial fibrillation, 50 to 100 J for atrial flutter, or 25 to 100 J if a biphasic waveform is used. Anteroposterior patch positions (e.g., right parasternal–left paraspinal) are preferable for AF over the antero anterior positions (e.g., right parasternal–left apical), which are often used for ventricular defibrillation. Low-energy internal defibrillation has also been reported to be successful, using epicardial wire defibrillation electrodes placed during open heart surgery (182–185).

2. Pharmacological Antiarrhythmic Therapy

Trials testing the efficacy of class I or III antiarrhythmic drugs in the treatment of postoperative AF are summarized in Table 8. Pharmacological conversion can be attempted using intravenous or oral regimens. Reported efficacy and dosing regimens of antiarrhythmic agents used for the acute conversion of atrial fibrillation after cardiac surgery are summarized in Table 9. Antiarrhythmic drugs may be continued until a follow-up visit, typically at 4 to 6 weeks, particularly if atrial fibrillation is recurrent.

Agents with intravenous forms are used most commonly after surgery; these currently include procainamide, ibutilide, and amiodarone. Use of quinidine is limited by proarrhythmia concerns, particularly in the postoper-ative setting, in which patients may be prone to electrolyte imbalances due to diuresis or fluid shifts. Disopyramide use has also been limited by side effects, including urinary retention. Oral flecainide and propafenone are usually reserved for patients with no coronary artery disease and with normal ventricular function, but they may be useful in patients after valve surgery who fit these criteria. Oral sotalol can be used in patients who can tolerate beta blockade, but with close attention to QT intervals and electrolyte balance because of the risk of proarrhythmia.

Availability of intravenous and oral forms makes procainamide a typical first-line choice after rate control has been achieved. A loading dose of 10 to 15 mg/kg IV at ≤50 mg/min is followed by a continuous infusion of 1 to 2 mg/min. Oral sustained-release preparations can subsequently be used, typically at 2 to 4 g/day in two to four divided doses, depending on the preparation. Doses should be adjusted according to serum levels, which should be checked daily during intravenous dosing. Levels of N-acetyl-procainamide (NAPA), an active metabolite of procainamide, can accumu-late to toxic levels with renal dysfunction. Potential side effects include hypotension, QRS widening, and proarrhythmia, including QT prolongation

Table 8 Class I or III Antiarrhythmic Drug Trials for the Treatment of Postoperative Atrial Arrhythmias

Author	Year	N	Design	Drug regimen 1	Drug regimen 2	% Conversion Drug 1	% Conversion Drug 2	p Value	Comments
Gavaghan (225)	1985	156	NR	Disopyramide IV 2 mg/kg, then 0.4 mg/kg/h or PO 600 mg qd		48			93% converted by discharge; 19% with side effects
Hjelms (226)	1992	30	R	Procainamide IV 25 mg/min, max 15 mg/kg	Digoxin IV 0.75–1 mg	87	60	0.05	
McAlister (227)	1990	80	R, C	Quinidine PO 400 mg, then 400 mg in 4 hr prn	Amiodarone IV 5 mg/kg × 20'	64	41	0.04	More side effects with quinidine
Gentili (86)	1992	50	NR	Propafenone IV 2 mg/kg × 10'		70			
Connolly (193)	1987	14	R, DB, P, C	Propafenone 2 mg/kg over 10'	Control	43	0	<0.001	Decreased VR, BP with propafenone
Geelen (228)	1999	62	R, DB	Propafenone IV 2 mg/kg × 10'	Procainamide IV 20 mg/kg at 30 mg/min to 1000 mg	76	61	NS	Propafenone better at 15', procainamide ↑, propafenone ↓ VR
Di Biasi (229)	1995	84	R, DB	Propafenone IV 2 mg/kg 15' then 10 mg/kg × 24 hr prn	Amiodarone IV 5 mg/kg × 15', then 15 mg/kg × 24 hr prn	68.4	82.6	NS	↓ VR with both; Propafenone better in 1st hr
Larbuisson (230)	1996	40	R	Propafenone IV 1–2 mg/kg × 10', then 420 mg/24 hr	Amiodarone IV 2.5–5 mg/kg × 10', then 900 mg × 24 hr	67	77	NS	Propafenone effective earlier

Table 8 Continued

Author	Year	N	Design	Drug regimen 1	Drug regimen 2	% Conversion Drug 1	Drug 2	p Value	Comments
Soucier (178)	2003	42	R	Propafenone 600 mg PO Ibutilide 1 mg up to 2 doses	Rate control	35 100	66	NS 0.01	
Wafa (231)	1989	29	R	Flecainide IV 1 mg/kg × 10', 1.5 mg/kg/hr × 1 hr, 0.25 mg/kg/h × 23 hr	Digoxin 0.5 mg, then 0.25 mg q 6 hr × 2 doses	60	0	<0.01	
Gavaghan (232)	1988	56	R	Flecainide IV 2 mg/kg × 2', 0.2 mg/kg/h × 12 hr, then PO	Digoxin 0.75 mg IV, then after 2 hr disopyramide 2 mg/kg IV, 0.4mg/kg/hr × 10 hr	86	89	NS	Time to conversion shorter with flecainide; 1 death, intractable ventricular arrhythmia in patient with toxic flecainide, poor ventricular and hepatic function day 5
Campbell (233)	1985	40	R	Sotalol IV 1 mg/kg, then 0.2 mg/kg × 12 hr	Digoxin 0.75 mg IV, 2 hr later disopyramide 2 mg/kg IV, then 0.4 mg/kg/hr × 10 hr	85	85	NS	Drug 1 effective earlier; acute urinary retention with Drug 2
Installe (234)	1981	90	NR	Amiodarone IV 2.5–5 mg/kg IV		61			Hypotension in 18%, transient unless ↓ LV

Study	Year	N	Design	Treatment	Comparison			p	Comments
Cochrane (235)	1994	30	R, C	Amiodarone IV 5 mg/kg to 400 mg max over 30', then after 30' 25 mg/hr adjusted to 40 mg/hr if HR > 120 bpm until 24 hr after conversion to SR	Digoxin 0.5 mg IV × 30', 0.25 mg IV after 2 hr, 0.125 mg IV after 5 and 9 hr, then weight/renal adjusted PO after 12 hr	93	80	NS	Crossover to 1/2 dose alternate arm if in AF at 24 hr; 24 hr endpoint listed; 15/15 (100%) converted on amiodarone, 2 recurred, then converted on digoxin; 13 of 15 converted on digoxin, 3 recurred transiently
Frost (192)	1997	98	R, DB, P	Dofetilide IV × 15' 4 µg/kg 8 µg/kg	Placebo	36 44	24	0.27 0.11	Short runs aberrancy, VT: 9% at 8 µg/kg
VanderLugt (187)	1999	302	R, DB, P	Ibutilide 0.25 mg 0.5 mg 1 mg	Placebo	40 47 57	15	0.0001	
Bernard (188)	2003	40	R, DB	Ibutilide 0.008 mg/kg over 10 min For AF persisting >4 hr, added amiodarone 5 mg/kg over 30 min, then 15 mg/kg over 24 hr	Amiodarone 5 mg/kg over 30 min; then 15 mg/kg over 24 hr if AF persistent	45	50	NS	4-hr conversion rates

Key: N, number of patients; D, design; R, randomized; DB, double-blinded; P, placebo-controlled; C, crossover; BP, blood pressure; VR, ventricular rate; VT, ventricular tachycardia; LV, left ventricle.
Source: Modified from Ref. 235.

Table 9 Regimens for Pharmacological Conversion of Postoperative Atrial Arrhythmias

Drug	Route	Dose	Success rate	Adverse effects/comments
Quinidine	PO	400 mg, then 400 mg in 4 hr	64%	TdP, PMVT; GI side effects hypotension; enhanced AVN conduction; usually avoided postoperatively because of risk of proarrhythmia with diuresis/electrolyte imbalances
Disopyramide	IV	2 mg/kg, then 0.4 mg/kg/hr	48–85%	Urinary retention; enhanced AVN conduction; AFlutter 1:1; VT; hypotension, TdP
	PO	600 mg qd		
Procainamide	IV	1–1.5 g at 25–50 mg/min	61–87%	Fever; enhanced AVN conduction; accumulates in renal failure, TdP, PMVT
Propafenone	PO	600 mg	55–87%[a]	?Avoid in CAD, LV dysfunction
	IV	2 mg/kg over 10 min	43–76%	
Flecainide	PO	300 mg	90%[a]	Avoid in CAD, LV dysfunction
	IV	2 mg/kg over 10 min	65–90%	
	IV	1 mg/kg × 10′, 1.5 mg/kg/h × 1hr, 0.25 mg/kg/h × 23 hr	60%	

	IV	2 mg/kg × 2′, 0.2 mg/kg/hr × 12 hr	86%	
Amiodarone	IV	2.5–5 mg/kg IV over 20 min, 15 mg/kg over 24 hr; or 1.2 g over 24 hr	41–93%	Hypotension
Sotalol	PO	80–160 mg, then 160–360 mg/d	52%[a]	Bradycardia; hypotension; CHF; TdP
	IV	1 mg/kg, then 0.2 mg/kg × 12 hr	85%	
Dofetilide	IV	4–8 ug/kg over 15′	36–44%	TdP; VT; must adjust dose for renal function
	PO	125–500 µg bld	29–32%[a]	
Ibutilide	IV	1 mg over 10 min, repeat in 10′ if no conversion	57%	TdP; PMVT

Key: TdP, torsades de pointes; PMVT, polymorphic ventricular tachycardia; GI, gastrointestinal; AVN, atrioventricular node; AFlutter, atrial flutter; VT, ventricular tachycardia.

[a] Nonsurgical atrial arrhythmia studies.

Source: Modified from Ref. 235.

and torsades de pointes. Hemodynamic effects may be seen in patients with severe left ventricular dysfunction. Gastrointestinal problems can also be a limiting factor. Procainamide can also be a cause of postoperative fever (186). If the drug is continued long-term, arthralgias and a lupus-like syndrome may develop. However, if used only for postoperative atrial arrhythmias, procainamide often can be stopped by 4 to 6 weeks after surgery.

Intravenous ibutilide, a class III potassium channel blocker, may convert atrial arrhythmias after cardiac surgery, with success rates of up to 57% (187). One study showed ibutilide to be more efficacious than procainamide in the conversion of short-term atrial fibrillation/flutter (188). A randomized double-blind study of ibutilide and amiodarone after cardiac surgery showed similar conversion rates within 4 hr (45% ibutilide, 50% amiodarone) (189). Another study reported higher success rates for termination of atrial flutter using rapid atrial pacing with less acceleration to AF when using ibutilide or procainamide (190). Patients should be monitored for QT prolongation and torsades de pointes.

Intravenous amiodarone has frequently been used in postoperative patients. It may be particularly helpful in hemodynamically unstable patients, those with recurrent AF despite cardioversion or other antiarrhythmic drugs, those undergoing rate control but refractory to conventional AV-nodal blocking drugs, or patients intolerant to other standard antiarrhythmic or rate-controlling drugs that are negatively inotropic. Rapid oral loading can also usually be achieved in patients with intact gastrointestinal function (191).

Dofetilide, another class III antiarrhythmic agent, has been studied for termination of AF and atrial flutter after CABG. In a double-blind, placebo-controlled randomized trial of 98 patients, dofetilide 4 to 8 μg/kg intravenously converted 36 and 44% of patients to sinus rhythm within 3 hr, compared to 24% on placebo (192). Although short episodes of aberrancy and ventricular tachycardia occurred in 3 patients, dofetilide was generally well tolerated and no torsades de pointes was reported. Dosage should be reduced if renal dysfunction is present.

Intravenous propafenone has been studied for postoperative atrial arrhythmias, although it is not available in this form in the United States (86,193). Earlier times to conversion compared to intravenous amiodarone or procainamide and contribution to ventricular rate control have been reported.

D. Recurrent Atrial Fibrillation

Recurrent AF may be treated with a trial of a different antiarrhythmic drug, such as sotalol or amiodarone, or—in the absence of coronary artery disease or ventricular dysfunction—propafenone or flecainide, followed by repeat electrical cardioversion. Alternatively, if the arrhythmia is well tolerated, the patient may be discharged on anticoagulation followed by another attempt at cardioversion after recovery from surgery, often at 4 to 6 weeks. Patients who maintain sinus rhythm with the aid of an antiarrhythmic drug may be discharged on that medication, which may be discontinued at the 4- to 6-week follow-up visit if there is no evidence of recurrence.

E. Atrial Flutter

The management of postoperative atrial flutter presents special challenges, since medical treatment is often ineffective. Patients undergoing valve repair or replacement, particularly of the mitral valve, associated with right or left atriotomies, may be particularly prone to incisional atrial flutters. Electrical cardioversion or rapid atrial pacing via transthoracic epicardial wires has been successfully employed acutely (194). For recurrent typical atrial flutter, catheter ablation of the posterior right atrial isthmus between the tricuspid annulus and inferior vena cava has been successful in long-term management of isthmus-dependent atrial flutter (195). Catheter ablation with mapping has also been successful for recurrent scar or incisional atrial flutters.

F. Anticoagulation

As in nonsurgical AF, anticoagulation is an essential consideration for patients with postoperative AF, particularly those in whom AF persists > 48 hr or continues to recur after cardioversion. AF is known to increase the risk of stroke in nonsurgical settings as well as in the postoperative state (5,80,81). The available evidence favors anticoagulation if AF persists longer than 48 hr, particularly if cardioversion is anticipated after this time (196,197). Heparin may be used, but may not be feasible in the immediate postoperative period. During the subacute period after surgery, initiation of oral warfarin (target INR 2.0 to 3.0) without intravenous heparin may be preferred by some surgeons. However, data supporting the use of anticoagulation in the postoperative period are lacking.

The role of left atrial appendage resection, ligation, stapling, or occlusion is being studied (198,199). However, for postoperative patients who have undergone this type of procedure, data remain sparse in demonstrating any lower risk of thromboembolism or stroke or to support the ability to forego anticoagulation in these patients (200).

VII. VALVULAR SURGERY

Postoperative arrhythmias after valvular surgery have been less well studied than arrhythmias after CABG. In a prospective study of 50 consecutive patients undergoing cardiac valve replacement, AF was the most common postoperative arrhythmia, occurring in 21 of 66 arrhythmic episodes (32%) (201). Supraventricular arrhythmias were more common after mitral valve replacement than after aortic valve replacement (73 vs. 43%). In a study of 70 patients undergoing cardiac surgery, AF occurred in 9 of 15 patients (60%) undergoing valve surgery, whereas it occurred in only 19 of 50 patients (38%) undergoing CABG (p = NS) (202). The reported incidence of postoperative AF after valve surgery ranges from 37 to 64% (5,10,202), and many valve patients have persistent AF prior to surgery.

Predictors of AF after valve surgery have not been as well delineated as after CABG. However, one of the strongest independent predictors of postoperative AF after valve surgery is again age (203). The highest postoperative atrial arrhythmia incidence has been reported after combination of CABG with carotid endarterectomy (60.0%), aortic valve replacement (60.1%), mitral valve repair (62.2%), or mitral valve replacement (63.6%) (5). Other predictors have included mitral stenosis, left atrial enlargement, use of systemic hypothermia, prior surgery, prior paroxysmal AF, postoperative electrolyte imbalance, and presence of frequent atrial ectopy (10,203,204).

A trend toward a decrease in incidence of AF after minimally invasive valve surgery has been reported compared to conventional mitral valve surgery (26.3% minimally invasive vs. 38.0% midline sternotomy, p = 0.08) (57,59). No difference in AF incidence has been reported after left atrial vs. extended transseptal approaches to mitral valve surgery (205).

Patients with valvular disease may be more difficult to maintain in sinus rhythm. Recurrence or persistence of AF was observed frequently in a retrospective study of 376 patients referred to an early postoperative rehabilitation program and in a prospective study of 232 patients who underwent valve procedures (206). AF persisted in 9% of the study population. Postdischarge AF occurred more frequently in patients who were older, had enlarged left atria, and had lower left ventricular ejection fraction; it was less frequent in patients taking beta blockers. One early study suggested that success in maintaining sinus rhythm is limited when the duration of AF is greater than 3 years or the left atrial size is more than 5.2 cm (207). However, achievement and maintenance of sinus rhythm can often be obtained with a reasonable expectation of success after valve surgery (208).

An issue in patients with valvular heart disease is whether it is worthwhile to attempt to restore sinus rhythm after valve replacement or repair in those with chronic persistent AF preoperatively. In 40 patients with pure mitral stenosis and chronic AF who underwent mitral valve replacement or commissurotomy, DC cardioversion with quinidine or disopyramide was performed less than 6 months after surgery (207). Twenty-four patients (60%) remained in sinus rhythm for more than 3 months after cardioversion and were therefore considered successes. These patients were younger (mean 38 vs. 47 years), had symptoms for a shorter period of time (3.0 vs 6.4 years), and had a smaller preoperative left atrial size (4.9 vs. 5.5 cm) by echocardiography. Following multivariate analysis, the authors concluded that for patients with preoperative left atrial sizes of >5.2 cm and symptoms for more than 3 years, the likelihood of successful cardioversion was too low to justify any attempt. In a more recent study (209), the probability of return to sinus rhythm after mitral valve repair was 94% when sinus rhythm was present preoperatively and 80% when AF was intermittent or less than 1 year's duration, but markedly lower for durations over 1 year. Postoperative return to sinus rhythm was associated with better 1- and 4-year survival compared to postoperative AF.

Late recurrence of AF after mitral valve repair was studied in 189 patients, 72 with preoperative chronic or paroxysmal AF followed for 12.2 ± 10 years (210). Predictors of late AF included older age, preoperative AF, preoperative antiarrhythmic drug treatment, elevated pulmonary artery pressure and heart rate, and low left ventricular ejection fraction. The authors suggested that patients with these risk factors might be candidates for combined mitral valve repair and surgery for AF (e.g., Maze operation; intraoperative pulmonary vein isolation). Other groups have also reported successful use of concomitant Maze surgery or intraoperative pulmonary vein isolation for patients undergoing valve surgery with a history of significant preoperative significant paroxysmal or persistent AF (211–214).

REFERENCES

1. Goldman L. Supraventricular tachyarrhythmias in hospitalized adults after surgery. Clinical correlates in patients over 40 years of age after major noncardiac surgery. Chest 1978; 73(4):450–454.
2. Nielsen J, Sorensen H, Alstrup P. Atrial fibrillation following thoracotomy for non-cardiac diseases, in particular cancer of the lung. Acta Med Scand 1973; 193:425–429.
3. Dyszkiewicz W, Skrzypczak M. Atrial fibrillation after surgery of the lung: clinical analysis of risk factors. Eur J Cardiothorac Surg 1998; 13(6):625–628.
4. Vecht RJ, Nicolaides EP, Ikweuke JK, Liassides C, Cleary J, Cooper WB. Incidence and prevention of supraventricular tachyarrhythmias after coronary bypass surgery. Int J Cardiol 1986; 13(2):125–134.
5. Creswell LL, Schuessler RB, Rosenbloom M, Cox JL. Hazards of postoperative atrial arrhythmias. Ann Thorac Surg 1993; 56(3):539–549.
6. Leitch JW, Thomson D, Baird DK, Harris PJ. The importance of age as a predictor of atrial fibrillation and flutter after coronary artery bypass grafting. J Thorac Cardiovasc Surg 1990; 100(3):338–342.

7. Fuller JA, Adams GG, Buxton B. Atrial fibrillation after coronary artery bypass grafting. Is it a disorder of the elderly? J Thorac Cardiovasc Surg 1989; 97(6):821–825.

8. Aranki SF, Shaw DP, Adams DH, et al. Predictors of atrial fibrillation after coronary artery surgery. Current trends and impact on hospital resources. Circulation 1996; 94(3):390–397.

9. Maisel WH, Rawn JD, Stevenson WG. Atrial fibrillation after cardiac surgery. Ann Intern Med 2001; 135(12):1061–1073.

10. Asher CR, Miller DP, Grimm RA, Cosgrove DM III, Chung MK. Analysis of risk factors for development of atrial fibrillation early after cardiac valvular surgery. Am J Cardiol 1998; 82(7):892–895.

11. Haissaguerre M, Jais P, Shah DC, et al. Spontaneous initiation of atrial fibrillation by ectopic beats originating in the pulmonary veins. N Engl J Med 1998; 339(10):659–666.

12. Saad EB, Saliba WI, Marrouche NF, Natale A. Pulmonary vein firing triggering atrial fibrillation after open heart surgery. J Cardiovasc Electrophysiol 2002; 13(12):1300–1302.

13. Bush HL Jr, Gelband H, Hoffman BF, Malm JR. Electrophysiological basis for supraventricular arrhythmias: following surgical procedures for aortic stenosis. Arch Surg 1971; 103(5):620–625.

14. Buxton AE, Josephson ME. The role of P wave duration as a predictor of postoperative atrial arrhythmias. Chest 1981; 80(1):68–73.

15. Tamis JE, Steinberg JS. Value of the signal-averaged P wave analysis in predicting atrial fibrillation after cardiac surgery. J Electrocardiol 1998; 30(suppl):36–43.

16. Lowe JE, Hendry PJ, Hendrickson SC, Wells R. Intraoperative identification of cardiac patients at risk to develop postoperative atrial fibrillation. Ann Surg 1991; 213(5):388–391. discussion 391–382.

17. Mathew JP, Parks R, Savino JS, et al. Atrial fibrillation following coronary artery bypass graft surgery: predictors, outcomes, and resource utilization. MultiCenter Study of Perioperative Ischemia Research Group. JAMA 1996; 276(4):300–306.

18. Frost L, Molgaard H, Christiansen EH, Hjortholm K, Paulsen PK, Thomsen PE. Atrial fibrillation and flutter after coronary artery bypass surgery: epidemiology, risk factors and preventive trials. Int J Cardiol 1992; 36(3):253–261.

19. Kecskemeti V, Kelemen K, Solti F, Szabo Z. Physiological and pharmacological analysis of transmembrane action potentials of human atrial fibers. Adv Myocardiol 1985; 6:37–47.

20. Hogue CW Jr, Domitrovich PP, Stein PK, et al. RR interval dynamics before atrial fibrillation in patients after coronary artery bypass graft surgery. Circulation 1998; 98(5):429–434.

21. Dimmer C, Tavernier R, Gjorgov N, Van Nooten G, Clement DL, Jordaens L. Variations of autonomic tone preceding onset of atrial fibrillation after coronary artery bypass grafting. Am J Cardiol 1998; 82(1):22–25.

22. Pichlmaier AM, Lang V, Harringer W, Heublein B, Schaldach M, Haverich A. Prediction of the onset of atrial fibrillation after cardiac surgery using the monophasic action potential. Heart 1998; 80(5):467–472.

23. Tittelbach V, Schwab M, Vollf JN, et al. Atrial fibrillation after coronary artery bypass surgery: association with changes in G protein levels in mononuclear leukocytes. Naunyn Schmiedebergs Arch Pharmacol 1999; 359(3):204–211.

24. Sato S, Yamauchi S, Schuessler RB, Boineau JP, Matsunaga Y, Cox JL. The effect of augmented atrial hypothermia on atrial refractory period, conduction, and atrial flutter/fibrillation in the canine heart. J Thorac Cardiovasc Surg 1992; 104(2):297–306.

25. Smith PK, Buhrman WC, Levett JM, Ferguson TB Jr, Holman WL, Cox JL. Supraventricular conduction abnormalities following cardiac operations. A complication of inadequate atrial preservation. J Thorac Cardiovasc Surg 1983; 85(1):105–115.

26. Tchervenkov CI, Wynands JE, Symes JF, Malcolm ID, Dobell AR, Morin JE. Persistent atrial activity during cardioplegic arrest: a possible factor in the etiology of postoperative supraventricular tachyarrhythmias. Ann Thorac Surg 1983; 36(4):437–443.

27. St Rammos K, Koullias GJ, Hassan MO, et al. Low preoperative HSP70 atrial myocardial levels correlate significantly with high incidence of postoperative atrial fibrillation after cardiac surgery. Cardiovasc Surg 2002; 10(3):228–232.

28. Bruins P, te Velthuis H, Yazdanbakhsh AP, et al. Activation of the complement system during and after cardiopulmonary bypass surgery: postsurgery activation involves C-reactive protein and is associated with postoperative arrhythmia. Circulation 1997; 96(10):3542–3548.

29. Angelini GD, Penny WJ, el-Ghamary F, et al. The incidence and significance of early pericardial effusion after open heart surgery. Eur J Cardiothorac Surg 1987; 1(3):165–168.

30. Mayr A, Knotzer H, Pajk W, et al. Risk factors associated with new onset tachyarrhythmias after cardiac surgery—a retrospective analysis. Acta Anaesthesiol Scand 2001; 45(5):543–549.

31. Van Wagoner DR, Pond AL, Lamorgese M, Rossie SS, McCarthy PM, Nerbonne JM. Atrial L-type Ca^{2+} currents and human atrial fibrillation. Circ Res 1999; 85(5):428–436.

32. Dobrev D, Wettwer E, Kortner A, Knaut M, Schuler S, Ravens U. Human inward rectifier potassium channels in chronic and postoperative atrial fibrillation. Cardiovasc Res 2002; 54(2):397–404.

33. Dupont E, Ko Y, Rothery S, et al. The gap-junctional protein connexin40 is elevated in patients susceptible to postoperative atrial fibrillation. Circulation 2001; 103(6):842–849.

34. Hashimoto K, Ilstrup DM, Schaff HV. Influence of clinical and hemodynamic variables on risk of supraventricular tachycardia after coronary artery bypass. J Thorac Cardiovasc Surg 1991; 101(1):56–65.

35. Dixon FE, Genton E, Vacek JL, Moore CB, Landry J. Factors predisposing to

supraventricular tachyarrhythmias after coronary artery bypass grafting. Am J Cardiol 1986; 58(6):476–478.

36. Nakai T, Lee RJ, Schiller NB, et al. The relative importance of left atrial function versus dimension in predicting atrial fibrillation after coronary artery bypass graft surgery. Am Heart J 2002; 143(1):181–186.

37. Kolvekar S, D'Souza A, Akhtar P, et al. Role of atrial ischaemia in development of atrial fibrillation following coronary artery bypass surgery. Eur J Cardiothorac Surg 1997; 11(1):70–75.

38. Loponen P, Taskinen P, Laakkonen E, et al. Peripheral vascular disease as predictor of outcome after coronary artery bypass grafting. Scand J Surg 2002; 91(2):160–165.

39. Mooe T, Gullsby S, Rabben T, Eriksson P. Sleep-disordered breathing: a novel predictor of atrial fibrillation after coronary artery bypass surgery. Coron Artery Dis 1996; 7(6):475–478.

40. Mendes LA, Connelly GP, McKenney PA, et al. Right coronary artery stenosis: an independent predictor of atrial fibrillation after coronary artery bypass surgery. J Am Coll Cardiol 1995; 25(1):198–202.

41. Pehkonen E. Rhythm and conduction disturbances after coronary artery bypass grafting. The role of ischemia and myocardial protection. Ann Chir Gynaecol 1998; 87(1):83.

42. Terada Y, Mitsui T, Matsushita S, et al. Atrial fibrillation after coronary artery bypass grafting. An increase in high-frequency atrial activity in patients with right coronary artery revascularization. Jpn J Thorac Cardiovasc Surg 1999; 47(1):6–13.

43. Hammon JW Jr, Wood AJ, Prager RL, Wood M, Muirhead J, Bender HW Jr. Perioperative beta blockade with propranolol: reduction in myocardial oxygen demands and incidence of atrial and ventricular arrhythmias. Ann Thorac Surg 1984; 38(4):363–367.

44. Salazar C, Frishman W, Friedman S, et al. beta-Blockade therapy for supraventricular tachyarrhythmias after coronary surgery: a propranolol withdrawal syndrome? Angiology 1979; 30(12):816–819.

45. Chang CM, Lee SH, Lu MJ, et al. The role of P wave in prediction of atrial fibrillation after coronary artery surgery. Int J Cardiol 1999; 68(3):303–308.

46. Steinberg JS, Zelenkofske S, Wong SC, Gelernt M, Sciacca R, Menchavez E. Value of the P-wave signal-averaged ECG for predicting atrial fibrillation after cardiac surgery. Circulation 1993; 88(6):2618–2622.

47. Klein M, Evans SJ, Blumberg S, Cataldo L, Bodenheimer MM. Use of P-wave-triggered, P-wave signal-averaged electrocardiogram to predict atrial fibrillation after coronary artery bypass surgery. Am Heart J 1995; 129(5):895–901.

48. Zaman AG, Alamgir F, Richens T, Williams R, Rothman MT, Mills PG. The role of signal averaged P wave duration and serum magnesium as a combined predictor of atrial fibrillation after elective coronary artery bypass surgery. Heart 1997; 77(6):527–531.

49. Stafford PJ, Kolvekar S, Cooper J, et al. Signal averaged P wave compared

with standard electrocardiography or echocardiography for prediction of atrial fibrillation after coronary bypass grafting. Heart 1997; 77(5):417–422.

50. Dimmer C, Jordaens L, Gorgov N, et al. Analysis of the P wave with signal averaging to assess the risk of atrial fibrillation after coronary artery bypass surgery. Cardiology 1998; 89(1):19–24.

51. Aytemir K, Aksoyek S, Ozer N, Aslamaci S, Oto A. Atrial fibrillation after coronary artery bypass surgery: P wave signal averaged ECG, clinical and angiographic variables in risk assessment. Int J Cardiol 1999; 69(1):49–56.

52. Hakala T, Berg E, Hartikainen JE, Hippelainen MJ. Intraoperative high-rate atrial pacing test as a predictor of atrial fibrillation after coronary artery bypass surgery. Ann Thorac Surg 2002; 74(6):2072–2075.

53. Frost L, Lund B, Pilegaard H, Christiansen EH. Re-evaluation of the role of P-wave duration and morphology as predictors of atrial fibrillation and flutter after coronary artery bypass surgery. Eur Heart J 1996; 17(7):1065–1071.

54. England MR, Gordon G, Salem M, Chernow B. Magnesium administration and dysrhythmias after cardiac surgery. A placebo-controlled, double-blind, randomized trial. JAMA 1992; 268(17):2395–2402.

55. Abreu JE, Reilly J, Salzano RP, Khachane VB, Jekel JF, Clyne CA. Comparison of frequencies of atrial fibrillation after coronary artery bypass grafting with and without the use of cardiopulmonary bypass. Am J Cardiol 1999; 83(5):775–776, A779.

56. Kilger E, Weis FC, Goetz AE, et al. Intensive care after minimally invasive and conventional coronary surgery: a prospective comparison. Intens Care Med 2001; 27(3):534–539.

57. Asher CR, DiMengo JM, Arheart KL, et al. Atrial fibrillation early postoperatively following minimally invasive cardiac valvular surgery. Am J Cardiol 1999; 84(6):744–747, A749.

58. Cohn LH, Adams DH, Couper GS, et al. Minimally invasive cardiac valve surgery improves patient satisfaction while reducing costs of cardiac valve replacement and repair. Ann Surg 1997; 226(4):421–426. discussion 427–428.

59. Cohn LH. Minimally invasive valve surgery. J Card Surg 2001; 16(3):260–265.

60. Stamou SC, Dangas G, Hill PC, et al. Atrial fibrillation after beating heart surgery. Am J Cardiol 2000; 86(1):64–67.

61. Angelini GD, Taylor FC, Reeves BC, Ascione R. Early and midterm outcome after off-pump and on-pump surgery in Beating Heart Against Cardioplegic Arrest Studies (BHACAS 1 and 2): a pooled analysis of two randomised controlled trials. Lancet 2002; 359(9313):1194–1199.

62. Zamvar VY, Khan NU, Madhavan A, Kulatilake N, Butchart EG. Clinical outcomes in coronary artery bypass graft surgery: comparison of off-pump and on-pump techniques. Heart Surg Forum 2002; 5(2):109–113.

63. Van Belleghem Y, Caes F, Maene L, Van Overbeke H, Moerman A, Van Nooten G. Off-pump coronary surgery: surgical strategy for the high-risk patient. Cardiovasc Surg 2003; 11(1):75–79.

64. Saatvedt K, Fiane AE, Sellevold O, Nordstrand K. Is atrial fibrillation caused by extracorporeal circulation? Ann Thorac Surg 1999; 68(3):931–933.

65. Lancey RA, Soller BR, Vander Salm TJ. Off-pump versus on-pump coronary artery bypass surgery: a case-matched comparison of clinical outcomes and costs. Heart Surg Forum 2000; 3(4):277–281.
66. Siebert J, Rogowski J, Jagielak D, Anisimowicz L, Lango R, Narkiewicz M. Atrial fibrillation after coronary artery bypass grafting without cardiopulmonary bypass. Eur J Cardiothorac Surg 2000; 17(5):520–523.
67. Chavanon O, Durand M, Hacini R, et al. Coronary artery bypass grafting with left internal mammary artery and right gastroepiploic artery, with and without bypass. Ann Thorac Surg 2002; 73(2):499–504.
68. Cartier R. Current trends and technique in OPCAB surgery. J Card Surg 2003; 18(1):32–46.
69. Siebert J, Lewicki L, Mlodnicki M, et al. Atrial fibrillation after conventional and off-pump coronary artery bypass grafting: two opposite trends in timing of atrial fibrillation occurrence? Med Sci Monit 2003; 9(3):CR137–CR141.
70. Brandt M, Harringer W, Hirt SW, et al. Influence of bicaval anastomoses on late occurrence of atrial arrhythmia after heart transplantation. Ann Thorac Surg 1997; 64(1):70–72.
71. Salem Bl, Chaudhry A, Haikal M, et al. Sustained supraventricular tachyarrhythmias following coronary artery bypass surgery comparing mammary versus saphenous vein grafts. Angiology 1991; 42(6):441–446.
72. Jensen BM, Alstrup P, Klitgard NA. Postoperative arrhythmias and myocardial electrolytes in patients undergoing coronary artery bypass grafting. Scand J Thorac Cardiovasc Surg 1996; 30(3–4):133–140.
73. Wahr JA, Parks R, Boisvert D, et al. Preoperative serum potassium levels and perioperative outcomes in cardiac surgery patients. Mutticenter Study of Perioperative Ischemia Research Group. JAMA 1999; 281(23):2203–2210.
74. Aglio LS, Stanford GG, Maddi R, Boyd JLd, Nussbaum S, Chernow B. Hypomagnesemia is common following cardiac surgery. J Cardiothorac Vasc Anesth 1991; 5(3):201–208.
75. Engelman RM, Haag B, Lemeshow S, Angelo A, Rousou JH. Mechanism of plasma catecholamine increases during coronary artery bypass and valve procedures. J Thorac Cardiovasc Surg 1983; 86(4):608–615.
76. Mohr R, Smolinsky A, Goor DA. Prevention of supraventricular tachyarrhythmia with low-dose propranolol after coronary bypass. J Thorac Cardiovasc Surg 1981; 81(6):840–845.
77. Daudon P, Corcos T, Gandjbakhch I, Levasseur JP, Cabrol A, Cabrol C. Prevention of atrial fibrillation or flutter by acebutolol after coronary bypass grafting. Am J Cardiol 1986; 58(10):933–936.
78. Rubin DA, Nieminski KE, Reed GE, Herman MV. Predictors, prevention, and long-term prognosis of atrial fibrillation after coronary artery bypass graft operations. J Thorac Cardiovasc Surg 1987; 94(3):331–335.
79. Crosby LH, Pifalo WB, Woll KR, Burkholder JA. Risk factors for atrial fibrillation after coronary artery bypass grafting. Am J Cardiol 1990; 66(20):1520–1522.
80. Taylor GJ, Malik SA, Colliver JA, et al. Usefulness of atrial fibrillation as a

predictor of stroke after isolated coronary artery bypass grafting. Am J Cardiol 1987; 60(10):905–907.

81. Reed GLD, Singer DE, Picard EH, DeSanctis RW. Stroke following coronary-artery bypass surgery. A case-control estimate of the risk from carotid bruits. N Engl J Med 1988; 319(19):1246–1250.

82. Almassi GH, Schowalter T, Nicolosi AC, et al. Atrial fibrillation after cardiac surgery: a major morbid event? Ann Surg 1997; 226(4):501–511. discussion 511–503.

83. D'Agostino RS, Svensson LG, Neumann DJ, Balkhy HH, Williamson WA, Shahian DM. Screening carotid ultrasonography and risk factors for stroke in coronary artery surgery patients. Ann Thorac Surg 1996; 62(6):1714–1723.

84. Stanley TO, Mackensen GB, Grocott HP, et al. The impact of postoperative atrial fibrillation on neurocognitive outcome after coronary artery bypass graft surgery. Anesth Analg 2002; 94(2):290–295.

85. Hogue CW Jr, Murphy SF, Schechtman KB, Davila-Roman VG. Risk factors for early or delayed stroke after cardiac surgery. Circulation 1999; 100(6):642–647.

86. Gentili C, Giordano F, Alois A, Massa E, Bianconi L. Efficacy of intravenous propafenone in acute atrial fibrillation complicating open-heart surgery. Am Heart J 1992; 123(5):1225–1228.

87. Yilmaz AT, Demirkilic U, Arstan M, et al. Long-term prevention of atrial fibrillation after coronary artery bypass surgery: comparison of quinidine, verapamil, and amiodarone in maintaining sinus rhythm. J Card Surg 1996; 11(1):61–64.

88. Yilmaz AT, Demirkilic U, Kuralay E, et al. Long-term prevention of atrial fibrillation after coronary artery surgery. Panminerva Med 1997; 39(2):103–105.

89. Loubani M, Hickey MS, Spyt TJ, Galinanes M. Residual atrial fibrillation and clinical consequences following postoperative supraventricular arrhythmias. Int J Cardiol 2000; 74(2–3):125–132.

90. Brathwaite D, Weissman C. The new onset of atrial arrhythmias following major noncardiothoracic surgery is associated with increased mortality. Chest 1998; 114(2):462–468.

91. Borzak S, Tisdale JE, Amin NB, et al. Atrial fibrillation after bypass surgery: does the arrhythmia or the characteristics of the patients prolong hospital stay? Chest 1998; 113(6):1489–1491.

92. Kim MH, Deeb GM, Morady F, et al. Effect of postoperative atrial fibrillation on length of stay after cardiac surgery (The Postoperative Atrial Fibrillation in Cardiac Surgery study [PACS(2)]. Am J Cardiol 2001; 87(7):881–885.

93. Paone G, Higgins RS, Havstad SL, Silverman NA. Does age limit the effectiveness of clinical pathways after coronory artery bypass graft surgery? Circulation 1998; 98(suppl 19):II41–II45.

94. Kowey PR, Taylor JE, Rials SJ, Marinchak RA. Meta-analysis of the effectiveness of prophylactic drug therapy in preventing supraventricular arrhythmia early after coronary artery bypass grafting. Am J Cardiol 1992; 69(9):963–965.

95. Chee TP, Prakash NS, Desser KB, Benchimol A. Postoperative supraventricular arrhythmias and the role of prophylactic digoxin in cardiac surgery. Am Heart J 1982; 104(5 Pt 1):974–977.

96. Weiner B, Rheinlander HF, Decker EL, Cleveland RJ. Digoxin prophylaxis following coronary artery bypass surgery. Clin Pharm 1986; 5(1):55–58.

97. Csicsko JF, Schatzlein MH, King RD. Immediate postoperative digitalization in the prophylaxis of supraventricular arrhythmias following coronary artery bypass. J Thorac Cardiovasc Surg 1981; 81(3):419–422.

98. Johnson LW, Dickstein RA, Fruehan CT, et al. Prophylactic digitalization for coronary artery bypass surgery. Circulation 1976; 53(5):819–822.

99. Tyras DH, Stothert JC Jr, Kaiser GC, Barner HB, Codd JE, Willman VL. Supraventricular tachyarrhythmias after myocardial revascularization: a randomized trial of prophylactic digitalization. J Thorac Cardiovasc Surg 1979; 77(2):310–314.

100. Parker FB Jr, Greiner-Hayes C, Bove EL, Marvasti MA, Johnson LW, Eich RH. Supraventricular arrhythmias following coronary artery bypass. The effect of preoperative digitalis. J Thorac Cardiovasc Surg 1983; 86(4):594–600.

101. Andrews TC, Reimold SC, Berlin JA, Antman EM. Prevention of supraventricular arrhythmias after coronary artery bypass surgery. A meta-analysis of randomized control trials. Circulation 1991; 84(suppl 5):III236–III244.

102. Silverman NA, Wright R, Levitsky S. Efficacy of low-dose propranolol in preventing postoperative supraventricular tachyarrhythmias: a prospective, randomized study. Ann Surg 1982; 196(2):194–197.

103. Matangi MF, Neutze JM, Graham KJ, Hill DG, Kerr AR, Barratt-Boyes BG. Arrhythmia prophylaxis after aorta-coronary bypass. The effect of minidose propranolol. J Thorac Cardiovasc Surg 1985; 89(3):439–443.

104. Stephenson LW, MacVaugh Hd, Tomasello DN, Josephson ME. Propranolol for prevention of postoperative cardiac arrhythmias: a randomized study. Ann Thorac Surg 1980; 29(2):113–116.

105. Khuri SF, Okike ON, Josa M, et al. Efficacy of nadolol in preventing supraventricular tachycardia after coronary artery bypass grafting. Am J Cardiol 1987; 60(6):51D–58D.

106. Abel RM, van Gelder HM, Pores IH, Liguori J, Gielchinsky I, Parsonnet V. Continued propranolol administration following coronary bypass surgery. Antiarrhythmic effects. Arch Surg 1983; 118(6):727–731.

107. Kowey PR, Dalessandro DA, Herbertson R, et al. Effectiveness of digitalis with or without acebutolol in preventing atrial arrhythmias after coronary artery surgery. Am J Cardiol 1997; 79(8):1114–1117.

108. Ivey MF, Ivey TD, Bailey WW, Williams DB, Hessel EAd, Miller DW Jr. Influence of propranolol on supraventricular tachycardia early after coronary artery revascularization. A randomized trial. J Thorac Cardiovasc Surg 1983; 85(2):214–218.

109. Crystal E, Connolly SJ, Sleik K, Ginger TJ, Yusuf S. Interventions on prevention of postoperative atrial fibrillation in patients undergoing heart surgery: a meta-analysis. Circulation 2002; 106(1):75–80.

110. Roffman JA, Fieldman A. Digoxin and propranolol in the prophylaxis of

supraventricular tachydysrhythmias after coronary artery bypass surgery. Ann Thorac Surg 1981; 31(6):496–501.

111. Mills SA, Poole GV Jr, Breyer RH, et al. Digoxin and propranolol in the prophylaxis of dysrhythmias after coronary artery bypass grafting. Circulation 1983; 68(3 Pt 2):II222–II225.

112. Davison R, Hartz R, Kaplan K, Parker M, Feiereisel P, Michaelis L. Prophylaxis of supraventricular tachyarrhythmia after coronary bypass surgery with oral verapamil: a randomized, double-blind trial. Ann Thorac Surg 1985; 39(4):336–339.

113. Smith EE, Shore DF, Monro JL, Ross JK. Oral verapamil fails to prevent supraventricular tachycardia following coronary artery surgery. Int J Cardiol 1985; 9(1):37–44.

114. Van Mieghem W, Tits G, Demuynck K, et al. Verapamil as prophylactic treatment for atrial fibrillation after lung operations. Ann Thorac Surg 1996; 61(4):1083–1085. discussion 1086.

115. Seitelberger R, Hannes W, Gleichauf M, Keilich M, Christoph M, Fasol R. Effects of diltiazem on perioperative ischemia, arrhythmias, and myocardial function in patients undergoing elective coronary bypass grafting. J Thorac Cardiovasc Surg 1994; 107(3):811–821.

116. el-Sadek M, Krause E. Postoperative antiarrhythmic effects of diltiazem in patients undergoing coronary bypass grafting. Cardiology 1994; 85(5):290–297.

117. Laub GW, Janeira L, Muralidharan S, et al. Prophylactic procainamide for prevention of atrial fibrillation after coronary artery bypass grafting: a prospective, double-blind, randomized, placebo-controlled pilot study. Crit Care Med 1993; 21(10):1474–1478.

118. Gold MR, O'Gara PT, Buckley MJ, DeSanctis RW. Efficacy and safety of procainamide in preventing arrhythmias after coronary artery bypass surgery. Am J Cardiol 1996; 78(9):975–979.

119. McCarty RJ, Jahnke EJ, Walker WJ. Ineffectiveness of quinidine in preventing atrial fibrillation following mitral valvotomy. Circulation 1966; 34(5):792–794.

120. Echt DS, Liebson PR, Mitchell LB, et al. Mortality and morbidity in patients receiving encainide, flecainide, or placebo. The Cardiac Arrhythmia Suppression Trial. N Engl J Med 1991; 324(12):781–788.

121. Merrick AF, Odom NJ, Keenan DJ, Grotte GJ. Comparison of propafenone to atenolol for the prophylaxis of postcardiotomy supraventricular tachyarrhythmias: a prospective trial. Eur J Cardiothorac Surg 1995; 9(3):146–149.

122. Borgeat A, Petropoulos P, Cavin R, Biollaz J, Munafo A, Schwander D. Prevention of arrhythmias after noncardiac thoracic operations: flecainide versus digoxin. Ann Thorac Surg 1991; 51(6):964–967 (discussion 967–968).

123. Suttorp MJ, Kingma JH, Peels HO, et al. Effectiveness of sotalol in preventing supraventricular tachyarrhythmias shortly after coronary artery bypass grafting. Am J Cardiol 1991; 68(11):1163–1169.

124. Gomes JA, Ip J, Santoni-Rugiu F, et al. Oral d,l sotalol reduces the incidence of postoperative atrial fibrillation in coronary artery bypass surgery patients: a randomized, double-blind, placebo-controlled study. J Am Coll Cardiol 1999; 34(2):334–339.

125. Nystrom U, Edvardsson N, Berggren H, Pizzarelli GP, Radegran K. Oral sotalol reduces the incidence of atrial fibrillation after coronary artery bypass surgery. Thorac Cardiovasc Surg 1993; 41(1):34–37.

126. Pfisterer ME, Kloter-Weber UC, Huber M, et al. Prevention of supraventricular tachyarrhythmias after open heart operation by low-dose sotalol: a prospective, double-blind, randomized, placebo-controlled study. Ann Thorac Surg 1997; 64(4):1113–1119.

127. Parikka H, Toivonen L, Heikkila L, Virtanen K, Jarvinen A. Comparison of sotalol and metoprolol in the prevention of atrial fibrillation after coronary artery bypass surgery. J Cardiovasc Pharmacol 1998; 31(1):67–73.

128. Suttorp MJ, Kingma JH, Tjon Joe Gin RM, et al. Efficacy and safety of low- and high-dose sotalol versus propranolol in the prevention of supraventricular tachyarrhythmias early after coronary artery bypass operations. J Thorac Cardiovasc Surg 1990; 100(6):921–926.

129. Forlani S, De Paulis R, de Notaris S, et al. Combination of sotalol and magnesium prevents atrial fibrillation after coronary artery bypass grafting. Ann Thorac Surg 2002; 74(3):720–725. discussion 725–726.

130. Jacquet L, Evenepoel M, Marenne F, et al. Hemodynamic effects and safety of sotalol in the prevention of supraventricular arrhythmias after coronary artery bypass surgery. J Cardiothorac Vasc Anesth 1994; 8(4):431–436.

131. Hohnloser SH, Meinertz T, Dammbacher T, et al. Electrocardiographic and antiarrhythmic effects of intravenous amiodarone: results of a prospective, placebo-controlled study. Am Heart J 1991; 121(1 Pt 1):89–95.

132. Butler J, Harriss DR, Sinclair M, Westaby S. Amiodarone prophylaxis for tachycardias after coronary artery surgery: a randomised, double blind, placebo controlled trial. Br Heart J 1993; 70(1):56–60.

133. Daoud EG, Strickberger SA, Man KC, et al. Preoperative amiodarone as prophylaxis against atrial fibrillation after heart surgery. N Engl J Med 1997; 337(25):1785–1791.

134. Redle JD, Khurana S, Marzan R, et al. Prophylactic oral amiodarone compared with placebo for prevention of atrial fibrillation after coronary artery bypass surgery. Am Heart J 1999; 138(1 Pt 1):144–150.

135. Guarnieri T, Nolan S, Gottlieb SO, Dudek A, Lowry DR. Intravenous amiodarone for the prevention of atrial fibrillation after open heart surgery: the Amiodarone Reduction in Coronary Heart (ARCH) trial. J Am Coll Cardiol 1999; 34(2):343–347.

136. Lee SH, Chang CM, Lu MJ, et al. Intravenous amiodarone for prevention of atrial fibrillation after coronary artery bypass grafting. Ann Thorac Surg 2000; 70(1):157–161.

137. Dorge H, Schoendube FA, Schoberer M, Stellbrink C, Voss M, Messmer BJ. Intraoperative amiodarone as prophylaxis against atrial fibrillation after coronary operations. Ann Thorac Surg 2000; 69(5):1358–1362.

138. Giri S, White CM, Dunn AB, et al. Oral amiodarone for prevention of atrial fibrillation after open heart surgery, the Atrial Fibrillation Suppression Trial (AFIST): a randomised placebo-controlled trial. Lancet 2001; 357(9259):830–836.

139. Maras D, Boskovic SD, Popovic Z, et al. Single-day loading dose of oral amiodarone for the prevention of new-onset atrial fibrillation after coronary artery bypass surgery. Am Heart J 2001; 141(5):E8.

140. Yazigi A, Rahbani P, Zeid HA, Madi-Jebara S, Haddad F, Hayek G. Postoperative oral amiodarone as prophylaxis against atrial fibrillation after coronary artery surgery. J Cardiothorac Vasc Anesth 2002; 16(5):603–606.

141. Tokmakoglu H, Kandemir O, Gunaydin S, Catav Z, Yorgancioglu C, Zorlutuna Y. Amiodarone versus digoxin and metoprolol combination for the prevention of postcoronary bypass atrial fibrillation. Eur J Cardiothorac Surg 2002; 21(3):401–405.

142. Solomon AJ, Greenberg MD, Kilborn MJ, Katz NM. Amiodarone versus a beta-blocker to prevent atrial fibrillation after cardiovascular surgery. Am Heart J 2001; 142(5):811–815.

143. Treggiari-Venzi MM, Waeber JL, Perneger TV, Suter PM, Adamec R, Romand JA. Intravenous amiodarone or magnesium sulphate is not cost-beneficial prophylaxis for atrial fibrillation after coronary artery bypass surgery. Br J Anaesth 2000; 85(5):690–695.

144. Mahoney EM, Thompson TD, Veledar E, Williams J, Weintraub WS. Cost-effectiveness of targeting patients undergoing cardiac surgery for therapy with intravenous amiodarone to prevent atrial fibrillation. J Am Coll Cardiol 2002; 40(4):737–745.

145. Reddy P, Dunn AB, White CM, Tsikouris JP, Giri S, Kluger J. An economic analysis of amiodarone versus placebo for the prevention of atrial fibrillation after open heart surgery. Pharmacotherapy 2002; 22(1):75–80.

146. Wurdeman RL, Mooss AN, Mohiuddin SM, Lenz TL. Amiodarone vs. sotalol as prophylaxis against atrial fibrillation/flutter after heart surgery: a meta-analysis. Chest 2002; 121(4):1203–1210.

147. Zimmer J, Pezzullo J, Choucair W, et al. Meta-analysis of antiarrhythmic therapy in the prevention of postoperative atrial fibrillation and the effect on hospital length of stay, costs, cerebrovascular accidents, and mortality in patients undergoing cardiac surgery. Am J Cardiol 2003; 91(9):1137–1140.

148. Fanning WJ, Thomas CS Jr, Roach A, Tomichek R, Alford WC, Stoney WS Jr. Prophylaxis of atrial fibrillation with magnesium sulfate after coronary artery bypass grafting. Ann Thorac Surg 1991; 52(3):529–533.

149. Speziale G, Ruvolo G, Fattouch K, et al. Arrhythmia prophylaxis after coronary artery bypass grafting: regimens of magnesium sulfate administration. Thorac Cardiovasc Surg 2000; 48(1):22–26.

150. Katholi R, Taylor G, Woods W, et al. $MgCl_2$ replacement after bypass surgery to prevent atrial fibrillation: a double blind, randomized trial. Circulation 1990; 82(suppl III):III-58.

151. Casthely PA, Yoganathan T, Komer C, Kelly M. Magnesium and arrhythmias after coronary artery bypass surgery. J Cardiothorac Vasc Anesth 1994; 8(2):188–191.

152. Jensen BM, Alstrup P, Klitgard NA. Magnesium substitution and postoperative arrhythmias in patients undergoing coronary artery bypass grafting. Scand Cardiovasc J 1997; 31(5):265–269.

153. Parikka H, Toivonen L, Pellinen T, Verkkala K, Jarvinen A, Nieminen MS. The influence of intravenous magnesium sulphate on the occurrence of atrial fibrillation after coronary artery by-pass operation. Eur Heart J 1993; 14(2):251–258.

154. Wistbacka JO, Koistinen J, Karlqvist KE, et al. Magnesium substitution in elective coronary artery surgery: a double- blind clinical study. J Cardiothorac Vasc Anesth 1995; 9(2):140–146.

155. Yeatman M, Caputo M, Narayan P, et al. Magnesium-supplemented warm blood cardioplegia in patients undergoing coronary artery revascularization. Ann Thorac Surg 2002; 73(1):112–118.

156. Gerstenfeld EP, Hill MR, French SN, et al. Evaluation of right atrial and biatrial temporary pacing for the prevention of atrial fibrillation after coronary artery bypass surgery. J Am Coll Cardiol 1999; 33(7):1981–1988.

157. Kurz DJ, Naegeli B, Kunz M, Genoni M, Niederhauser U, Bertel O. Epicardial, biatrial synchronous pacing for prevention of atrial fibrillation after cardiac surgery. Pacing Clin Electrophysiol 1999; 22(5):721–726.

158. Greenberg MD, Katz NM, Luliano S, Tempesta BJ, Solomon AJ. Atrial pacing for the prevention of atrial fibrillation after cardiovascular surgery [see comments]. J Am Coll Cardiol 2000; 35(6):1416–1422.

159. Chung MK, Augostini RS, Asher CR, et al. Ineffectiveness and potential proarrhythmia of atrial pacing for atrial fibrillation prevention after coronary artery bypass grafting. Ann Thorac Surg 2000; 69(4):1057–1063.

160. Blommaert D, Gonzalez M, Mucumbitsi J, et al. Effective prevention of atrial fibrillation by continuous atrial overdrive pacing after coronary artery bypass surgery [see comments]. J Am Coll Cardiol 2000; 35(6):1411–1415.

161. Fan K, Lee KL, Chiu CS, et al. Effects of biatrial pacing in prevention of postoperative atrial fibrillation after coronary artery bypass surgery. Circulation 2000; 102(7):755–760.

162. Goette A, Mittag J, Friedl A, et al. Pacing of Bachmann's bundle after coronary artery bypass grafting. Pacing Clin Electrophysiol 2002; 25(7):1072–1078.

163. Levy T, Fotopoulos G, Walker S, et al. Randomized controlled study investigating the effect of biatrial pacing in prevention of atrial fibrillation after coronary artery bypass grafting. Circulation 2000; 102(12):1382–1387.

164. Daoud EG, Dabir R, Archambeau M, Morady F, Strickberger SA. Randomized, double-blind trial of simultaneous right and left atrial epicardial pacing for prevention of post–open heart surgery atrial fibrillation. Circulation 2000; 102(7):761–765.

165. Klemperer JD, Klein IL, Ojamaa K, et al. Triiodothyronine therapy lowers the incidence of atrial fibrillation after cardiac operations. Ann Thorac Surg 1996; 61(5):1323–1327. discussion 1328–1329.

166. Chaney MA, Nikolov MP, Blakeman B, Bakhos M, Slogoff S. Pulmonary effects of methylprednisolone in patients undergoing coronary artery bypass grafting and early tracheal extubation. Anesth Analg 1998; 87(1):27–33.

167. Halvorsen P, Raeder J, White PF, et al. The effect of dexamethasone on side effects after coronary revascularization procedures. Anesth Analg 2003; 96(6):1578–1583.

168. Yared JP, Starr NJ, Torres FK, et al. Effects of single dose, postinduction dexamethasone on recovery after cardiac surgery. Ann Thorac Surg 2000; 69(5):1420–1424.

169. Kuralay E, Ozal E, Demirkili U, Tatar H. Effect of posterior pericardiotomy on postoperative supraventricular arrhythmias and late pericardial effusion (posterior pericardiotomy). J Thorac Cardiovasc Surg 1999; 118(3): 492–495.

170. Asimakopoulos G, Della Santa R, Taggart DP. Effects of posterior pericardiotomy on the incidence of atrial fibrillation and chest drainage after coronary revascularization: a prospective randomized trial. J Thorac Cardiovasc Surg 1997; 113(4):797–799.

171. Farsak B, Gunaydin S, Tokmakoglu H, Kandemir O, Yorgancioglu C, Zorlutuna Y. Posterior pericardiotomy reduces the incidence of supraventricular arrhythmias and pericardial effusion after coronary artery bypass grafting. Eur J Cardiothorac Surg 2002; 22(2):278–281.

172. Landymore RW, Howell F. Recurrent atrial arrhythmias following treatment for postoperative atrial fibrillation after coronary bypass operations. Eur J Cardiothorac Surg 1991; 5(8):436–439.

173. Myers MG, Alnemri K. Rate control therapy for atrial fibrillation following coronary artery bypass surgery. Can J Cardiol 1998; 14(11):1363–1366.

174. Lee JK, Klein GJ, Krahn AD, et al. Rate-control versus conversion strategy in postoperative atrial fibrillation: a prospective, randomized pilot study. Am Heart J 2000; 140(6):871–877.

175. Kowey PR, Stebbins D, Igidbashian L, et al. Clinical outcome of patients who develop PAF after CABG surgery. Pacing Clin Electrophysiol 2001; 24(2):191–193.

176. Cioffi G, Cemin C, Russo TE, Pellegrini A, Terrasi F, Ferrario G. Post-discharge recurrences of new-onset atrial fibrillation following cardiac surgery: impact of low-dose amiodarone and beta-blocker prophylaxis. Ital Heart J 2000; 1(10):691–697.

177. Solomon AJ, Kouretas PC, Hopkins RA, Katz NM, Wallace RB, Hannan RL. Early discharge of patients with new-onset atrial fibrillation after cardiovascular surgery. Am Heart J 1998; 135(4):555–563.

178. Soucier R, Silverman D, Abordo M, et al. Propafenone versus ibutilide for post operative atrial fibrillation following cardiac surgery: neither strategy improves outcomes compared to rate control alone (the PIPAF study). Med Sci Monit 2003; 9(3):PI19–PI23.

179. Tisdale JE, Padhi ID, Goldberg AD, et al. A randomized, double-blind comparison of intravenous diltiazem and digoxin for atrial fibrillation after coronary artery bypass surgery. Am Heart J 1998; 135(5 Pt 1):739–747.

180. Mooss AN, Wurdeman RL, Mohiuddin SM, et al. Esmolol versus diltiazem in the treatment of postoperative atrial fibrillation/atrial flutter after open heart surgery. Am Heart J 2000; 140(1):176–180.

181. Ommen SR, Odell JA, Stanton MS. Atrial arrhythmias after cardiothoracic surgery. N Engl J Med 1997; 336(20):1429–1434.

182. Liebold A, Haisch G, Rosada B, Kleine P. Internal atrial defibrillation—a new

treatment of postoperative atrial fibrillation. Thorac Cardiovasc Surg 1998; 46(6):323–326.

183. Kleine P, Blommaert D, van Nooten G, et al. Multicenter results of TADpole heart wire system used to treat postoperative atrial fibrillation. Eur J Cardiothorac Surg 1999; 15(4):525–526. discussion 527.

184. Liebold A, Rodig G, Birnbaum DE. Performance of temporary epicardial stainless steel wire electrodes used to treat atrial fibrillation: a study in patients following open heart surgery. Pacing Clin Electrophysiol 1999; 22(2):315–319.

185. Bechtel JF, Christiansen JF, Sievers HH, Bartels C. Low-energy cardioversion versus medical treatment for the termination of atrial fibrillation after CABG. Ann Thorac Surg 2003; 75(4):1185–1188.

186. Murray KD, Vlasnik JJ. Procainamide-induced postoperative pyrexia. Ann Thorac Surg 1999; 68(3):1072–1074.

187. VanderLugt JT, Mattioni T, Denker S, et al. Efficacy and safety of ibutilide fumarate for the conversion of atrial arrhythmias after cardiac surgery. Circulation 1999; 100(4):369–375.

188. Volgman AS, Carberry PA, Stambler B, et al. Conversion efficacy and safety of intravenous ibutilide compared with intravenous procainamide in patients with atrial flutter or fibrillation. J Am Coll Cardiol 1998; 31(6):1414–1419.

189. Bernard EO, Schmid ER, Schmidlin D, Scharf C, Candinas R, Germann R. Ibutilide versus amiodarone in atrial fibrillation: a double-blinded, randomized study. Crit Care Med 2003; 31(4):1031–1034.

190. Stambler BS, Wood MA, Ellenbogen KA. Comparative efficacy of intravenous ibutilide versus procainamide for enhancing termination of atrial flutter by atrial overdrive pacing. Am J Cardiol 1996; 77(11):960–966.

191. Mostow ND, Vrobel TR, Noon D, Rakita L. Rapid control of refractory atrial tachyarrhythmias with high-dose oral amiodarone. Am Heart J 1990; 120(6 Pt 1):1356–1363.

192. Frost L, Mortensen PE, Tingleff J, Platou ES, Christiansen EH, Christiansen N. Efficacy and safety of dofetilide, a new class III antiarrhythmic agent, in acute termination of atrial fibrillation or flutter after coronary artery bypass surgery. Dofetilide Post-CABG Study Group. Int J Cardiol 1997; 58(2): 135–140.

193. Connolly SJ, Mulji AS, Hoffert DL, Davis C, Shragge BW. Randomized placebo-controlled trial of propafenone for treatment of atrial tachyarrhythmias after cardiac surgery. J Am Coll Cardiol 1987; 10(5):1145–1148.

194. Waldo AL, MacLean WA, Cooper TB, Kouchoukos NT, Karp RB. Use of temporarily placed epicardial atrial wire electrodes for the diagnosis and treatment of cardiac arrhythmias following open-heart surgery. J Thorac Cardiovasc Surg 1978; 76(4):500–505.

195. Feld GK, Fleck RP, Chen PS, et al. Radiofrequency catheter ablation for the treatment of human type 1 atrial flutter. Identification of a critical zone in the reentrant circuit by endocardial mapping techniques. Circulation 1992; 86(4):1233–1240.

196. Laupacis A, Albers G, Dalen J, Dunn MI, Jacobson AK, Singer DE.

Antithrombotic therapy in atrial fibrillation. Chest 1998; 114(suppl 5):579S–589S.

197. Arnold AZ, Mick MJ, Mazurek RP, Loop FD, Trohman RG. Role of prophylactic anticoagulation for direct current cardioversion in patients with atrial fibrillation or atrial flutter. J Am Coll Cardiol 1992; 19(4):851–855.

198. Johnson WD, Ganjoo AK, Stone CD, Srivyas RC, Howard M. The left atrial appendage: our most lethal human attachment! Surgical implications. Eur J Cardiothorac Surg 2000; 17(6):718–722.

199. Crystal E, Lamy A, Connolly SJ, et al. Left Atrial Appendage Occlusion Study (LAAOS): a randomized clinical trial of left atrial appendage occlusion during routine coronary artery bypass graft surgery for long-term stroke prevention. Am Heart J 2003; 145(1):174–178.

200. Blackshear JL, Odell JA. Appendage obliteration to reduce stroke in cardiac surgical patients with atrial fibrillation. Ann Thorac Surg 1996; 61(2):755–759.

201. Smith R, Grossman W, Johnson L, Segal H, Collins J, Dalen J. Arrhythmias following cardiac valve replacement. Circulation 1972; 45(5):1018–1023.

202. Michelson MJE, MacVaugh H. Postoperative arrhythmias after coronary artery and cardiac valvular surgery detected by long-term electrocardiographic monitoring. Am Heart J 1979; 97:442–448.

203. Ducceschi V, D'Andrea A, Galderisi M, et al. Risk predictors of paroxysmal atrial fibrillation following aortic valve replacement. Ital Heart J 2001; 2(7):507–512.

204. Orlowska-Baranowska E, Baranowski R, Michalek P, Hoffman P, Rywik T, Rawczylska-Englert I. Prediction of paroxysmal atrial fibrillation after aortic valve replacement in patients with aortic stenosis: identification of potential risk factors. J Heart Valve Dis 2003; 12(2):136–141.

205. Tambeur L, Meyns B, Flameng W, Daenen W. Rhythm disturbances after mitral valve surgery: comparison between left atrial and extended trans-septal approach. Cardiovasc Surg 1996; 4(6):820–824.

206. Cioffi G, Mureddu G, Cemin C, et al. Characterization of post-discharge atrial fibrillation following open-heart surgery in uncomplicated patients referred to an early rehabilitation program. Ital Heart J 2001; 2(7):519–528.

207. Flugelman MY, Hasin Y, Katznelson N, Kriwisky M, Shefer A, Gotsman MS. Restoration and maintenance of sinus rhythm after mitral valve surgery for mitral stenosis. Am J Cardiol 1984; 54(6):617–619.

208. Skoularigis J, Rothlisberger C, Skudicky D, Essop MR, Wisenbaugh T, Sareli P. Effectiveness of amiodarone and electrical cardioversion for chronic rheumatic atrial fibrillation after mitral valve surgery. Am J Cardiol 1993; 72(5):423–427.

209. Obadia JF, el Farra M, Bastien OH, Lievre M, Martelloni Y, Chassignolle JF. Outcome of atrial fibrillation after mitral valve repair. J Thorac Cardiovasc Surg 1997; 114(2):179–185.

210. Vogt PR, Brunner-LaRocca HP, Rist M, et al. Preoperative predictors of recurrent atrial fibrillation late after successful mitral valve reconstruction. Eur J Cardiothorac Surg 1998; 13(6):619–624.

211. Cox JL, Ad N, Palazzo T, et al. The Maze-III procedure combined with valve surgery. Semin Thorac Cardiovasc Surg 2000; 12(1):53–55.
212. McCarthy PM, Gillinov AM, Castle L, Chung M, Cosgrove D III. The Cox-Maze procedure: the Cleveland Clinic experience. Semin Thorac Cardiovasc Surg 2000; 12(1):25–29.
213. Ad N, Cox JL. Combined mitral valve surgery and the Maze III procedure. Semin Thorac Cardiovasc Surg 2002; 14(3):206–209.
214. Bando K, Kobayashi J, Kosakai Y, et al. Impact of Cox Maze procedure on outcome in patients with atrial fibrillation and mitral valve disease. J Thorac Cardiovasc Surg 2002; 124(3):575–583.
215. Ali IM, Sanalla AA, Clark V. Beta-blocker effects on postoperative atrial fibrillation. Eur J Cardiothorac Surg 1997; 11(6):1154–1157.
216. Paull DL, Tidwell SL, Guyton SW, et al. Beta blockade to prevent atrial dysrhythmias following coronary bypass surgery. Am J Surg 1997; 173(5):419–421.
217. Connolly SJ, Cybulsky I, Lamy A, et al. Double-blind, placebo-controlled, randomized trial of prophylactic metoprolol for reduction of hospital length of stay after heart surgery: the beta-Blocker Length Of Stay (BLOS) study. Am Heart J 2003; 145(2):226–232.
218. Solomon AJ, Berger AK, Trivedi KK, Hannan RL, Katz NM. The combination of propranolol and magnesium does not prevent postoperative atrial fibrillation. Ann Thorac Surg 2000; 69(1):126–129.
219. Yazicioglu L, Eryilmaz S, Sirlak M, et al. The effect of preoperative digitalis and atenolol combination on postoperative atrial fibrillation incidence. Eur J Cardiothorac Surg 2002; 22(3):397–401.
220. Janssen J, Loomans L, Harink J, et al. Prevention and treatment of supraventricular tachycardia shortly after coronary artery bypass grafting: a randomized open trial. Angiology 1986; 37(8):601–609.
221. Evrard P, Gonzalez M, Jamart J, et al. Prophylaxis of supraventricular and ventricular arrhythmias after coronary artery bypass grafting with low-dose sotalol. Ann Thorac Surg 2000; 70(1):151–156.
222. Matsuura K, Takahara Y, Sudo Y, Ishida K. Effect of Sotalol in the prevention of atrial fibrillation following coronary artery bypass grafting. Jpn J Thorac Cardiovasc Surg 2001; 49(10):614–617.
223. White CM, Giri S, Tsikouris JP, et al. A comparison of two individual amiodarone regimens to placebo in open heart surgery patients. Ann Thorac Surg 2002; 74(1):69–74.
224. Gerstenfeld EP, Khoo M, Martin RC, et al. Effectiveness of bi-atrial pacing for reducing atrial fibrillation after coronary artery bypass graft surgery. J Interv Card Electrophysiol 2001; 5(3):275–283.
225. Gavaghan TP, Fenetey MP, Campbell TJ, Morgan JJ. Atrial tachyarrhythmias after cardiac surgery: results of disopyramide therapy. Aust N Z J Med 1985; 15(1):27–32.
226. Hjelms E. Procainamide conversion of acute atrial fibrillation after open-heart surgery compared with digoxin treatment. Scand J Thorac Cardiovasc Surg 1992; 26(3):193–196.

227. McAlister HF, Luke RA, Whitlock RM, Smith WM. Intravenous amiodarone bolus versus oral quinidine for atrial flutter and fibrillation after cardiac operations. J Thorac Cardiovasc Surg 1990; 99(5):911–918.

228. Geelen P, O'Hara GE, Roy N, et al. Comparison of propafenone versus procainamide for the acute treatment of atrial fibrillation after cardiac surgery. Am J Cardiol 1999; 84(3):345–347, A348–A349.

229. Di Biasi P, Scrofani R, Paje A, Cappiello E, Mangini A, Santoli C. Intravenous amiodarone vs propafenone for atrial fibrillation and flutter after cardiac operation. Eur J Cardiothorac Surg 1995; 9(10):587–591.

230. Larbuisson R, Venneman I, Stiels B. The efficacy and safety of intravenous propafenone versus intravenous amiodarone in the conversion of atrial fibrillation or flutter after cardiac surgery. J Cardiothorac Vasc Anesth 1996; 10(2):229–234.

231. Wafa SS, Ward DE, Parker DJ, Camm AJ. Efficacy of flecainide acetate for atrial arrhythmias following coronary artery bypass grafting. Am J Cardiol 1989; 63(15):1058–1064.

232. Gavaghan TP, Koegh AM, Kelly RP, Campbell TJ, Thorburn C, Morgan JJ. Flecainide compared with a combination of digoxin and disopyramide for acute atrial arrhythmias after cardiopulmonary bypass. Br Heart J 1988; 60(6):497–501.

233. Campbell TJ, Gavaghan TP, Morgan JJ. Intravenous sotalol for the treatment of atrial fibrillation and flutter after cardiopulmonary bypass. Comparison with disopyramide and digoxin in a randomised trial. Br Heart J 1985; 54(1):86–90.

234. Installe E, Schoevaerdts JC, Gadisseux P, Charles S, Tremouroux J. Intravenous amiodarone in the treatment of various arrhythmias following cardiac operations. J Thorac Cardiovasc Surg 1981; 81(2):302–308.

235. Cochrane AD, Siddins M, Rosenfeldt FL, et al. A comparison of amiodarone and digoxin for treatment of supraventricular arrhythmias after cardiac surgery. Eur J Cardiothorac Surg 1994; 8(4):194–198.

236. Chung MK, Asher CR, Yamada D, Eagle KA. Arrhythmias after cardiac and noncardiac surgery. In: Podrid PJ, Kowey PR, eds. Arrhythmia: Mechanisms, Diagnosis and Management. 2d ed. Philadelphia: Lippincott Williams & Wilkins, 2001.

237. Asher CR, Chung MK, Eagle KA, Lauer MS. Atrial fibrillation following cardiac surgery. In: Falk R, Podrid P, eds. Atrial Fibrillation: Mechanisms and Management. 2d ed. New York: Lippincott-Raven, 1997.

238. Chung MK. Proarrhythmic effects of post-operative pacing intended to prevent atrial fibrillation: evidence from a clinical trial. Cardiac Electrophysiology Rev. Submitted.

14

The Last Word: Treatment of Atrial Fibrillation in the Recent Past and in the Future

Gerald V. Naccarelli
Pennsylvania State University College of Medicine and the Milton S. Hershey Medical Center, Hershey, Pennsylvania, U.S.A.

Peter Kowey
Jefferson Medical College, Philadelphia, and The Lankenau Hospital and Main Line Health System, Wynnewood, Pennsylvania, U.S.A.

New therapies and the results of clinical trials have dramatically altered the treatment of atrial fibrillation. Recent advances have improved our understanding of rate-control strategies, conversion modalities, the maintenance of sinus rhythm, nonpharmacological prevention, and antiembolic measures. The authors who have contributed to this state-of-the-art update on atrial fibrillation have helped us to offer our readers a contemporary overview of this common disease.

For rate control, once-a-day beta blockers and calcium channel blockers have replaced digoxin as front-line rate-control agents for several reasons. Trials have demonstrated that beta blockers and calcium channel blockers are more effective and achieve rate control more rapidly than digoxin. In addition, multiple trials have shown that beta blockers prolong survival in patients with left ventricular dysfunction. There is an increasing volume of data from basic experiments suggesting that calcium channel blockers may attenuate early atrial electrical remodeling (see Chaps. 3 and 4). In the critical care setting, intravenous amiodarone has been added to the armamentarium of more traditional intravenous rate-control therapies. In refractory patients,

AV junction ablation, with ablate-and-pace strategies, has improved symptoms and reversed tachycardia-induced cardiomyopathy. As reviewed by Wyse (Chap. 5), the results of the PIAF, AFFIRM, RACE, and STAF studies have leveled the playing field by making chronic rate control a reasonable option in the treatment of atrial fibrillation instead of more aggressive strategies to maintain sinus rhythm. These trials were limited in that they compared two strategies. No data exist to prove that patients remaining in atrial fibrillation have a prognosis as good as that of patients who effectively maintain sinus rhythm.

Multiple trials and new therapies have improved our understanding of cost-effective strategies to manage atrial fibrillation acutely. Intravenous ibutilide, oral dofetilide, and oral bolus class IC antiarrhythmics are now routinely used in appropriate patients to convert atrial fibrillation to sinus rhythm. Like implantable devices, biphasic shock external cardioversion is replacing internal direct-current cardioversion as the method of choice for converting persistent atrial fibrillation to sinus rhythm. The ACUTE trial has helped us adopt an alternative tranesophageal echocardiographic approach to safely convert patients while minimizing the risk of thromboembolic events in patients who have persistent atrial fibrillation. An update on cardioversion is presented by Timmerman and Crijns (Chap. 8).

Chung extensively reviews efficient approaches to the management of patients with postthoracotomy atrial fibrillation (Chap. 13). Although there are some effective prophylactic approaches that can minimize postthoracotomy atrial fibrillation, the frequency of this arrhythmia in this setting presents a challenge to clinicians.

Over the last decade, commercial approval of DL-sotalol and dofetilide has provided useful additions to our pharmacological armamentarium for maintaining sinus rhythm. Data from multiple safety trials—including CAST, SWORD, EMIAT, CAMIAT, DIAMOND-MI, ALIVE, GESICA, CHF-STAT, and DIAMOND-CHF—have guided us in developing algorithms for choosing safe antiarrhythmic agents in the treatment of patients with and without structural heart disease.

Other new drug therapies with novel mechanisms of action are forthcoming. Drugs that are in clinical development (see Chap. 9) include azimilide (a once-a-day I_{Kr} and I_{Ks} blocker), dronedarone (an amiodarone-like drug without the iodine moiety), piboserod (a 5-HT4 receptor antagonist); RSD 1235 (an atrial-selective potassium inhibitor), ZP123 (which facilitates conduction in the gap junction), and two intravenous drugs that are longer-acting A-1 adenosine agonists. Several new drugs under development have used our understanding of molecular biology to develop more atrial-selective agents that might be efficacious in atrial tissue yet minimize drug-induced ventricular arrhythmias. Some of the new antiarrhythmic agents, with novel mechanisms of action, may be useful alone or in combination with more traditional anti-arrhythmic agents.

As reviewed by Chen (Chap. 12), mapping and ablation/isolation of pulmonary vein triggers promises to change the landscape as a front-line treatment for the suppression of atrial fibrillation. Nonpharmacological treatment (see Chaps. 11 and 12) will have added benefit in combination with anti-arrhythmic drugs (hybrid therapy) that had previously been ineffective when used alone. In addition, the use of angiotensin-converting enzyme (ACE) inhibitors and angiotensin-receptor blockers appears to be useful in preventing atrial fibrillation with and without antiarrhythmic drugs by counteracting stretch-activated channels and directly by blocking angiotensin II, among other mechanisms of benefit.

Significant advances in decreasing morbidity and mortality from atrial fibrillation have come from multiple trials delineating risk factors for embolic stroke and that have proven that therapeutic levels of warfarin can significantly reduce embolic stroke rates. The results of AFFIRM and RACE suggest that chronic therapeutic anticoagulation must be maintained even in patients controlled on antiarrhythmic drugs if such patients have ongoing risk factors for thromboembolic events, such as hypertension and diabetes. As discussed by Flaker, the development of oral antithrombin inhibitors, such as ximelgatran, offers the possibility of therapeutic anticoagulation without the need for checking INR status. In both Sportif III and V, ximelagatran was demonstrated not to be inferior to warfarin in preventing embolic events.

Atrial fibrillation continues to be a difficult condition to treat. We struggle to understand the multiple mechanisms (stretch and ischemia, as well as hormonal, metabolic, inflammatory, structural, and autonomic effects) that trigger the substrate sustaining this arrhythmia (see Chaps. 3 and 4). Given multiple mechanisms, it is naïve to think that one therapy could be useful for all patients with atrial fibrillation. The application of molecular biology and mapping techniques offers hope that these will help us to treat this condition in the future. With the aging of the population (see Chap. 1), it is particularly important to develop therapies that will help us in our battle to control and hopefully cure atrial fibrillation.

Index